The
Law of
Hospital and
Health Care Administration:
Cases and Materials

The
Law of
Hospital and
Health Care Administration:
Cases and Materials

Compiled and Edited by
J. Stuart Showalter
Bernard D. Reams, Jr.

Foreword by Arthur F. Southwick

Health Administration Press
Ann Arbor, Michigan   1993

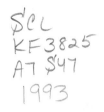
97 96 95 94   5 4 3 2

Library of Congress Cataloging-in-Publication Data

Showalter, J. Stuart.
    The law of hospital and health care administration : cases and materials / J. Stuart
Showalter and Bernard D. Reams, Jr.
        p.   cm.
    ISBN 0-910701-94-6 (alk. paper)
    1. Hospitals—Law and legislation—United States—Cases. 2. Medical care—Law and
legislation—United States—Cases. I. Reams, Bernard D. II. Title.
KF3825.A7S47 1993 344.73'03211—dc20 [347.3043211] 93-14239 CIP

The paper used in this publication meets the minimum requirements of American National
Standard for Information Sciences—Permanence of Paper for Printed Library Materials,
ANSI Z39.48-1984. ⊗™

Health Administration Press
A division of the Foundation of the
    American College of Healthcare Executives
1021 East Huron Street
Ann Arbor, Michigan 48104-9990
(313) 764-1380

Contents

Foreword

As the principal author of *The Law of Hospital and Health Care Administration,* Second Edition (with Debora A. Slee), I am delighted that Stuart Showalter and Bernard Reams have undertaken the editing of these cases to accompany my text. Each case is followed by suggested discussion questions, which individual instructors using the text and cases together can add to or subtract from at their discretion when leading discussions in the classroom. Further, each chapter is introduced by comments placing both the text and the cases in perspective.

Misters Showalter and Reams have selected the cases with care based on their classroom teaching in the health administration program at Washington University School of Medicine, St. Louis. In a sense each case is a "landmark" decision announcing trends in state common law or in the interpretation of statutory or constitutional materials. Accordingly, some of these judicial decisions have provided precedent for other courts to follow pursuant to the doctrine of *stare decisis.* On the other hand, several of the cases have rejected previous precedent, thus reversing a rule of the common law or interpretation of formal, "written" law materials.

In my opinion the most effective method for instruction in law is the study of cases. The facts of the particular situation determine both the outcome of litigation and the policy of governmental administrative agencies. In short, the facts generate the rule of law. Persons studying law for the first time seldom realize this fundamental underpinning of the Anglo-American legal system. They need to read cases, as well as constitutional and statutory materials, to appreciate how and why rules of law are developed and how they can be applied to solve particular problems. Case instruction also provides opportunities to stress that rules of law are constantly being changed, modified, and expanded to conform to society's current expectations; that not all jurisdictions follow the same rules; that courts as well as administrative agencies play an active role in the development of law; and that there is constant interaction between judicial and legislative bodies. This book provides the materials for attaining these goals.

Throughout my own teaching of graduate students in the Department of Health Services Management and Policy at the University of Michigan School of Public Health, I required that students read actual legal decisions as well as the text. I revised the list of cases annually and made it available to faculty using the text. However, the cases were not edited, and the students often found it difficult to pinpoint the essence of the decisions and to identify with precision the legal issues being decided. Mr. Showalter and Mr. Reams experienced the same reaction from students at Washington University and decided that the judicial decisions should be edited. I readily agreed.

I wish good fortune to faculty and students who use these cases and materials.

Arthur F. Southwick
Professor Emeritus of Business Law and
    Health Services Management and Policy
University of Michigan

Preface

This book is compiled from the actual opinions of various federal and state courts. They illustrate the legal principles discussed in Arthur F. Southwick's *The Law of Hospital and Health Care Administration*, Second Edition (Ann Arbor, MI: Health Administration Press, 1988), and the chapter numbering follows that text.

Each chapter contains excerpts from published cases. Deletions made by the editors from the original texts of the opinions are generally indicated by ellipsis (. . .); in some instances, however, lengthy omissions are summarized in bracketed material written by the editors. Omissions found in published versions of cases are shown with asterisks (* * *). Except where pedagogic purposes require their retention, all footnotes and in-text citations to cases have been omitted from the opinions without notation.

In addition to the judicial opinions, this book contains discussion questions and commentary prepared by the editors. Because learning is not a spectator sport, it is hoped that the combination of opinions, discussion questions, and commentary will allow for active classroom discussion. Instructors are encouraged to use these materials in that manner, and students are encouraged to read and consider the cases from the standpoint of their application to material described in the textbook.

In preparing for class discussions, the student must understand where each case stands in the hierarchy of the legal system, how it got to the court considering it, and the implications of the ultimate decision. Students must be able to discuss how the principles involved in the cases relate not only to the particular facts involved at the time of the decision but also to health care administration today. In this manner the case materials will be most beneficial to a full understanding of the U.S. legal system.

The following outline may be a helpful way of structuring the student's analysis of the cases:

1. *Procedure.* Who are the parties? Who brought the action? In what court did the case originate? Who won at the trial court level? What is the appellate history of the case?

2. *Facts.* What are the relevant facts as recited by this court? Are there any facts that you would like to know but that are not revealed in the opinion?

3. *Issues.* What are the precise issues being litigated, as stated by the court? Do you agree with the way the court has framed those issues?

4. *Holding.* What is the court's decision? What is its rationale for that decision? Do you agree with that rationale?

5. *Implications.* What does the case mean for health care today? What were its implications when the decision was announced? How should health care administrators prepare to deal with these implications? What would be different today if the case had been decided differently?

This is not the only framework with which to analyze legal cases, and students are advised to determine their own instructor's methodology, but whatever technique is used, the point is that a structured analysis will result in the best learning.

The editors wish to acknowledge the work of Cheryl Caponegro, a student at Washington University School of Law, for her valuable research assistance, without which these materials could not have been collected in a timely fashion. In addition, we wish to thank Ann O'Keeffe, who spent late nights and many weekends in the law library running LEXIS searches and converting electronic bits and bytes into the printed word. Our sincere thanks go to both of these fine, professional women.

Finally, thanks are extended as well to our families for their understanding of our late hours and preoccupied attitudes during the preparation of the manuscript.

1

Introduction to the Anglo-American Legal System

The legal system of this country has fascinated scholars for over two hundred years. The subject can be approached as one solely of legal theory, but for a full understanding, one must also consider such subjects as history, sociology, politics, economics, and ethics. And the choice of analytical method is only the first challenge for the student, for the roots of our legal tradition can be traced not just to the American War for Independence but as far back as the Norman conquest of England in 1066. It is little wonder, then, that many view the richness of the U.S. legal tradition with emotions approaching reverence.

Stated in the most basic (and most important) way, the purpose of the Anglo-American legal system is to provide an alternative to self-help and personal conflict as a way of resolving disputes between individuals, organizations, or governments within this society. Considering the size and complexity of our nation, the litigiousness of our people, and the wide range of possible disputes, our judicial system is remarkably successful in achieving its purpose.

It is essential that the student of health care administration gain a level of familiarity with law and the legal system, for law is one of the most common threads in the fabric of the health care industry today. Virtually every decision made and every action taken by health care administrators has legal implications; and *all* such decisions and actions are explicitly or implicitly based on some legal principle.

Having emphasized the importance of the subject, however, we must also admit that many health administration students find the topic frustrating. Law is far from an exact science. It has none of the precision of mathematics or the empiricism of science or even medicine. It is a social science, and its imprecision frustrates some students.

Yet the uncertainty and flexibility of the law are what give it its strength and its appeal. It is based on a set of general rules that must be applied to the infinite variety of human behavior. The basic principles have evolved over centuries of experience, and they continue to change to meet the emerging needs of society. Thus the courts not only determine the facts of a particular situation, apply a legal principle, and determine the outcome as though some sort of sociological calculus existed; they also interpret those fundamental doctrines and adapt them in light of changing times.

Viewed in its proper light, the law is a beautiful and constantly (albeit slowly) changing tapestry that generally reflects the beliefs of society at any given location or point in time.

Adding to the complexity of the tapestry is the federal nature of our governmental system. This means that to study the U.S. legal system one must study

fifty-two court systems in the United States, since each state and the District of Columbia has its own separate system, in addition to the federal courts. The large number of different courts makes study of law in the United States extremely complex, especially when courts in different states use divergent approaches in deciding cases. Nevertheless, although law students must often study a "majority" approach and several "minority" approaches to the same legal issue, the complexity also adds a great deal of strength and vitality to the American system because a wide number of resolutions to a particular problem may be tested in individual states before a consensus is reached regarding the most desirable solution. (Southwick, 12)

The cases chosen for this chapter reflect some of this complexity and diversity. Although there may be (and are) various sources of law in this country, no legal principle is much more than a theory until one or another court interprets and applies it in deciding real-life disputes between real-life people. It is in this manner that our society has chosen to bring order out of anarchy.

The cases in this chapter (and, indeed, in the entire book) can be studied at various levels. For example, they illustrate what used to be referred to as civics and is now more widely known as American government; thus, they can be evaluated at the level of what they say about the theory and structure of U.S. government.

Certainly, this is a worthwhile perspective. But it is hoped that in addition to the political science aspects involved, the student will see in these cases some distinctly human and sociological aspects. For example, consider the difficult situation experienced by Catherine Jackson that led to her power being cut off; consider the implications of the decision for thousands of other Catherine Jacksons and, indeed, for tens of thousands of businesses, small and large, who might stand in similar relation to the issues as did Metropolitan Edison. Consider, also, the medical and sociological aspects of *Woods v. Lancet*, the basic facts of what happened to Mr. Tompkins in *Erie R.R. Co. v. Tompkins*, the public policy issues relating to drug testing exemplified by *Secretary of Transp. v. Railway Labor Executives' Ass'n.*, or the extremely divisive and emotional aspects of the abortion controversy as represented by *Planned Parenthood v. Casey*.

The practical questions and larger social issues underlying these cases are the kinds of topics that it is hoped the materials in this book will elicit. The point is usually not so much that the questions are answered but that they are asked.

Jackson v. Metropolitan Edison Co.
419 U.S. 345 (1974)

Rehnquist, J.

Respondent Metropolitan Edison Co. is a privately owned and operated Pennsylvania corporation which holds a certificate of public convenience issued by the Pennsylvania Public Utility Commission empowering it to deliver electricity to a service area which includes the city of York, PA. As a condition of holding its certificate, it is subject to extensive regulation by the Commission. Under a provision of its general tariff filed with the Commission, it has the right to discontinue service to any customer on reasonable notice of nonpayment of bills.

Petitioner Catherine Jackson is a resident of York, who has received electricity in the past from respondent. Until September 1970, petitioner received electric service to her home in York under an account with respondent in her own name. When her account was terminated because of asserted delinquency in payments due for service, a new account with respondent was opened in the name of one James Dodson,

another occupant of the residence, and service to the residence was resumed. . . . In August 1971, Dodson left the residence. Service continued thereafter but concededly no payments were made. Petitioner states that no bills were received during this period.

On October 7, 1971, employees of Metropolitan came to the residence and inquired as to Dodson's present address. Petitioner stated that it was unknown to her. On the following day, another employee visited the residence and informed petitioner that the meter had been tampered with so as not to register amounts used. She disclaimed knowledge of this and requested that the service account for her home be shifted from Dodson's name to that one of Robert Jackson, later identified as her 12-year-old son. Four days later on October 11, 1971, without further notice to petitioner, Metropolitan employees disconnected her service.

Petitioner then filed suit against Metropolitan in the United States District Court for the Middle District of Pennsylvania under the Civil Rights Act of 1871, 42 U.S.C. § 1983, seeking damages for the termination and an injunction requiring Metropolitan to continue providing power to her residence until she had been afforded notice, a hearing, and an opportunity to pay any amounts found due. She urged that . . . Metropolitan's termination of her service for alleged nonpayment . . . constituted "state action" depriving her of property in violation of the Fourteenth Amendment's guarantee of due process of law.

The District Court granted Metropolitan's motion to dismiss petitioner's complaint on the ground that the termination did not constitute state action and hence was not subject to judicial scrutiny under the Fourteenth Amendment. On appeal, the United States Court of Appeals for the Third Circuit affirmed, also finding an absence of state action. We granted certiorari to review this judgment.

The Due Process Clause of the Fourteenth Amendment provides: "[N]or shall any State deprive any person of life, liberty, or property, without due process of law." In 1883, this Court in the Civil Rights Cases affirmed the essential dichotomy set forth in that Amendment between deprivation by the State, subject to scrutiny under its provisions, and private conduct, "however discriminatory or wrongful," against which the Fourteenth Amendment offers no shield.

We have reiterated that distinction on more than one occasion since then. While the principle that private action is immune from the restrictions of the Fourteenth Amendment is well established and easily stated, the question whether particular conduct is "private," on the one hand, or "state action," on the other, frequently admits of no easy answer.

Here the action complained of was taken by a utility company which is privately owned and operated, but which in many particulars of its business is subject to extensive state regulation. The mere fact that a business is subject to state regulation does not by itself convert its action into that of the State for purposes of the Fourteenth Amendment. Nor does the fact that the regulation is extensive and detailed, as in the case of most public utilities, do so. . . . [T]he inquiry must be whether there is a sufficiently close nexus between the State and the challenged action of the regulated entity so that the action of the latter may be fairly treated as that of the State itself. The true nature of the State's involvement may not be immediately obvious, and detailed inquiry may be required in order to determine whether the test is met.

Petitioner advances a series of contentions which, in her view, lead to the conclusion that this case should fall on the [state action] side of the line . . . rather than on the [private action] side of that line. We find none of them persuasive.

[The Court here embarks on a lengthy discussion of each of the petitioner's arguments. First, she argued that there was state action because Metropolitan was a state-recognized monopoly. The Court doubted that Metropolitan had been granted a monopoly, but even if it had, the Court found this fact did not make Metropolitan's actions state action because the actions complained of had no relationship to whether it was or was not a monopoly. Next, she argued that Metropolitan supplied an "essential public service" that state law required it to provide and that it was therefore performing a public function that amounted to state action. The Court dismissed this argument, saying that there is a difference between providing a utility service and performing a function traditionally exercised only by government (such as eminent domain). The Court continued:]

Perhaps in recognition of the fact that the supplying of utility service is not traditionally the exclusive prerogative of the State, petitioner invites the expansion of the doctrine of this limited line of cases [on state action] into a broad principle that all businesses "affected with the public interest" are state actors in all their actions.

We decline the invitation for [these] reasons . . . :

"It is clear that there is no closed class or category of businesses affected with a public interest * * * . The phrase 'affected with a public interest' can, in the nature of things, mean no more than that an industry, for adequate reason, is subject to control for the public good. . . ."

Doctors, optometrists, lawyers, Metropolitan, and [a] grocery selling a quart of milk are all in regulated businesses, providing arguably essential goods and services, "affected with a public interest." We do not believe that such a status converts their every action, absent more, into that of the State.

. . . .

We also find absent in the instant case the symbiotic relationship presented in *Burton v. Wilmington Parking Authority*. There where a private lessee, who practiced racial discrimination, leased space for a restaurant from a state parking authority in a publicly owned building, the Court held that the State had so far insinuated itself into a position

of interdependence with the restaurant that it was a joint participant in the enterprise. We cautioned, however, that while a "multitude of relationships might appear to some to fall within the Amendment's embrace," differences in circumstances beget differences in law, limiting the actual holding to lessees of public property.

. . . .

All of petitioner's arguments taken together show no more than that Metropolitan was a heavily regulated, privately owned utility, enjoying at least a partial monopoly in the providing of electrical service within its territory, and that it elected to terminate service to petitioner in a manner which the Pennsylvania Public Utility Commission found permissible under state law. Under our decision this is not sufficient to connect the State of Pennsylvania with respondent's action so as to make the latter's conduct attributable to the State for purposes of the Fourteenth Amendment.

. . . We therefore have no occasion to decide whether petitioner's claim to continued service was "property" for purposes of that Amendment, or whether "due process of law" would require a State [that took] similar action to accord petitioner the procedural rights for which she contends. The judgment of the Court of Appeals for the Third Circuit is therefore

Affirmed.

Discussion Questions

1. What are the facts of this case? What is the issue?

2. In what court was it decided, and how did it get to that court?

3. What did the court below decide, and why? What did this court decide, and why?

4. What is *certiorari*? What is an *injunction*?

5. How do your feel about Catherine Jackson?

6. What does it mean to be "affected with the public interest"?

7. What is the significance of the Fourteenth Amendment to the U.S. Constitution in this case? What does one have to prove to establish a "due process" claim under the Fourteenth Amendment?

8. What is the *Burton* case? Why is it important for this decision? What was the key factor in *Burton*, and why was the result in that case different than in *Jackson*?

9. What would have been the implications of the opposite result in this case (for hospitals, for example)?

10. What does this case tell you about the operation of the judicial system?

Woods v. Lancet
303 N.Y. 349, 102 N.E.2d 691 (1951)

Desmond, J.

[The case involves negligence and resulting injuries to a fetus during the ninth month of pregnancy. The injuries caused the baby to be born with permanent disabilities. Based on an earlier New York case, *Drobner v. Peters*, decided in 1921, the trial court dismissed the child's lawsuit for "failure to state a cause of action." The Appellate Division (the intermediate appellate court) voted to affirm, notwithstanding what one justice termed "the obvious injustice of the rule" of *Drobner*. Another said that although he felt bound by the earlier case he would allow the child to recover if it were an open issue in the state. Against this background, the highest court of New York proceeded to consider its earlier precedent.]

. . . It will hardly be disputed that justice (not emotionalism or sentimentality) dictates the enforcement of such a cause of action. The trend in decisions of other courts, and the writings of learned commentators . . . is strongly toward making such a recovery possible. The precise question for us on this appeal is: shall we follow *Drobner v. Peters*, or shall we bring the common law of this State, on this question, into accord with justice? I think, as New York State's court of last resort, we should make the law conform to right.

. . . . There is . . . no material distinction between [the *Drobner*] case and the one we are passing on now. However, *Drobner v. Peters* must be examined against a background of history and of the legal thought of its time and of the thirty years that have passed since it was handed down.

[The court points out that *Drobner* was the first case of its time and, hence, was decided without the benefit of precedent. In addition, "the practical difficulties of proof" and "the theoretical lack of separate human existence of an infant *in utero*" were factors in the outcome of *Drobner*. However, the opinion points out that since 1921 "numerous and impressive affirmative precedents have been developed." It cites cases in California, Ohio, Canada, and New Jersey, plus a law review article in England and the legal treatise, *Prosser on Torts*.]

What, then, stands in the way of a reversal here? Surely, as an original proposition, we would, today, be hard put to it to find a sound reason for the old rule. Following *Drobner v. Peters* would call for an affirmance, but the chief basis for that holding (lack of precedent) no longer exists. And it is not a very strong reason, anyhow, in a case like this. . . . Negligence law is common law, and the common law has been molded and changed and brought up-to-date in many another case. Our court said, long ago, that it had not only the right, but the duty to re-examine a question where justice demands it . . . . No reason appears why there should not be the same approach when traditional common-law rules of negligence result in injustice. . . . We act in the finest common-law tradi-tion when we adapt and alter decisional law to produce common-sense justice.

The same answer goes to the argument that the change we here propose should come from the Legislature, not the courts. Legislative action there could, of course, be, but we abdicate our own function, in a field peculiarly nonstatutory, when we refuse to reconsider an old and unsatisfactory court-made rule. . . .

Two other reasons for dismissal (besides lack of precedent) are given in *Drobner v. Peters* . . . . The first of those, discussed in many of the other writings on the subject herein cited, has to do with the supposed difficulty of proving or disproving that certain injuries befell the unborn child, or that they produced the defects discovered at birth, or later. Such difficulties there are, of course, and, indeed, it seems to be commonly accepted that only a blow of tremendous force will ordinarily injure a foetus [*sic*], so carefully does nature insulate it. But such difficulty of proof or finding is not special to this particular kind of lawsuit . . . . Every day in all our trial courts (and before administrative tribunals, particularly the Workmen's Compensation Board), such issues are disposed of, and it is an inadmissible concept that uncertainty of proof can ever destroy a legal right. The questions of causation, reasonable certainty, etc., which will arise in these cases are no different, in kind, from the ones which have arisen in thousands of other negligence cases decided in this State, in the past.

The other objection to recovery here is the purely theoretical one that a foetus *in utero* has no existence of its own separate from that of its mother . . . . We need not deal here with so large a subject. It is to be remembered that we are passing on the sufficiency of a complaint which alleges that this injury occurred during the ninth month of the mother's pregnancy, in other words, to a viable foetus, later born. Therefore, we confine our holding in this case to prepartum injuries to such viable children. . . . This child, when injured, was in fact, alive and capable of being delivered and of remaining alive, separate from its mother. We agree with the dissenting Justice below that "To deny the infant relief in this case is not only a harsh result, but its effect is to do reverence to an outmoded, timeworn fiction not founded on fact and within common knowledge untrue and unjustified."

The judgments should be reversed, and the motion denied, with costs in all courts.

Discussion Questions

1. What is the issue in this case? How was it decided? Do you agree with the result?

2. How is this case a good example of stare decisis?

3. Why does the court refer to cases in other jurisdictions and even other countries? How are those cases relevant?

4. When is it appropriate for the court to let the legislature decide issues of first impression, and when is it appropri-

ate for the court to do so? What about the oft-heard complaint of judge-made law?

5. About 20 years after this decision, the U.S. Supreme Court decided *Roe v. Wade*, the abortion case. Is *Woods* consistent or inconsistent with the *Roe* holding? Why?

6. What does this case teach you about the workings of the judicial system?

Planned Parenthood of S.E. Pa. v. Casey
112 S. Ct. 2791 (1992)

[This is the abortion case that upheld the Supreme Court's 1973 decision in *Roe v. Wade*, upheld numerous provisions of a Pennsylvania law restricting abortions, and invalidated a portion of that law. The following excerpt—a portion of the opinion of the Court announced by Justices O'Connor, Kennedy, and Souter—is provided for its insights into the concept of stare decisis. The remainder of the case is presented in Chapter 11.]

The examination of the conditions justifying the repudiation of *Adkins* by *West Coast Hotel* and *Plessy* by *Brown* is enough to suggest the terrible price that would have been paid if the Court had not overruled as it did. In the present case, however, as our analysis to this point makes clear, the terrible price would be paid for overruling. Our analysis would not be complete, however, without explaining why overruling *Roe*'s central holding would not only reach an unjustifiable result under principles of stare decisis, but would seriously weaken the Court's capacity to exercise the judicial power and to function as the Supreme Court of a Nation dedicated to the rule of law. To understand why this would be so it is necessary to understand the source of this Court's authority, the conditions necessary for its preservation, and its relationship to the country's understanding of itself as a constitutional Republic.

The root of American governmental powers is revealed most clearly in the instance of the power conferred by the Constitution upon the Judiciary of the United States and specifically upon this Court. As Americans of each succeeding generation are rightly told, the Court cannot buy support for its decisions by spending money and, except to a minor degree, it cannot independently coerce obedience to its decrees. The Court's power lies, rather, in its legitimacy, a product of substance and perception that shows itself in the people's acceptance of the Judiciary as fit to determine what the Nation's law means and to declare what it demands.

The underlying substance of this legitimacy is of course the warrant for the Court's decisions in the Constitution and the lesser sources of legal principle on which the Court draws. That substance is expressed in the Court's opinions, and our contemporary understanding is such that a decision without principled justification would be no judicial act at all. But even when justification is furnished by apposite legal principle, something more is required. Because not every conscientious claim of principled justification will be accepted as such, the justification claimed must be beyond dispute. The Court must take care to speak and act in ways that allow people to accept its decision on the terms the Court claims for them, as grounded truly in principle, not as compromises with social and political pressures having, as such, no bearing on the principled choices that the Court is obliged to make. Thus, the Court's legitimacy depends on making legally principled decisions under circumstances in which their principled character is sufficiently plausible to be accepted by the Nation.

The need for principled action to be perceived as such is implicated to some degree whenever this, or any other appellate court, overrules a prior case. This is not to say, of course, that this Court cannot give a perfectly satisfactory explanation in most cases. People understand that some of the Constitution's language is hard to fathom and that the Court's Justices are sometimes able to perceive significant facts or to understand principles of law that eluded their predecessors and that justify departures from existing decisions. However upsetting it may be to those most directly affected when one judicially derived rule replaces another, the country can accept some correction of error without necessarily questioning the legitimacy of the Court.

In two circumstances, however, the Court would almost certainly fail to receive the benefit of the doubt in overruling prior cases. There is, first, a point beyond which frequent overruling would overtax the country's belief in the Court's good faith. Despite the variety of reasons that may inform and justify a decision to overrule, we cannot forget that such a decision is usually perceived (and perceived correctly) as, at the least, a statement that a prior decision was wrong. There is a limit to the amount of error that can plausibly be imputed to prior courts. If that limit should be exceeded, disturbance of prior rulings would be taken as evidence that justifiable reexamination of principle had given way to drives for particular results in the short term. The legitimacy of the Court would fade with the frequency of its vacillation.

That first circumstance can be described as hypothetical; the second is to the point here and now. Where, in the performance of its judicial duties, the Court decides a case in such a way as to resolve the sort of intensely divisive controversy reflected in *Roe* and those rare, comparable cases, its decision has a dimension that the resolution of the normal case does not carry. It is the dimension present whenever the Court's interpretation of the Constitution calls the contending sides of a national controversy to end their national division by accepting a common mandate rooted in the Constitution.

The Court is not asked to do this very often, having thus addressed the Nation only twice in our lifetime, in the decisions of *Brown* and *Roe*. But when the Court does act in this way, its decision requires an equally rare precedential force to counter the inevitable efforts to overturn it and to thwart its implementation. Some of those efforts may be mere unprincipled emotional reactions; others may proceed from principles worthy of profound respect. But whatever the premises of opposition may be, only the most convincing justification under accepted standards of precedent could suffice to demonstrate that a later decision overruling the first was anything but a surrender to political pressure, and an unjustified repudiation of the principle on which the Court staked its authority in the first instance. So to overrule under fire in the absence of the most compelling reason to reexamine a watershed decision would subvert the Court's legitimacy beyond any serious question. . . .

The country's loss of confidence in the judiciary would be underscored by an equally certain and equally reasonable condemnation for another failing in overruling unnecessarily and under pressure. Some cost will be paid by anyone who approves or implements a constitutional decision where it is unpopular, or who refuses to work to undermine the decision or to force its reversal. The price may be criticism or ostracism, or it may be violence. An extra price will be paid by those who themselves disapprove of the decision's results when viewed outside of constitutional terms, but who nevertheless struggle to accept it, because they respect the rule of law. To all those who will be so tested by following, the Court implicitly undertakes to remain steadfast, lest in the end a price be paid for nothing. The promise of constancy, once given, binds its maker for as long as the power to stand by the decision survives and the understanding of the issue has not changed so fundamentally as to render the commitment obsolete. From the obligation of this promise this Court cannot and should not assume any exemption when duty requires it to decide a case in conformance with the Constitution. A willing breach of it would be nothing less than a breach of faith, and no Court that broke its faith with the people could sensibly expect credit for principle in the decision by which it did that.

It is true that diminished legitimacy may be restored, but only slowly. Unlike the political branches, a Court thus weakened could not seek to regain its position with a new mandate from the voters, and even if the Court could somehow go to the polls, the loss of its principled character could not be retrieved by the casting of so many votes. Like the character of an individual, the legitimacy of the Court must be earned over time. So, indeed, must be the character of a Nation of people who aspire to live according to the rule of law. Their belief in themselves as such a people is not readily separable from their understanding of the Court invested with the authority to decide their constitutional cases and speak before all others for their constitutional ideals. If the Court's legitimacy should be undermined, then, so would the country be in its very ability to see itself through its constitutional ideals. The Court's concern with legitimacy is not for the sake of the Court but for the sake of the Nation to which it is responsible.

The Court's duty in the present case is clear. In 1973, it confronted the already divisive issue of governmental power to limit personal choice to undergo abortion, for which it provided a new resolution based on the due process guaranteed by the Fourteenth Amendment. Whether or not a new social consensus is developing on that issue, its divisiveness no less today than in 1973, and pressure to overrule the decision, like pressure to retain it, has grown only more intense. A decision to overrule *Roe*'s essential holding under the existing circumstances would address error, if error there was, at the cost of both profound and unnecessary damage to the Court's legitimacy, and to the Nation's commitment to the rule of law. It is therefore imperative to adhere to the essence of *Roe*'s original decision, and we do so today.

Discussion Questions

1. What does this excerpt tell you about stare decisis?

2. How would you compare and contrast this description of stare decisis with that of *Woods v. Lancet*? Are there any substantial differences?

3. How do you think the judges in *Planned Parenthood* would have decided *Woods*, and vice versa?

4. In the first paragraph of this excerpt, the Court refers to two pairs of cases in which prior Supreme Court decisions were overruled. Do you know what those cases were about?

Erie R.R. Co. v. Tompkins
304 U.S. 64 (1938)

Brandeis, J.

The question for decision is whether the oft-challenged doctrine of *Swift v. Tyson* shall now be disapproved.

Tompkins, a citizen of Pennsylvania, was injured on a dark night by a passing freight train of the Erie Railroad Company while walking along its right of way at Hughestown in that state. He claimed that the accident occurred through negligence in the operation, or maintenance, of the train; that he was rightfully on the premises as licensee because on a commonly used beaten footpath which ran for a short distance alongside the tracks; and that he was struck by something which looked like a door projecting from one of the moving cars. To enforce that claim he brought an action in the federal court for Southern New York, which had jurisdiction because the company is a corporation of that state. It denied liability; and the case was tried by a jury.

The Erie insisted that its duty to Tompkins was no greater than that owed to a trespasser. It contended, among other things, that its duty to Tompkins, and hence its liability, should be determined in accordance with the Pennsylvania law; that under the law of Pennsylvania, as declared by its highest court, persons who use pathways along the railroad right of way . . . are to be deemed trespassers; and that the railroad is not liable for injuries to undiscovered trespassers resulting from its negligence, unless it be wanton or willful. Tompkins denied that any such rule had been established by the decisions of the Pennsylvania courts; and contended that, since there was no statute of the state on the subject, the railroad's duty and liability is to be determined in federal courts as a matter of general law.

The trial judge refused to rule that the applicable law precluded recovery. The jury brought in a verdict of $30,000; and the judgment entered thereon was affirmed by the Circuit Court of Appeals, which held that it was unnecessary to consider whether the law of Pennsylvania was as contended, because the question was one not of local, but of general, law, and that "upon questions of general law the federal courts are free, in absence of a local statute, to exercise their independent judgment as to what the law is . . . ."

The Erie had contended that application of the Pennsylvania rule was required, among other things, by section 34 of the Federal Judiciary Act of September 24, 1789, which provides, "The laws of the several States, except where the Constitution, treaties, or statutes of the United States otherwise require or provide, shall be regarded as rules of decision in trials at common law, in the courts of the United States, in cases where they apply."

Because of the importance of the question whether the federal court was free to disregard the alleged rule of the Pennsylvania common law, we granted certiorari.

First. Swift v. Tyson held that federal courts exercising jurisdiction on the ground of diversity of citizenship need not, in matters of general jurisprudence, apply the unwritten law of the state as declared by its highest court; that they are free to exercise an independent judgment as to what the common law of the state is—or should be; and that, as there stated by Mr. Justice Story, "the true interpretation of the 34th section limited its application to state laws, strictly local, that is to say, to the positive statutes of the state, and the construction thereof adopted by the local tribunals, and to rights and titles to things having a permanent locality, such as the rights and titles to real estate, and other matters immovable and intra-territorial in their nature and character. It never has been supposed by us, that the section did apply, or was designed to apply, to questions of a more general nature . . . ."

[The opinion then goes on to point out that after *Swift,* much doubt was expressed about whether that interpretation of § 34 was correct, and it commented that scholars had recently established "that the [original] purpose of the section was merely to make certain that, in all matters except those in which some federal law is controlling, the federal courts exercising jurisdiction in diversity of citizenship cases *would apply as their rules of decision the law of the state, unwritten as well as written*" (emphasis added). The court then pro-

ceeds to discuss a case that brought the criticism of *Swift* to a head.]

[In that case, the Brown & Yellow Taxicab & Transfer Co.,] a Kentucky corporation owned by Kentuckians, and the Louisville Nashville Railroad, also a Kentucky corporation, wished that the former should have the exclusive privilege of soliciting passenger and baggage transportation at the Bowling Green, Ky., railroad station; and [also wished that] that the Black & White [cab company] should be prevented from interfering with that privilege. Knowing that such a contract would be void under the common law of Kentucky, it was arranged that the Brown & Yellow reincorporate under the law of Tennessee, and that the contract with the railroad should be executed there. The suit was then brought by the Tennessee corporation in the federal court for Western Kentucky to enjoin competition by the Black & White; an injunction issued by the District Court was sustained by the Court of Appeals; and this Court, citing many decision in which the doctrine of *Swift v. Tyson* had been applied, affirmed the decree.

Second. Experience in applying the doctrine of *Swift v. Tyson,* had revealed its defects, political and social; and the benefits expected to flow from the rule did not accrue. Persistence of state courts in their own opinions on questions of common law prevented uniformity; and the impossibility of discovering a satisfactory line of demarcation between the province of general law and that of local law developed a new well of uncertainties.

On the other hand, the mischievous results of the doctrine had become apparent. Diversity of citizenship jurisdiction was conferred in order to prevent apprehended discrimination in state courts against those not citizens of the state. *Swift v. Tyson* introduced grave discrimination by noncitizens against citizens. It made rights enjoyed under the unwritten "general law" vary according to whether enforcement was sought in the state or in the federal court; and the privilege of selecting the court in which the right should be determined was conferred upon the noncitizen. Thus the doctrine rendered impossible equal protection of the law. In attempting to promote uniformity of law throughout the United States, the doctrine had prevented uniformity in the administration of the law of the state.

. . . .

In part the discrimination resulted from the wide range of persons held entitled to avail themselves of the federal rule by resort to the diversity of citizenship jurisdiction. Through this jurisdiction individual citizens willing to remove from their own state and become citizens of another might avail themselves of the federal rule. And, without even change of residence, a corporate citizen of the state could avail itself of the federal rule by reincorporating under the laws of another state, as was done in the *Taxicab* Case.

The injustice and confusion incident to the doctrine of *Swift v. Tyson* have been repeatedly urged as reasons for abolishing or limiting diversity of citizenship jurisdiction. Other legislative relief has been proposed. If only a question of statutory construction were involved, we should not be prepared to abandon a doctrine so widely applied throughout nearly a century. But the unconstitutionality of the course pursued has now been made clear, and compels us to do so.

Third. Except in matters governed by the Federal Constitution or by acts of Congress, the law to be applied in any case is the law of the state. And whether the law of the state shall be declared by its Legislature in a statute or by its highest court in a decision is not a matter of federal concern. There is no federal general common law. Congress has no power to declare substantive rules of common law applicable in a state whether they be local in their nature or "general," be they commercial law or a part of the law of torts. And no clause in the Constitution purports to confer such a power upon the federal courts. . . .

The fallacy underlying the rule declared in *Swift v. Tyson* is made clear by Mr. Justice Holmes. The doctrine rests upon the assumption that there is "a transcendental body of law outside of any particular State but obligatory within it unless and until changed by statute," that federal courts have the power to use their judgment as to what the rules of common law are; [*sic*] and that in the federal courts "the parties are entitled to an independent judgment on matters of general law":

"But law in the sense in which courts speak of it today does not exist without some definite authority behind it. The common law so far as it is enforced in a State, whether called common law or not, is not the common law generally but the law of that State existing by the authority of that State without regard to what it may have been in England or anywhere else. . . .

"The authority and only authority is the State, and if that be so, the voice adopted by the State as its own [whether it be of its Legislature or of its Supreme Court] should utter the last word."

Thus the doctrine of *Swift v. Tyson* is, as Mr. Justice Holmes said, "an unconstitutional assumption of powers by the Courts of the United States which no lapse of time or respectable array of opinion should make us hesitate to correct." In disapproving that doctrine we do not hold unconstitutional section 34 . . . . We merely declare that in applying the doctrine this Court and the lower courts have invaded rights which in our opinion are reserved by the Constitution to the several states.

Fourth. The defendant contended that by the common law of Pennsylvania . . . the only duty owed to the plaintiff was to refrain from willful or wanton injury. The plaintiff denied that such is the Pennsylvania law. In support of their respective contentions the parties discussed and cited many decisions of the Supreme Court of the state. The Circuit Court of Appeals ruled that the question of liability is one of general law[,] and on that ground [it] declined to decide the issue of state law. As we hold this was error, the judgment is reversed and the case remanded to it for further proceedings in conformity with our opinion.

Reversed.

Discussion Questions

1. Why is the law of Pennsylvania important for a case in a court located in New York?

2. What is the significance of the concepts of *duty* and *trespass*?

3. In the Judiciary Act, quoted in the opinion, there is reference to "the laws of the several states . . . ." What does this mean? Why does careful interpretation of this statute become important for this opinion?

4. Why did criticism of the *Swift* doctrine become widespread after the decision in *Black & White Taxicab*? What happened in that case?

5. What is the purpose of diversity jurisdiction of the federal courts?

6. What further proceedings are necessary?

7. How does this case deepen your understanding of the role of the federal courts and their relationship to state courts and other branches of government?

Skinner v. Ry. Labor Executives' Ass'n.
489 U.S. 602 (1989)

Kennedy, J.

The Federal Railroad Safety Act of 1970 authorizes the Secretary of Transportation to "prescribe, as necessary, appropriate rules, regulations, orders, and standards for all areas of railroad safety." Finding that alcohol and drug abuse by railroad employees poses a serious threat to safety, the Federal Railroad Administration (FRA) has promulgated regulations that mandate blood and urine tests of employees who are involved in certain train accidents. The FRA also has adopted regulations that do not require, but do authorize, railroads to administer breath and urine tests to employees who violate certain safety rules. The question presented by this case is whether these regulations violate the Fourth Amendment.

[In part I of the opinion, the Supreme Court reviews the railroad industry's attempts to curtail drug and alcohol use by personnel while on duty. A voluntary standard known as "Rule G," published by the Association of American Railroads, had been found inadequate, so in 1983 the FRA promulgated federal regulations.

These regulations, which supplement Rule G, prohibited covered railroad employees from possessing or being under the influence of drugs or alcohol while on duty. They provide, in a section known as "Subpart C," for *mandatory* blood and urine testing of any employee involved in a serious accident; in Subpart D they authorize railroads to require blood and urine testing when impairment by drugs or alcohol is suspected.

The regulations were challenged by the Railway Labor Executives' Association. The U.S. District Court for the District of Columbia upheld the regulations saying that the railroad employees' interest in the integrity of their own bodies was outweighed by the "public and governmental interest in the . . . promotion . . . of railroad safety."

The U.S. Court of Appeals for the D.C. Circuit reversed. It concluded that blood and urine tests amount to "searches" under the Fourth Amendment to the U.S. Constitution. To be valid under the Fourth Amendment, a search must be reasonable. The court held that these searches are not reasonable because, except for Subpart D, they do not require "individualized suspicion" of any person; instead, Subpart C seems to authorize blanket testing of employees without probable cause.

On petition by the government, the U.S. Supreme Court granted certiorari. In part II of the opinion the court reviews and affirms prior courts' rulings that blood and urine testing under color of government regulation must be considered searches under the Fourth Amendment.]

III

A

To hold that the Fourth Amendment is applicable to the drug and alcohol testing prescribed by the FRA regulations is only to begin the inquiry into the standards governing such intrusions. For the Fourth Amendment does not proscribe all searches and seizures, but only those that are unreasonable. What is reasonable, of course, "depends on all of the circumstances surrounding the search or seizure and the nature of the search or seizure itself." Thus, the permissibility of a particular practice "is judged by balancing its intrusion on the individual's Fourth Amendment interests against its promotion of legitimate governmental interests."

In most criminal cases, we strike this balance in favor of the procedures described by the Warrant Clause of the Fourth Amendment. [Therefore,] except in certain well-defined circumstances, a search or seizure in such a case is not reasonable unless it is accomplished pursuant to a judicial warrant issued upon probable cause. We have recognized exceptions to this rule, however, "when 'special needs, beyond the normal need for law enforcement, make the warrant and probable-cause requirement impracticable.' " When faced with such special needs, we have not hesitated to balance the governmental and privacy interests to assess the practicality of the warrant and probable cause requirements in the particular context.

The Government's interest in regulating the conduct of railroad employees to ensure safety, like its supervision of probationers or regulated industries, or its operation of a government office, school, or prison, "likewise presents 'special needs' beyond normal law enforcement that may justify departures from the usual warrant and probable-cause requirements." The hours of service employees covered by the FRA regulations include persons engaged in handling orders concerning train movements, operating crews, and those engaged in the maintenance and repair of signal systems. It is undisputed that these and other covered employees are engaged in safety-sensitive tasks. The FRA so found, and respondents conceded the point at oral argument. As we have recognized, the whole premise of the Hours of Service Act is that "the length of hours of service has direct relation to the efficiency of the human agencies upon which protection [of] life and property necessarily depends." . . .

The FRA has prescribed toxicological tests, not to assist in the prosecution of employees, but rather "to prevent accidents and casualties in railroad operations that result from impairment of employees by alcohol or drugs." This governmental interest in ensuring the safety of the traveling public and of the employees themselves plainly justifies prohibiting covered employees from using alcohol or drugs on duty, or while subject to being called for duty. This interest also "require[s] and justifies the exercise of supervision to assure that the restrictions are in fact observed." The question that remains, then, is whether the Government's need to monitor compliance with these restrictions justifies the privacy intrusions at issue absent a warrant or individualized suspicion.

B

An essential purpose of a warrant requirement is to protect privacy interests by assuring citizens subject to a search or seizure that such intrusions are not the random or arbitrary acts of government agents. A warrant assures the citizen that the intrusion is authorized by law, and that it is narrowly limited in its objectives and scope. A warrant also provides the detached scrutiny of a neutral magistrate, and thus ensures an objective determination whether an intrusion is justified in any given case. In the present context, however, a warrant would do little to further these aims. Both the circumstances justifying toxicological testing and the permissible limits of such intrusions are defined narrowly and specifically in the regulations that authorize them, and doubtless are well known to covered employees. Indeed, in light of the standardized nature of the tests and the minimal discretion vested in those charged with administering the program, there are virtually no facts for a neutral magistrate to evaluate.

We have recognized, moreover, that the Government's interest in dispensing with the warrant requirement is at its strongest when, as here, "the burden of obtaining a warrant is likely to frustrate the governmental purpose behind the search." As the FRA recognized, alcohol and other drugs are eliminated from the bloodstream at a constant rate, and blood and breath samples taken to measure whether these substances were in the bloodstream when a triggering event occurred must be obtained as soon as possible. Although the metabolites of some drugs remain in the urine for longer periods of time and may enable the FRA to estimate whether the employee was impaired by those drugs at the time of a covered accident, incident, or rule violation, the delay necessary to procure a warrant nevertheless may result in the destruction of valuable evidence.

The Government's need to rely on private railroads to set the testing process in motion also indicates that insistence on a warrant requirement would impede the achievement of the Government's objective. Railroad supervisors, like school officials and hospital administrators, are not in the business of investigating violations of the criminal laws or enforcing administrative codes, and otherwise have little occasion to become familiar with the intricacies of this Court's Fourth Amendment jurisprudence. "Imposing unwieldy warrant procedures . . . upon supervisors, who would otherwise have no reason to be familiar with such procedures, is simply unreasonable."

In sum, imposing a warrant requirement in the present context would add little to the assurances of certainty and regularity already afforded by the regulations, while significantly hindering, and in many cases frustrating, the objectives of the Government's testing program. We do not believe that a warrant is essential to render the intrusions here at issue reasonable under the Fourth Amendment.

C

Our cases indicate that even a search that may be performed without a warrant must be based, as a general matter, on probable cause to believe that the person to be searched has violated the law. When the balance of interests precludes insistence on a showing of probable cause, we have usually required "some quantum of individualized suspicion" before concluding that a search is reasonable. We made it clear, however, that a showing of individualized suspicion is not a constitutional floor, below which a search must be presumed unreasonable. In limited circumstances, where the privacy interests implicated by the search are minimal, and where an important governmental interest furthered by the intrusion would be placed in jeopardy by a requirement of individualized suspicion, a search may be reasonable despite the absence of such suspicion. We believe this is true of the intrusions in question here.

By and large, intrusions on privacy under the FRA regulations are limited. To the extent transportation and like restrictions are necessary to procure the requisite blood, breath, and urine samples for testing, this interference alone is minimal given the employment context in which it takes place. Ordinarily, an employee consents to significant restrictions in his freedom of movement where necessary for his employment, and few are free to come and go as they please during working hours. Any additional interference with a railroad employee's freedom of movement that occurs in the time it takes to procure a blood, breath, or urine sample for testing cannot, by itself, be said to infringe significant privacy interests.

. . . .

The breath tests authorized by Subpart D of the regulations are even less intrusive than the blood tests prescribed by Subpart C. Unlike blood tests, breath tests do not require piercing the skin and may be conducted safely outside a hospital environment and with a minimum of inconvenience or embarrassment. Further, breath tests reveal the level of alcohol in the employee's bloodstream and nothing more. Like the blood-testing procedures mandated by Subpart C, which can be used only to ascertain the presence of alcohol or controlled substances in the bloodstream, breath tests reveal no other facts in which the employee has a substantial privacy interest. In all the circumstances, we cannot conclude that the administration of a breath test implicates significant privacy concerns.

A more difficult question is presented by urine tests. Like breath tests, urine tests are not invasive of the body and, under the regulations, may not be used as an occasion for inquiring into private facts unrelated to alcohol or drug use. We recognize, however, that the procedures for collecting the necessary samples, which require employees to perform an excretory function traditionally shielded by great privacy, raise concerns not implicated by blood or breath tests. While we would not characterize these additional privacy concerns as minimal in most contexts, we note that the regulations endeavor to reduce the intrusiveness of the collection process. The regulations do not require that samples be furnished under the direct observation of a monitor, despite the desirability of such a procedure to ensure the integrity of the sample. The sample is also collected in a medical environment, by personnel unrelated to the railroad employer, and is thus not unlike similar procedures encountered often in the context of a regular physical examination.

More importantly, the expectations of privacy of covered employees are diminished by reason of their participation in an industry that is regulated pervasively to ensure safety, a goal dependent, in substantial part, on the health and fitness of covered employees. This relation between safety and employee fitness was recognized by Congress when it enacted the Hours of Service Act in 1907, and also when it authorized the Secretary to "test . . . railroad facilities, equipment, rolling stock, operations, or persons, as he deems necessary to carry out the provisions" of the Federal Railroad Safety Act of 1970. It has also been recognized by state governments, and has long been reflected in industry practice, as evidenced by the industry's promulgation and enforcement of Rule G. Indeed, the FRA found, and the Court of Appeals acknowledged, that "most railroads require periodic physical examinations for train and engine employees and certain other employees."

We do not suggest, of course, that the interest in bodily security enjoyed by those employed in a regulated industry must always be considered minimal. Here, however, the covered employees have long been a principal focus of regulatory concern. As the dissenting judge below noted: "The reason is obvious. An idle locomotive, sitting in the roundhouse, is harmless. It becomes lethal when operated negligently by persons who are under the influence of alcohol or drugs." Though some of the privacy interests implicated by the toxicological testing at issue reasonably might be viewed as significant in other contexts, logic and history show that a diminished expectation of privacy attaches to information relating to the physical condition of covered employees and to this reasonable means of procuring such information. We conclude, therefore, that the testing procedures contemplated by Subparts C and D pose only limited threats to the justifiable expectations of privacy of covered employees.

By contrast, the Government interest in testing without a showing of individualized suspicion is compelling. Employees subject to the tests discharge duties fraught with such risks of injury to others that even a momentary lapse of attention can have disastrous consequences. . . .

While no procedure can identify all impaired employees with ease and perfect accuracy, the FRA regulations supply an effective means of deterring employees engaged in safety-sensitive tasks from using controlled substances or alcohol in the first place. . . .

The testing procedures contemplated by Subpart C also help railroads obtain invaluable information about the causes of major accidents, and to take appropriate measures to safeguard the general public. . . .

A requirement of particularized suspicion of drug or alcohol use would seriously impede an employer's ability to obtain this information, despite its obvious importance. . . .

. . . .

We conclude that the compelling Government interests served by the FRA's regulations would be significantly hindered if railroads were required to point to specific facts giving rise to a reasonable suspicion of impairment before testing a given employee. In view of our conclusion that, on the present record, the toxicological testing contemplated by the regulations is not an undue infringement on the justifiable expectations of privacy of covered employees, the Government's compelling interests outweigh privacy concerns.

IV

The possession of unlawful drugs is a criminal offense that the Government may punish, but it is a separate and far more dangerous wrong to perform certain sensitive tasks while under the influence of those substances. Performing those tasks while impaired by alcohol is, of course, equally danger-ous, though consumption of alcohol is legal in most other contexts. The Government may take all necessary and reasonable regulatory steps to prevent or deter that hazardous conduct, and since the gravamen of the evil is performing certain functions while concealing the substance in the body, it may be necessary, as in the case before us, to examine the body or its fluids to accomplish the regulatory purpose. The necessity to perform that regulatory function with respect to railroad employees engaged in safety-sensitive tasks, and the reasonableness of the system for doing so, have been established in this case.

Alcohol and drug tests conducted in reliance on the authority of Subpart D cannot be viewed as private action outside the reach of the Fourth Amendment. Because the testing procedures mandated or authorized by Subparts C and D effect searches of the person, they must meet the Fourth Amendment's reasonableness requirement. In light of the limited discretion exercised by the railroad employers under the regulations, the surpassing safety interests served by toxicological tests in this context, and the diminished expectation of privacy that attaches to information pertaining to the fitness of covered employees, we believe that it is reasonable to conduct such tests in the absence of a warrant or reasonable suspicion that any particular employee may be impaired. We hold that the alcohol and drug tests contemplated by Subparts C and D of the FRA's regulations are reasonable within the meaning of the Fourth Amendment. The judgment of the Court of Appeals is accordingly reversed.

. . . .

JUSTICE MARSHALL, with whom JUSTICE BRENNAN joins, dissenting.

The issue in this case is not whether declaring a war on illegal drugs is good public policy. The importance of ridding our society of such drugs is, by now, apparent to all. Rather, the issue here is whether the Government's deployment in that war of a particularly draconian weapon—the compulsory collection and chemical testing of railroad workers' blood and urine—comports with the Fourth Amendment. Precisely because the need for action against the drug scourge is manifest, the need for vigilance against unconstitutional excess is great. History teaches that grave threats to liberty often come in times of urgency, when constitutional rights seem too extravagant to endure. The World War II relocation-camp cases, and the Red scare and McCarthy-era internal subversion cases, are only the most extreme reminders that when we allow fundamental freedoms to be sacrificed in the name of real or perceived exigency, we invariably come to regret it.

In permitting the Government to force entire railroad crews to submit to invasive blood and urine tests, even when it lacks any evidence of drug or alcohol use or other wrongdoing, the majority today joins those shortsighted courts which have allowed basic constitutional rights to fall prey to momentary emergencies. The majority holds that the need of the Federal Railroad Administration (FRA) to deter and diagnose train accidents outweighs any "minimal" intrusions on personal dignity and privacy posed by mass toxicological testing of persons who have given no indication whatsoever of impairment. In reaching this result, the majority ignores the text and doctrinal history of the Fourth Amendment, which require that highly intrusive searches of this type be based on probable cause, not on the evanescent cost-benefit calculations of agencies or judges. But the majority errs even under its own utilitarian standards, trivializing the raw intrusiveness of, and overlooking serious conceptual and operational flaws in, the FRA's testing program. These flaws cast grave doubts on whether that program, though born of good intentions, will do more than ineffectually symbolize the Government's opposition to drug use.

The majority purports to limit its decision to postaccident testing of workers in "safety-sensitive" jobs, much as it limits its holding in the companion case to the testing of transferees to jobs involving drug interdiction or the use of firearms. But the damage done to the Fourth Amendment is not so easily cabined. The majority's acceptance of dragnet blood and urine testing ensures that the first, and worst, casualty of the war on drugs will be the precious liberties of our citizens. I therefore dissent. . . .

. . . .

In his first dissenting opinion as a Member of this Court, Oliver Wendell Holmes observed:

"Great cases, like hard cases, make bad law. For great cases are called great, not by reason of their real importance in shaping the law of the future, but because of some accident of immediate overwhelming interest which appeals to the feelings and distorts the judgment. These immediate interests exercise a kind of hydraulic pressure which makes what previously was clear seem doubtful, and before which even well settled principles of law will bend."

A majority of this Court, swept away by society's obsession with stopping the scourge of illegal drugs, today succumbs to the popular pressures described by Justice Holmes. In upholding the FRA's plan for blood and urine testing, the majority bends time-honored and textually based principles of the Fourth Amendment—principles the Framers of the Bill of Rights designed to ensure that the Government has a strong and individualized justification when it seeks to invade an individual's privacy. I believe the Framers would be appalled by the vision of mass governmental intrusions upon the integrity of the human body that the majority allows to become reality. The immediate victims of the majority's constitutional timorousness will be those railroad workers whose bodily fluids the Government may now forcibly collect and analyze. But ultimately, today's decision will reduce the privacy all citizens may enjoy, for, as Justice Holmes understood, principles of law, once bent, do not snap back easily. I dissent.

Discussion Questions

1. What does this case teach about principles of constitutional law and their application to current issues?

2. Why does the Fourth Amendment not apply to actions of private parties? Why are the railroads, when they comply with these regulations, considered to be something other than private parties?

3. Can you define what reasonable searches and seizures are? How would you know one if you saw one?

4. What kinds of special needs would justify bypassing the requirement of a search warrant? Do you agree that the problem of substance abuse among railroad employees is a serious enough need? How about among surgeons? Pediatricians? Internists? Nurses? How about human immunodeficiency virus (HIV) seropositivity or active acquired immunodeficiency syndrome (AIDS)?

5. Do you agree with the concerns raised by the dissenting opinion?

2

Breach of Contract and Intentional Tort

Having begun to sense the purpose and function of the courts and how different courts relate to each other (vertically and horizontally within a jurisdiction and also between state or federal jurisdictions), the student must now consider the substantive subjects of the law: contracts, intentional torts, negligence, and the like.

In this chapter we take up the general principles of contract law—the elements of a valid contract, defenses to contract actions, and remedies—and relate those principles to various aspects of the physician-patient and hospital-patient relationships. We also discuss the nature of intentional torts and their application to health care administration.

A contract is generally defined as an agreement between two or more persons that creates an obligation to do or refrain from doing a particular thing. Contracts articulate the conditions to which the parties have agreed and state their rights and duties in accordance with these conditions. The role of the court is to enforce a valid contract as the parties agreed unless grounds exist to bar its enforcement. The elements necessary to create a valid contract are explained in Southwick's text.

Although contract principles may help delineate both the nature and scope of the parties' rights and responsibilities, they usually cannot do so completely. For example, the nature of the traditional offer and acceptance required for an ordinary contract, express or implied, may vary in a health care setting due to the medical exigencies of a given situation. Additionally, while the parties to a commercial contract bargain on relatively equal footing to reach agreeable terms, in health care situations the patient is usually at a relative disadvantage for a variety of reasons.

Patients go to a doctor or hospital in need of care, sometimes urgent care, and the health care provider alone possesses the unique and specialized knowledge required for successful patient treatment. Thus, protracted bargaining usually does not occur in health care settings, due to both the disparities in medical knowledge between the parties and the overriding need for prompt medical treatment.

As a result, doctor-patient or hospital-patient contracts might not be as clear as their commercial counterparts might be. Add to this that physicians are ethically bound by fiduciary obligations to their patients, and the analogy of the traditional contract becomes even weaker. Nonetheless, contract principles remain applicable to health care, even if only to determine when or if they should ever apply.

In reading the following cases the student should continue to be aware of procedural aspects (the particular court involved, the prior history of the case, the facts and legal issues being addressed, etc.), but the cases should also be read for their substantive content and what lessons they provide for health care providers.

Oliver v. Brock
342 So. 2d 1 (Ala. 1976)

Shores, J.

Anita Oliver, through her mother, Cathy Oliver, brought suit against Bryan Whitfield Memorial Hospital of Demopolis, Dr. F.S. Whitfield, Dr. Paul Ketcham, and Dr. E.C. Brock, alleging that the plaintiffs had retained Drs. Whitfield, Ketcham and Brock to treat her for injuries received as a result of an automobile accident. [The allegations were that Drs. Whitfield and Ketcham had called Dr. Brock in on a consultation "for the diagnosis, care and treatment of the Plaintiff, Anita Oliver."]

The trial court granted Dr. Brock's motion for summary judgment and the plaintiffs appealed.

[The essential evidence in the case was a set of affidavits by the doctors and one by Mrs. Oliver. The affidavit of Dr. Brock stated, in part:]

. . . I have never seen or talked to Anita Oliver or Cathy Oliver; I have never had Anita Oliver and Cathy Oliver as a patient. I have never been engaged or requested to serve as a consultant in the treatment of Anita Oliver. I was not employed or engaged in consult with the doctors treating Anita Oliver concerning her complaints or medical problems.

I have never had Anita Oliver as a patient of mine; there has never been the doctor-patient relationship between Anita Oliver and myself; I have never been employed by the parents or guardians of Anita Oliver to treat, diagnose, or assist in any way in the care and treatment of Anita Oliver.

I know Dr. F. S. Whitfield . . . and I have talked to him on the telephone on occasions in the past. During the year 1974 and the early part of 1975, Dr. Whitfield did not mention Anita Oliver's name to me on the phone and I was not employed by him to assist in the treatment of Anita Oliver, or to act as a consultant with him in the treatment of Anita Oliver.

[Dr. Whitfield's affidavit admitted that Anita Oliver was his patient, then confirmed that he had talked to Dr. Brock about Anita Oliver:]

[I] had the occasion to and did call Dr. Ernest C. Brock, a practicing physician in Tuscaloosa, Alabama, with reference to Dr. Brock's recommendations concerning the care and treatment of *another* patient [and] during the course of such conversation [I] did describe generally the injuries of plaintiff and the type of treatment [I] was then giving plaintiff, and Dr. Brock did indicate to [me] that under the circumstances described he thought the treatment to be correct; [I] did not disclose to Dr. Brock the name of the patient; [my] discussion with Dr. Brock was gratuitous on his part and for [my] guidance in connection with the treatment of plaintiff; [I] did not employ Dr. Brock to care for or treat plaintiff and Dr. Brock did not care for or treat plaintiff to [my] knowledge. In the discharge summary . . . [I] did make note of the telephone conversation with Dr. Brock and of the suggestions made to [me] by Dr. Brock but did not suggest . . . that Dr. Brock was in any way employed . . . in the care and treatment of plaintiff . . . .

[The only evidence for the plaintiffs was Mrs. Cathy Oliver's affidavit, which said that she had been concerned about Dr. Whitfield's and Dr. Ketcham's treatment and that Dr. Whitfield told her that he would call Dr. Brock to get some advice. The affidavit went on to say that she saw in the medical records that Dr. Brock had been consulted, and it concluded, "I sincerely believe that Dr. Brock took part in the treatment of my daughter and that he is at fault for the serious injuries suffered by my daughter as a result of this treatment."]

The question before us is whether, based upon the supporting affidavits, Dr. Brock has carried the burden placed upon a movant for summary judgment to demonstrate that there is no genuine issue of material fact and that he is entitled to prevail on the motion as a matter of law. . . .

A physician owes his patient the duty of due care in his treatment of that patient. That is not controverted. The question is whether there is any evidence to suggest that a physician-patient relationship was ever created between Dr. Brock and the plaintiff patient. The general rule is stated in 61 Am. Jur. 2d, Physicians, Surgeons and Other Healers, § 96:

"A physician is under no obligation to engage in practice or to accept professional employment . . . . The relation is a consensual one wherein the patient knowingly seeks the assistance of a physician and the physician knowingly accepts him as a patient. The relationship between a physician and patient may result from an express or implied contract . . . and the rights and liabilities of the parties thereto are governed by the general law of contract . . . . [T]he voluntary acceptance of the physician-patient relationship by the affected parties creates a prima facie presumption of a contractual relationship between them. A physician may accept a patient and thereby incur the consequent duties although his services are performed gratuitously or at the solicitation and on the guaranty of a third person. * * * "

. . . .

We fail to see any evidence from which it could be concluded that Dr. Brock has consented to treat the child, or any from which it could be inferred that he consented to act in a consulting capacity. . . .

. . . Mrs. Oliver states in her affidavit that she "sincerely believes" that Dr. Brock took part in the treatment of her daughter. However, it has been held that belief, no matter how sincere, is not equivalent to knowledge [and] that a statement in an affidavit that the affiant verily believes does not satisfy the requirements of the [rules of evidence]. Apart from her belief that Dr. Brock took part in the treatment of her daughter, Mrs. Oliver offers only the hearsay statements of Dr. Whitfield, who told her that Dr. Brock told him that he was treating the child correctly. . . . Whether or not a physician-patient relationship exists depends upon the facts in each case, but some facts must be supplied to support a conclusion that the relationship has been created. In this case, there are no facts which can support the conclusion that the relationship ever existed between Dr. Brock and the patient. [The court goes on to point out that the medical record is not a part of the record but is only referred to in two of the affidavits.]

There is nothing in this record to support the allegation that Dr. Brock took any part in the treatment of Anita Oliver. . . . The judgment of the trial court in granting motion for summary judgment on his behalf is, therefore, affirmed.

BEATTY, Justice (concurring specially):

The mere discussion between professional people of hypothetical situations cannot be viewed as a basis for liability. To hold otherwise would tend to adversely affect the quality of the services they offer to members of the public. Physicians, lawyers, dentists, engineers, and other professionals, by comparing problem-solving approaches with other members of their disciplines, have the opportunity to learn from one another. Possessing this freedom, they are better positioned to bring theory into practice for the benefit of those whom they serve. Our decision in this case preserves these essential learning situations for all professional people.

Discussion Questions

1. What other facts would you like to know that this opinion does not tell you?

2. What factors did the court use in determining whether Dr. Brock had a doctor-patient relationship with Mrs. Oliver? Do you agree with those factors? Are there others? Which are most significant for you?

3. Where should one draw a firm line between "mere discussion . . . of hypothetical situations" and an actual physician-patient relationship? Or should there even be such a line?

4. Does the "hallway consultation" exemplified by this case pose any new risks for physicians in this era of AIDS and HIV seropositivity?

5. Must a physician accept a new patient who is suffering from AIDS?

Guilmet v. Campbell
385 Mich. 57, 188 N.W.2d 601 (1971)

Kavanagh, J.

This appeal presents a very simple question, but it is fraught with great danger for the public weal.

The question is: Was the trial court in error in refusing to grant defendants' motion for a judgment notwithstanding the jury's verdict for the plaintiffs?

The defendants are skilled surgeons who performed a relatively complicated operation on plaintiff Richard Guilmet, and after such operation the plaintiffs suffered very great damages.

The danger attendant upon the decision here is that on one hand if we sanction the award of damages to the plaintiffs we may foster suits which threaten the freedom physicians and surgeons must have in the practice of their vital profession, and on the other hand if we deprive these plaintiffs of their award we not only may do them an injustice but impair the very process by which we seek to administer justice.

[The facts of the case involved Richard Guilmet's serious peptic ulcer and the conversations he had with Dr. Campbell before the first in a series of surgeries for the condition. The plaintiff's essentially uncontradicted testimony was that Dr. Campbell told him, "Once you have an operation, it takes care of all of your troubles. You can eat as you want to, you can drink as you want to, you can go as you please." In response to further questioning, the plaintiff testified:]

A. Well, he explained to me how they do this operation, and that at that time he told me that him and his associate, Dr. Arena, were specialists, *and there was nothing to it at all. It was a very simple operation according to them.*

Q. Did he talk at all about whether he had performed these [surgeries] before?

A. Yes, he did. . . . I asked him how often. He said, *"Very often."*

Q. Any discussion as to complications or problems that may arise, that may result?

A. I asked him about it, how long I'd be out of work. He said, "approximately *three to four weeks at the most,"* and I asked him about any complications, anything dangerous. He said, *"No, there is no danger at all in this operation."*

. . . .

Q. What was the discussion about the future use of medication?

A. Well, he said, *"after this operation, you can throw your pillbox away, your Maalox you can throw away"* . . . . [Emphasis in the opinion.]

[Following this conversation, Mr. Guilmet had the operation, a vagotomy, and as a result suffered "ruptured esophagus due to surgical trauma in doing the vagotomy with bilateral effusion and mediastinal emphysema and mediastinitis." It was estimated that the mortality rate from a ruptured esophagus was 50 to 75 percent. This led to three subsequent operations, transfusion-related hepatitis, loss of about 80 pounds, sleep disorders, scarring, loss of his job, recurrent infections, physical weakness, and social inactivity.

The plaintiff filed suit on two theories: negligence in performing the operation and breach of contract. The contract count alleged that "Defendants in furtherance of their contract jointly undertook to examine, diagnose, treat and operate upon and care for Plaintiff so as to cure him of the stomach disorder from which he was then suffering."

After the evidence was in, the defense moved for a directed verdict, and that motion was denied. The jury found no negligence in performing the operation but awarded damages of $50,000 on the breach of contract count. The defendants then moved for judgment notwithstanding the verdict, but the trial court denied this motion as well. The intermediate court affirmed this decision, and the Supreme Court of Michigan accepted it for review.]

The gravamen of the plaintiffs' breach of contract complaint is that: (1) The . . . gist of what the defendant told him . . . (2) . . . amounted to an offer of a contract to achieve by the operation the condition described. (3) That in reliance on the description, the plaintiff accepted the offer, and [(4)] in breach of the contract the condition described did not result.

In effect by their motion for judgment N.O.V., the defendants ask the court to rule as a matter of law that such statements by defendant *before the parties had contracted for the operation* as to the danger, convalescence, and result can *not* be regarded as a term of a contract between a physician and his patient.

This we will not do for we agree with Mr. Justice Cooley when he said:

[W]here the terms of a negotiation are left to oral proofs the question what the parties said and did, and what they intended should be understood thereby, is single and cannot be separated so as to refer one part to the jury and another part to the judge; but in its entirety the question is one of fact. * * *

We hold that the terms of a contract, when contested, are for the jury's determination. This is true even when the evidence of the terms is uncontradicted.

We recognize that what we hold is sometimes made clearer by stating what we do not hold. Here we do not say that [the doctor *promises* a cure] every time the doctor says to his patient prior to the formation of their contract, for example, "I recommend an immediate appendectomy. It will fix you up fine. You will be back at work in no time. Do not worry about it—I have done hundreds of these operations. It is really a very simple thing." . . .

What we are saying is that under some circumstances the trier of fact might conclude that a doctor so speaking did contract to "cure" his patient.

. . . .

Justice Talbot Smith in *Stewart v. Rudner* articulated our concern for the sensitivity of this area of engagement, when he said:

"A doctor and his patient, of course, have the same general liberty to contract with respect to their relationship as other parties entering into consensual relationship with one another, and a breach thereof will give rise to a cause of action. It is proper to note, with respect to the contracts of physicians, that certain qualitative differences should be observed, since the doctor's therapeutic reassurance that his patient will be all right, not to worry, must not be converted into a binding promise by the disappointed or quarrelsome."

This sound counsel, however, should not be read to import a different standard to this relationship than to any other. It merely stresses the importance of circumstances in determining the effect of words in establishing a contract. The qualitative differ-

ence between the relationship of a physician and his patient and the relationship between a shopkeeper and his customer is a significant circumstance the fact finder must remember in assaying their respective words of undertaking.

. . . .

We conclude that under the circumstances disclosed by this record the trial court was correct in sending this case to the jury to determine the offer, acceptance, breach and damages, and refusing to grant judgment notwithstanding their verdict.

As did the Court of Appeals, we affirm.

Discussion Questions

1. What is the real issue in this case? Has the court expressed it well?

2. Why should contract principles enter into this situation? Is this not really a malpractice case?

3. What is the significance of the word "undertook" in the breach-of-contract count filed by the plaintiff?

4. Why was there a finding of "no negligence"? If there was, in fact, no negligence, how can the plaintiff be awarded $50,000?

5. What is *judgment notwithstanding the verdict? Gravamen? N.O.V.?*

6. What procedural standard did the court use in deciding this appeal?

7. Can you describe what this opinion says about the relationship between courts in a state judicial system and between legal issues and factual issues in a trial?

8. According to Southwick (see 42–43), the Michigan legislature effectively overruled the *Guilmet* decision in 1974 by passing a statute that required alleged contracts for cure to be in writing and signed by the physician. What does this action say about the system of checks and balances in our government? What does it say about the political climate in the early 1970s?

9. As a matter of public policy, should agreements guaranteeing results be in writing?

Sullivan v. O'Connor
363 Mass. 579, 296 N.E.2d 183 (1973)

Kaplan, J.

The plaintiff patient secured a jury verdict of $13,500 against the defendant surgeon for breach of contract in respect to an operation upon the plaintiff's nose. The substituted consolidated bill of exceptions presents questions about the correctness of the judge's instructions on the issue of damages.

The declaration was in two counts. In the first count, the plaintiff alleged that she, as patient, entered into a contract with the defendant, a surgeon, wherein the defendant promised to perform plastic surgery on her nose and thereby to enhance her beauty and improve her appearance; that he performed the surgery but failed to achieve the promised result; rather the result of the surgery was to disfigure and deform her nose, to cause her pain in body and mind, and to subject her to other damage and expense. The second count, based on the same transaction, was in the conventional form for malpractice, charging that the defendant had been guilty of negligence in performing the surgery. Answering, the defendant entered a general denial.

On the plaintiff's demand, the case was tried by jury. At the close of the evidence, the judge put to the jury, as special questions, the issues of liability under the two counts, and instructed them accordingly. The jury returned a verdict for the plaintiff on the contract count, and for the defendant on the negligence count. The judge then instructed the jury on the issue of damages.

As background to the instructions and the parties' exceptions, we mention certain facts as the jury could find them. The plaintiff was a professional entertainer, and this was known to the defendant. The agreement was as alleged in the declaration. More particularly, judging from exhibits, the plaintiff's nose had been straight, but long and prominent; the defendant undertook by two operations to reduce its prominence and somewhat to shorten it, thus making it more pleasing in relation to the plaintiff's other features.

Actually the plaintiff was obliged to undergo three operations, and her appearance was worsened. Her nose now had a concave line to about the midpoint, at which it became bulbous; viewed frontally, the nose from bridge to midpoint was flattened and broadened, and the two sides of the tip had lost symmetry. This configuration evidently could not be improved by further surgery. The plaintiff did not demonstrate, however, that her change of appearance had resulted in loss of employment. Payments by the plaintiff covering the defendant's fee and hospital expenses were stipulated at $622.65.

The judge instructed the jury, first, that the plaintiff was entitled to recover her out-of-pocket expenses incident to the operations. Second, she could recover the damages flowing directly, naturally, proximately, and foreseeably from the defendant's breach of promise. These would comprehend damages for any disfigurement of the plaintiff's nose—that is, any change of appearance for the worse—including the effects of the consciousness of such disfigurement on the plaintiff's mind, and in this connection the jury should consider the nature of the plaintiff's profession. Also consequent upon the defendant's breach, and compensable, were the pain and suffering involved in the third operation, but not in the first two. As there was no proof that any loss of earnings by the plaintiff resulted from the breach, that element should not enter into the calculation of damages.

By his exceptions the defendant contends that the judge erred in allowing the jury to take into account anything but the plaintiff's out-of-pocket expenses (presumably at the stipulated amount). The defendant excepted to the judge's refusal of his request for a general charge to that effect, and, more specifically, to the judge's refusal of a charge that the plaintiff could not recover for pain and suffering connected with the third operation or for impairment of the plaintiff's appearance and associated mental distress.

The plaintiff on her part excepted to the judge's refusal of a request to charge that the plaintiff could recover the difference in value between the nose as promised and the nose as it appeared after the operations. However, the plaintiff in her brief expressly waives this exception and others made by her in case this court overrules the defendant's exceptions; thus she would be content to hold the jury's verdict in her favor.

We conclude that the defendant's exceptions should be overruled.

It has been suggested on occasion that agreements between patients and physicians by which the physician undertakes to effect a cure or to bring about a given result should be declared unenforceable on grounds of public policy. See *Guilmet v. Campell* (dissenting opinion). But there are many decisions recognizing and enforcing such contracts, and the law of Massachusetts has treated them as valid, although we have had no decision meeting head on the contention that they should be denied legal sanction. These causes of action are, however, considered a little suspect, and thus we find courts straining sometimes to read the pleadings as sounding only in tort for negligence, and not in contract for breach of promise, despite sedulous efforts by the pleaders to pursue the latter theory.

It is not hard to see why the courts should be unenthusiastic or skeptical about the contract theory. Considering the uncertainties of medical science and the variations in the physical and psychological conditions of individual patients, doctors can seldom in good faith promise specific results. Therefore it is unlikely that physicians of even average integrity will in fact make such promises. Statements of opinion by the physician with some optimistic coloring are a different thing, and may indeed have therapeutic value. But patients may transform such statements into firm promises in their own minds, especially when they have been disappointed in the event, and testify in that sense to sympathetic juries. If actions for breach of promise can be readily maintained, doctors, so it is said, will be frightened into practising "defensive medicine." On the other hand, if these actions were outlawed, leaving only the possibility of suits for malpractice, there is fear that the public might be exposed to the enticements of charlatans, and confidence in the profession might ultimately be shaken. The law has taken the middle of the road position of allowing actions based on alleged contract, but insisting on clear proof. Instructions to the jury may well stress this requirement and point to tests of truth, such as the complexity or difficulty of an operation as bearing on the probability that a given result was promised.

If an action on the basis of contract is allowed, we have next the question of the measure of damages to be applied where liability is found. Some cases have taken the simple view that the promise by the physician is to be treated like an ordinary commercial promise, and accordingly that the successful plaintiff is entitled to a standard measure of recovery for breach of contract—"compensatory" ("expectancy") damages, an amount intended to put the plaintiff in the position he would be in if the contract had been performed, or, presumably, at the plaintiff's election, "restitution" damages, an amount corresponding to any benefit conferred by the plaintiff upon the defendant in the performance of the contract disrupted by the defendant's breach.

Thus in [a New Hampshire case] the defendant doctor was taken to have promised the plaintiff to convert his damaged hand by means of an operation into a good or perfect hand, but the doctor so operated as to damage the hand still further. The court, following the usual expectancy formula, would have asked the jury to estimate and award to the plaintiff the difference between the value of a good or perfect hand, as promised, and the value of the hand after the operation. (The same formula would apply, although the dollar result would be less, if the operation had neither worsened nor improved the condition of the hand.) If the plaintiff had not yet paid the doctor his fee, that amount would be deducted from the recovery. There could be no recovery for the pain and suffering of the operation, since that detriment would have been incurred even if the operation had been successful; one can say that this detriment was not "caused" by the breach. But where the plaintiff by reason of the operation was put to more pain than he would have had to endure, had the doctor performed as promised, he should be compensated for that difference as a proper part of his expectancy recovery. It may be noted that on an alternative count for malpractice the plaintiff in the *Hawkins* case had been nonsuited; but on ordinary principles this could not affect the contract claim, for it is hardly a defence to a breach of contract that the promisor acted innocently and without negligence. . . .

Other cases, including a number in New York, without distinctly repudiating the *Hawkins* type of analysis, have indicated that a different and generally more lenient measure of damages is to be applied in patient-physician actions based on breach of alleged special agreements to effect a cure, attain a stated result, or employ a given medical method. This measure is expressed in somewhat variant ways, but the substance is that the plaintiff is to recover any expenditures made by him and for other detriment (usually not specifically described in the opinions) following proximately and foreseeably upon the defendant's failure to carry out his promise. This, be it noted, is not a "restitution" measure, for

it is not limited to restoration of the benefit conferred on the defendant (the fee paid) but includes other expenditures, for example, amounts paid for medicine and nurses; so also it would seem according to its logic to take in damages for any worsening of the plaintiff's condition due to the breach. Nor is it an "expectancy" measure, for it does not appear to contemplate recovery of the whole difference in value between the condition as promised and the condition actually resulting from the treatment. Rather the tendency of the formulation is to put the plaintiff back in the position he occupied just before the parties entered upon the agreement, to compensate him for the detriments he suffered in reliance upon the agreement. . . .

For breach of the patient-physician agreements under consideration, a recovery limited to restitution seems plainly too meager, if the agreements are to be enforced at all. On the other hand, an expectancy recovery may well be excessive. The factors, already mentioned, which have made the cause of action somewhat suspect, also suggest moderation as to the breadth of the recovery that should be permitted. Where, as in the case at bar and in a number of the reported cases, the doctor has been absolved of negligence by the trier, an expectancy measure may be thought harsh. We should recall here that the fee paid by the patient to the doctor for the alleged promise would usually be quite disproportionate to the putative expectancy recovery. To attempt, moreover, to put a value on the condition that would or might have resulted, had the treatment succeeded as promised, may sometimes put an exceptional strain on the imagination of the fact finder. As a general consideration, Fuller and Perdue argue that the reasons for granting damages for broken promises to the extent of the expectancy are at their strongest when the promises are made in a business context, when they have to do with the production or distribution of goods or the allocation of functions in the market place; they become weaker as the context shifts from a commercial to a noncommercial field.

There is much to be said, then, for applying a reliance measure to the present facts, and we have only to add that our cases are not unreceptive to the use of that formula in special situations. We have, however, had no previous occasion to apply it to patient-physician cases.

The question of recovery on a reliance basis for pain and suffering or mental distress requires further attention. We find expressions in the decisions that pain and suffering (or the like) are simply not compensable in actions for breach of contract. The defendant seemingly espouses this proposition in the present case. True, if the buyer under a contract for the purchase of a lot of merchandise, in suing for the seller's breach, should claim damages for mental anguish caused by his disappointment in the transaction, he would not succeed; he would be told, perhaps, that the asserted psychological injury was not fairly foreseeable by the defendant as a probable consequence of the breach of such a business contract. But there is no general rule barring such items of damage in actions for breach of contract. It is all a question of the subject matter and background of the contract, and when the contract calls for an operation on the person of the plaintiff, psychological as well as physical injury may be expected to figure somewhere in the recovery, depending on the particular circumstances. . . . Again, it is said in a few of the New York cases, concerned with the classification of actions for statute of limitations purposes, that the absence of allegations demanding recovery for pain and suffering is characteristic of a contract claim by a patient against a physician, that such allegations rather belong in a claim for malpractice. These remarks seem unduly sweeping. Suffering or distress resulting from the breach going beyond that which was envisaged by the treatment as agreed, should be compensable on the same ground as the worsening of the patient's conditions because of the breach. Indeed it can be argued that the very suffering or distress "contracted for"—that which would have been incurred if the treatment achieved the promised result—should also be compensable on the theory underlying the New York cases. For that suffering is "wasted" if the treatment fails. Otherwise stated, compensation for this waste is arguably required in order to complete the restoration of the status quo ante.

It would, however, be a mistake to think in terms of strict "formulas." For example, a jurisdiction which would apply a reliance measure to the present facts might impose a more severe damage sanction for the wilful use by the physician of a method of operation that he undertook not to employ.

In the light of the foregoing discussion, all the defendant's exceptions fail: the plaintiff was not confined to the recovery of her out-of-pocket expenditures; she was entitled to recover also for the worsening of her condition, and for the pain and suffering and mental distress involved in the third operation. These items were compensable on either an expectancy or a reliance view. We might have been required to elect between the two views if the pain and suffering connected with the first two operations contemplated by the agreement, or the whole difference in value between the present and the promised conditions, were being claimed as elements of damage. But the plaintiff waives her possible claim to the former element, and to so much of the latter as represents the difference in value between the promised condition and the condition before the operations.

Discussion Questions

1. What benefits exist for the plaintiff seeking relief in a contract action for breach of a promise to cure as opposed to a standard negligence actions?

2. How does the plaintiff measure damages in such a lawsuit?

3. What are the policy arguments for or against requiring that agreements guaranteeing therapeutic results be in writing?

Guy v. Arthur H. Thomas Co.
55 Ohio St. 2d 183, 378 N.E.2d 488 (1978)

Locher, J.

[This case involved a work-related injury suffered by a hospital employee who was subsequently treated for her injury at the hospital where she was employed. The issue involved the application of Ohio's workers' compensation law, which generally provides an employer's exclusive liability for an employee's injuries.]

Appellant does not contend that she has an action against appellee hospital for the original compensable injury, but does assert that her action against the appellee hospital for malpractice is not prohibited by [the workers' compensation law]. . . . Appellant thus raises the application of the dual-capacity doctrine, urging that, in the instant cause, appellee hospital appears in two capacities, *i.e.*, as an employer and as a hospital, and that, as an employer, appellee hospital is liable for workers' compensation benefits, and, as a hospital it is liable in tort.

The Court of Appeals rejected this argument . . . . The Court of Appeals . . . found that, since appellant's injury "was received or contracted in the course of her employment at the defendant hospital she is barred from proceeding against the hospital for aggravating the injury." . . .

We are not persuaded that the purpose of [workers' compensation laws] is to prohibit appellant's action against appellee hospital for its negligent treatment. The genesis of workers' compensation in the United States and Ohio was the inability of the common-law remedies to cope with modern industrialism and its inherent injuries to workers. Implicit therefrom is the concept that workers' compensation statutes related generally to the legal connection or relationship between employer and employee. . . .

Workmen's [*sic*] compensation legislation rests upon the idea of status, that is, upon the conception that an injured workman is entitled to compensation for an injury sustained in the service of an industry to whose operation he contributes his work as the owner contributes his capital—the one for the sake of the wages and the other for the sake of the profits. The act is based not upon any act or omission of the employer, but upon the existence of the relationship which the employee bears to the employment because of and in the course of which he has been injured. [Quoting the U.S. Supreme Court.]

. . . .

In juxtaposition, where the employer-employee relationship does not exist, workers' compensation has not been found to affect the right of a workman to sue a third-party tortfeasor for injuries received in the course of his employment through negligence.

[The court proceeds to summarize a California case with similar facts in which the dual-capacity doctrine was used to the employee's benefit. In the course of the California opinion are found the following words on the subject: "[W]here, as here, it is perfectly apparent that the person involved—Dr. Shane—bore towards his employee two relationships—that of employer and that of a doctor—there should be no hesitancy in recognizing this fact as fact. Such a conclusion, in this case, is in precise accord with the facts and is realistic and not legalistic." The Ohio court found this logic "compelling and applicable."]

. . . The anomalous result urged by appellee [the hospital] is that the workers' compensation laws of Ohio require appellee hospital's liability to be distinguished upon whether the malpractice that aggravates a compensable injury was bestowed upon its hospital employee or any other hospital's employee or, for that matter, another's employee. Appellant's need for protection from malpractice was neither more nor less than that of another's employee. The appellee hospital, with respect to its treatment of the appellant, did so as a hospital, not as an employer, and its relationship with the appellant was that of a hospital-patient with all the concomitant traditional obligations. Furthermore, it is not denied that, if appellant's compensable injury had been aggravated by any other hospital, appellant would have had a cause of action for malpractice. We find no compelling reason why an action should be less viable merely because the traditional obligations and duties of the tortfeasor spring from the extra-relational capacity of the employer, rather than a third party.

. . . .

Accordingly, the judgment of the Court of Appeals is reversed, and the cause is remanded to the trial court for further proceedings in accordance with this opinion.

Discussion Questions

1. Do you agree with the way the court has stated the issue in this case?

2. What does it matter whether the remedy is workers' compensation or a tort action for medical malpractice?

3. What is the purpose of workers' compensation statutes?

4. Are there any additional facts that you would like to know about this situation?

5. This case is an example of one of the exceptions to the general rule that workers' compensation laws are the exclusive remedy for an employee's injuries. What are the other exceptions?

6. What does the discussion of workers' compensation tell you about the physician-patient relationship?

7. What are the implications of this type of case for corporate medical departments?

Mohr v. Williams
95 Minn. 261, 104 N.W. 12 (1905)

Brown, J.

Defendant is a physician and surgeon of standing and character, making disorders of the ear a specialty, and having an extensive practice in the city of St. Paul. He was consulted by plaintiff, who complained to him of trouble with her right ear, and, at her request, made an examination of that organ for the purpose of ascertaining its condition. He also at the same time examined her left ear, but, owing to foreign substances therein, was unable to make a full and complete diagnosis at that time. The examination of her right ear disclosed a large perforation in the lower portion of the drum membrane, and a large polyp in the middle ear, which indicated that some of the small bones of the middle ear (ossicles) were probably diseased. He informed plaintiff of the result of his examination, and advised an operation for the purpose of removing the polyp and diseased ossicles. After consultation with her family physician, and one or two further consultations with defendant, plaintiff decided to submit to the proposed operation. She was not informed that her left ear was in any way diseased, and understood that the necessity for an operation applied to her right ear only. She repaired to the hospital, and was placed under the influence of anaesthetics; and, after being made unconscious, defendant made a thorough examination of her left ear, and found it in a more serious condition than her right one. . . . He called this discovery to the attention of Dr. Davis—plaintiff's family physician, who attended the operation at her request—who also examined the ear and confirmed defendant in his diagnosis. Defendant also further examined the right ear, and found its condition less serious than expected, and finally concluded that the left, instead of the right, should be operated upon; devoting to the right ear other treatment. He then performed the operation of ossiculectomy on plaintiff's left ear; removing a portion of the drum membrane, and scraping away the diseased portion of the inner wall of the ear. The operation was in every way successful and skillfully performed. It is claimed by plaintiff that the operation greatly impaired her hearing, seriously injured her person, and, not having been consented to by her, was wrongful and unlawful, constituting an assault and battery; and she brought this action to recover damages therefor.

The trial in the court below resulted in a verdict for plaintiff for $14,322.50. Defendant thereafter moved the court for judgment notwithstanding the verdict, on the ground that, on the evidence presented, plaintiff was not entitled to recover, or, if that relief was denied, for a new trial on the ground, among others, that the verdict was excessive; appearing to have been given under the influence of passion and prejudice. The trial court denied the motion for judgment, but granted a new trial on the ground, as stated in the order, that the damages were excessive. Defendant appealed from the order denying the motion for judgment, and plaintiff appealed from the order granting a new trial.

   . . . .

We shall consider first the question whether, under the circumstances shown in the record, the consent of plaintiff to the operation was necessary. If, under the particular facts of this case, such consent was unnecessary, no recovery can be had, for the evidence fairly shows that the operation complained of was skillfully performed and of a generally beneficial nature. But if the consent of plaintiff was necessary, then the further questions presented become important.

The evidence tends to show that, upon the first examination of plaintiff, defendant pronounced the left ear in good condition, and that, at the time plaintiff repaired to the hospital to submit to the operation on her right ear, she was under the impression that no difficulty existed as to the left. In fact, she testified that she had not previously experienced any trouble with that organ. It cannot be doubted that ordinarily the patient must be consulted, and his consent given, before a physician may operate upon him.

   . . . .

If the physician advises his patient to submit to a particular operation, and the patient weighs the dangers and risks incident to its performance, and finally consents, he thereby, in effect, enters into a contract authorizing his physician to operate to the extent of the consent given, but no further.

It is not, however, contended by defendant that under ordinary circumstances consent is unnecessary, but that, under the particular circumstances of this case, consent was implied; that it was an emergency case, such as to authorize the operation without express consent or permission.

But such is not the case at bar. The diseased condition of plaintiff's left ear was not discovered in the course of an operation on the right which was authorized, but upon an independent examination of that organ, made after the authorized operation was found unnecessary. Nor is the evidence such as to justify the court in holding, as a matter of law, that it was such an affection as would result immediately in the serious injury of plaintiff, or such an emergency as to justify proceeding without her consent. She had experienced no particular difficulty with that ear, and the questions as to when its diseased condition would become alarming or fatal, and whether there was an immediate necessity for an operation, were, under the evidence, questions of fact for the jury.

   . . . .

The last contention of defendant is that the act complained of did not amount to an assault and battery. This is based upon the theory that, as plaintiff's left ear was in fact diseased, in a condition dangerous and threatening to her health, the operation was necessary, and, having been skillfully performed at a time when plaintiff had requested a like operation on the other ear, the charge of assault and battery cannot be sustained; that, in view of these conditions, and the

claim that there was no negligence on the part of defendant, and an entire absence of any evidence tending to show an evil intent, the court should say, as a matter of law, that no assault and battery was committed, even though she did not consent to the operation. In other words, that the absence of a showing that defendant was actuated by a wrongful intent, or guilty of negligence, relieves the act of defendant from the charge of an unlawful assault and battery.

We are unable to reach that conclusion, though the contention is not without merit. It would seem to follow from what has been said on the other features of the case that the act of defendant amounted at least to a technical assault and battery. If the operation was performed without plaintiff's consent, and the circumstances were not such as to justify its performance without, it was wrongful; and, if it was wrongful, it was unlawful. . . . [E]very person has a right to complete immunity of his person from physical interference of others, except in so far as contact may be necessary under the general doctrine of privilege; and any unlawful or unauthorized touching of the person of another, except it be in the spirit of pleasantry, constitutes an assault and battery. In the case at bar, as we have already seen, the question whether defendant's act in performing the operation upon plaintiff was authorized was a question for the jury to determine. If it was unauthorized, then it was, within what we have said, unlawful. It was a violent assault, not a mere pleasantry; and, even though no negligence is shown, it was wrongful and unlawful. The case is unlike a criminal prosecution for assault and battery, for there an unlawful intent must be shown. But that rule does not apply to a civil action, to maintain which it is sufficient to show that the assault complained of was wrongful and unlawful or the result of negligence.

[The Supreme Court denies the doctor's motion for judgment notwithstanding the verdict.]

Discussion Questions

1. Discuss what the court means by "technical assault and battery."

2. When will a surgeon be justified in operating beyond the scope of the patient's consent?

3. How should consent forms be drafted to anticipate these kinds of difficulties?

Stowers v. Wolodzko
386 Mich. 119, 191 N.W.2d 355 (1971)

Swainson, J.

This case presents complicated issues concerning the liability of a doctor for actions taken subsequent to a person's confinement in a private mental hospital pursuant to a valid court order.

Plaintiff, a housewife, resided in Livonia, Michigan, with her husband and children. She and her husband had been experiencing a great deal of marital difficulties and she testified that she had informed her husband two months previous to the events giving rise to this cause of action that she intended to file for a divorce.

On December 6, 1963, defendant appeared at plaintiff's home and introduced himself as "Dr. Wolodzko." Dr. Wolodzko had never met either plaintiff or her husband before he came to the house. He stated that he had been called by the husband, who had asked him to examine plaintiff. Plaintiff testified that defendant told her that he was there to ask about her husband's back. She testified that she told him to ask her husband, and that she had no further conversation with him or her husband. She testified that he never told her that he was a psychiatrist.

Dr. Wolodzko stated in his deposition that he told plaintiff he was there to examine her. However, upon being questioned upon this point, he stated that he could "not specifically" recollect having told plaintiff that he was there to examine her. He stated in his deposition that he was sure that the fact he was a psychiatrist would have come out, but that he couldn't remember if he had told plaintiff that he was a psychiatrist.

Plaintiff subsequently spoke to Dr. Wolodzko at the suggestion of a Livonia policewoman, following a domestic quarrel with her husband. He did inform her at that time that he was a psychiatrist.

On December 30, 1963, defendant Wolodzko and Dr. Anthony Smyk, apparently at the request of plaintiff's husband and without the authorization, knowledge, or consent of plaintiff, signed a sworn statement certifying that they had examined plaintiff and found her to be mentally ill. Such certificate was filed with the Wayne County Probate Court on January 3, 1964, and on the same date an order was entered by the probate court for the temporary hospitalization of plaintiff until a sanity hearing could be held. The judge ordered plaintiff committed to Ardmore Acres, a privately operated institution, pursuant to the provisions of [Michigan law].

Plaintiff was transported to Ardmore Acres on January 4, 1964.

The parties are in substantial agreement as to what occurred at Ardmore Acres. Defendant requested permission to treat the plaintiff on several different occasions, and she refused. For six days, she was placed in the "security room," which was a bare room except for the bed. The windows of the room were covered with wire mesh. During five of the six days, plaintiff refused to eat, and at all times refused medication. Defendant telephoned orders to the hospital and prescribed certain medication. He visited her often during her stay.

When plaintiff arrived at the hospital she was refused permission to receive or place telephone calls, or to receive or write letters. Dr. Wolodzko conceded at the trial that plaintiff wished to contact her brother in Texas by telephone and that he forbade her to do so. After nine days, she was allowed to call her family, but no one else. Plaintiff testified on direct examination that once during her hospitalization she asked one of her children to call her relatives in Texas and that defendant took her to her room and told her, "Mrs. Stowers, don't try that again. If you do, you will never see your children again." It is undisputed that plaintiff repeatedly requested permission to call an attorney and that Dr. Wolodzko refused such permission.

At one point when plaintiff refused medication, on the written orders of defendant, she was held by three nurses and an attendant and was forcibly injected with the medication. Hospital personnel testified at the trial that the orders concerning medication and deprivation of communication were pursuant to defendant's instructions.

Plaintiff, by chance, found an unlocked telephone near the end of her hospitalization and made a call to her relatives in Texas. She was released by court order on January 27, 1964.

Plaintiff filed suit alleging false imprisonment, assault and battery, and malpractice, against defendant Wolodzko, Anthony Smyk and Ardmore Acres. Defendants Ardmore Acres and Smyk were dismissed prior to trial.... The court granted the motion as to the count of malpractice only, but allowed the counts of assault and battery and false imprisonment to go to the jury. At the conclusion of the trial, the jury returned a verdict for plaintiff in the sum of $40,000....

....

The second issue involves whether or not there was evidence from which a jury could find false imprisonment.

"False imprisonment is the unlawful restraint of an individual's personal liberty or freedom of locomotion." It is clear that plaintiff was restrained against her will. Defendant, however, contends that because the detention was pursuant to court order (and hence not unlawful), there can be no liability for false imprisonment. However, defendant was not found liable for admitting or keeping plaintiff in Ardmore Acres. His liability stems from the fact that after plaintiff was taken to Ardmore Acres, defendant held her incommunicado and prevented her from attempting to obtain her release, pursuant to law. Holding a person incommunicado is clearly a restraint of one's freedom, sufficient to allow a jury to find false imprisonment.

Defendant contends that it was proper for him to restrict plaintiff's communication with the outside world. Defendant's witness, Dr. Sidney Bolter, testified that orders restricting communications and visitors are customary in cases of this type. Hence, defendant contends these orders were lawful and could not constitute the basis for an action of false imprisonment. However, the testimony of Dr. Bolter is not conclusive on this point.

Psychiatry is a relatively new professional discipline and, as with all disciplines, there is a great deal of controversy within the profession as to precisely what methods of treatment should be used. Psychiatrists have a great deal of power over their patients. In the case of a person confined to an institution, this power is virtually unlimited. All professions (including the legal profession) contain unscrupulous individuals who use their position to injure others. The law must provide protection against the torts committed by these individuals. In the case of mental patients, in order to have this protection, they must be able to communicate with the outside world. In our country, even a person who has committed the most abominable crime has the right to consult with an attorney.

Our Court and the courts of our sister States have recognized that interference with attempts of persons incarcerated to obtain their freedom may constitute false imprisonment. Further, we have jealously protected the individual's rights by providing that a circuit judge "who wilfully or corruptly refuses or neglects to consider an application, action, or motion for habeas corpus, is guilty of malfeasance in office."

... [P]laintiff ... was attempting to communicate with a lawyer or relative in order to obtain her release. Defendant prevented her from doing so. We ... hold that the actions on the part of defendant constitute false imprisonment.

A person temporarily committed to an institution pursuant to statute certainly must have the right to make telephone calls to an attorney or relatives. We realize that it may be necessary to restrict visits to a patient confined to a mental institution. However, the same does not apply to the right of a patient to call an attorney or relative for aid in obtaining his release. This does not mean that an individual has an unlimited right to make numerous telephone calls, once he is confined pursuant to statute. Rather, it does mean that such an individual does have a right to communicate with an attorney and/or a relative in an attempt to obtain his release.

Dr. Bolter was unable to give any valid reason why a person should not be allowed to consult with an attorney. We do not believe there is such a reason. While problems may be caused in a few cases because of this requirement, the facts in the instant case provide cogent reasons as to why such a rule is necessary. Mrs. Stowers was able to obtain her release after she made the telephone call to her relatives and they, in turn, obtained an attorney for her. Prior to this, because of the order of no communications, she was virtually held a prisoner with no chance of redress. We, therefore, agree with the Court of Appeals that there was sufficient evidence from which a jury could find that Dr. Wolodzko had committed false imprisonment.

. . . .

As Chief Justice Cooley stated almost a century ago in *Van Deusen v. Newcomer* (1879):

"An insane person does not necessarily lose his sense of justice, or of his right to the protection of the law; and when he is seized without warning, and without the hearing of those whom he might believe would testify in his behalf, and delivered helpless into the hands of strangers, to be dealt with as they may decide within the limits of a large discretion, it is impossible that he should not feel keenly the seeming injustice and lawlessness of the proceeding."

The amount awarded was within the range of the evidence, does not "shock our judicial conscience," and should not be set aside. The Court of Appeals is affirmed. . . .

Discussion Questions

1. What other information would you like to have in order to fully evaluate this case?

2. What steps might Dr. Wolodzko have taken to avoid liability for the tort of false imprisonment?

3. How are these kinds of cases handled today, clinically and legally?

3

Negligence

Beneath the extraordinary complexity of modern U.S. law lies an equally extraordinary simplicity, "as clear and orderly as anatomy"[1]: people have certain obligations toward each other; these obligations may be in the form of criminal laws, standards of ordinary prudence, or duties voluntarily assumed, but wherever they are found, their breach can be remedied through legal action rather than self-help and personal conflict.

Nowhere else is this basic simplicity of the law more evident than in the field of negligence, the most common form of litigation and the field that probably owes more to our common-law roots than any other.

Negligence is a branch of torts. A tort, simply put, is a kind of wrong. Crimes and breaches of contract are wrongs as well, of course, but negligence is a civil wrong that is neither criminal nor contractual and involves the violation of an instinctual rule of behavior—one of those basic obligations we owe each other—the obligation to be careful and prudent in our relationships.

This concept seems self-evident, but until about 110 years ago it was caught in a hopeless tangle of rules of behavior without "any underlying principle to explain their diversity."[2] But in the summer of 1880, the giant of American jurisprudence, Oliver Wendell Holmes, Jr.,

saw a simple principle that seemed to bring order into the jumble.

The organizing principle of the law was not found in the rules themselves, which were hopelessly diverse, as disparate and varied as the circumstances of human behavior. People came into court because they had been injured in some way and not because someone had violated a rule of behavior. Was the injury being complained of an accident—of which the law took no notice—or was it someone's fault? Under the skin of modern law lay not rules of behavior but a primitive impulse: blame. "Even a dog distinguishes between being stumbled over and being kicked."

The law of torts was simply the line drawn between accidental and blameworthy injuries. The line had not been drawn all at once, but by inarticulate decisions in one case after another. The concept of blame had evolved from an instinctive impulse for retribution to a modern notion of fairness. People were now held accountable only for injuries they might have foreseen and forestalled. What a person of ordinary intelligence and foresight could not foresee was accidental and therefore blameless.[3]

Holmes developed these insights, never before understood or explained, as much like a philosopher as a legal scholar. In a series of 12 masterful lectures he explained how the law had developed through "the force of [society's] collective instinct,"[4] and he set the stage for the twentieth century's emphasis on substantive fairness. The lectures were then published as a book entitled *The Common Law*, perhaps the most important single volume in American jurisprudence before or since.

The Common Law begins with an oft-quoted paragraph that summarizes in a few eloquent words the reasons why so many respect and revere our legal system:

The life of the law has not been logic; it has been experience. The felt necessities of the time, the prevalent moral and political

1. S. Novick, *Honorable Justice: The Life of Oliver Wendell Holmes* 148 (1989).
2. *Id.* at 157.
3. *Id.* The quote in the first full paragraph is from a Holmes law review article written earlier that year.
4. *Id.* at 159.

theories, institutions of public policy, avowed or unconscious, even the prejudices which judges share with their fellow men, have had a good deal more to do than the syllogism in determining the rules by which men should be governed. The law embodies the story of a nation's development through many centuries, and it cannot be dealt with as if it contained only the axioms and corollaries of a book of mathematics.[5]

Experience, the "life of the law," teaches that negligence embodies four simple concepts: duty, breach, injury, and causation. These are the subject of Chapter 3 and the following case materials.

Perin v. Hayne
210 N.W.2d 609 (Ia. 1973)

McCormick, J.

This is an appeal from a directed verdict for a doctor in a malpractice action. We affirm.

The claim arose from an anterior approach cervical fusion performed on plaintiff Ilene Perin by defendant Robert A. Hayne . . . . The fusion was successful in eliminating pain, weakness and numbness in plaintiff's back, neck, right arm and hand caused by two protruded cervical discs, but plaintiff alleged she suffered paralysis of a vocal chord because of injury to the right recurrent laryngeal nerve during surgery. . . . The injury reduced her voice to a hoarse whisper.

She sought damages on four theories: specific negligence, res ipsa loquitur, breach of express warranty[,] and battery or trespass. After both parties has rested, trial court sustained defendant's motion for directed verdict, holding the evidence insufficient to support jury consideration of the case on any of the pleaded theories. Plaintiff assigns this ruling as error. We must review each of the pleaded bases for recovery in the light of applicable law and the evidence.

I. *Specific negligence.* Plaintiff alleges there was sufficient evidence to support jury submission of her charge defendant negligently cut or injured the recurrent laryngeal nerve. Plaintiff had protruded discs at the level of the fifth and sixth cervical interspaces. The purpose of surgery was to remove the protruded discs and fuse the vertebrae with bone dowels from her hip. Removal of a disc ends the pinching of the nerve in the spinal column which causes the patient's pain. The bone supplants the disc.

The procedure involves an incision in the front of the neck at one side of the midline at a level slightly below the "adam's apple." Four columns run through the neck. The vertebrae and spinal chord are in the axial or bone column at the rear. In order to get to the axial column the surgeon must retract the visceral column which lies in front of it. The visceral column, like the vascular columns on each side of it, is covered with a protective fibrous sheath, called fascia. It contains the esophagus and trachea. The recurrent laryngeal nerve, which supplies sensitivity to the muscles that move the vocal chords, is located between the esophagus and trachea.

The surgeon does not enter the visceral column during the cervical fusion procedure. The same pliancy which enables the neck to be turned enables the visceral column to be retracted to one side to permit access to the axial column. The retraction is accomplished by using a gauze-padded retractor specifically designed for retraction of the visceral column during this surgery.

The record shows the defendant used this procedure in the present case. Plaintiff was under general anesthetic. The anesthesia record is normal, and there is no evidence of any unusual occurrence during surgery. Defendant denied any possibility the laryngeal nerve was severed. He said it could not be severed unless the visceral fascia was entered, and it was not. He also believed it would be impossible to sever the nerve during such surgery without also severing the esophagus or trachea or both.

[An expert witness testifying for the plaintiff testified that it would be unusual to specifically encounter the laryngeal nerve during this surgery but that "the injury could occur despite the exercise of all proper skill and care."]

Defendant testified he did not know the cause of the injury but presumed it resulted from contusion of the nerve incident to retraction of the visceral column. He thought plaintiff's laryngeal nerve may have been peculiarly susceptible to such injury. He insisted the surgery was done just as it always was and if he were doing it again he would do it the same way. He said one study has shown the surgery will result in paralysis of a vocal chord in two or three-tenths of one percent of cases in which it is used. He also said there is no way to predict or prevent such instances.

. . . .

In considering the propriety of the verdict directed for defendant we give the evidence supporting plaintiff's claim the most favorable construction it will reasonably bear.

We recognize three possible means to establish specific negligence of a physician. One is through expert testimony, the second through evidence showing [that] the physician's lack of care is so obvious as to be within comprehension of the layman, and the third (actually an extension of the second) evidence that the physician injured a part of the body not involved in the treatment. The first means is the rule and the others are exceptions to it.

In this case plaintiff asserts [that] a jury question was generated by the first and third means. We do not agree.

Plaintiff alleges the laryngeal nerve was negligently cut or injured. The record is devoid of any evidence the nerve was severed during surgery . . . .

5. O. Holmes, *The Common Law* 1 (1881).

The doctors agree the technique employed by defendant was proper. The sole basis for suggesting the expert testimony would support a finding of specific negligence is that the nerve was injured during retraction. Where an injury may occur despite due care, a finding of negligence cannot be predicated solely on the fact it did occur.

. . . .

Plaintiff also maintains there is evidence of negligence from the fact this is a case of injury to a part of the body not involved in the treatment. However, that is not so. The surgical procedure did include retraction of the visceral column. It was very much in the surgical field.

. . . .

Trial court did not err in directing a verdict for defendant on the issue of specific negligence.

II. *Res ipsa loquitur.* Plaintiff also alleges the applicability of the doctrine of res ipsa loquitur. Our most recent statement of the doctrine appears in [a 1973 case]:

Under the doctrine of res ipsa loquitur, where (1) injury or damage is caused by an instrumentality under the exclusive control of defendant and (2) the occurrence is such as in the ordinary course of things would not happen if reasonable care had been used, the happening of the injury permits, but does not compel, and inference defendant was negligent.

The contest in this case concerns presence of the second foundation fact [from the quoted paragraph].

. . . Defendant argues the second foundation fact for res ipsa loquitur is absent because it does not lie in the common knowledge of laymen to say injury to the laryngeal nerve does not occur if due care is exercised in anterior approach cervical fusion surgery.

We must initially decide what has previously been an open question in this jurisdiction: may the common experience to establish the second foundation fact for res ipsa loquitur be shown by expert testimony?

[The court proceeds to review cases from Wisconsin, California, Oregon, and Washington, plus three legal treatises on the subject. It quotes with favor the following:]

In the usual case the basis of past experience from which this conclusion may be drawn is common to the community, and is a matter of general knowledge, which the court recognizes on much the same basis as when it takes judicial notice of facts which everyone knows. It may, however, be supplied by the evidence of the parties; and expert testimony that such an event usually does not occur without negligence may afford a sufficient basis for the inference.

Thus we disagree with defendant's contention [that] the second foundation fact must be based exclusively on the common knowledge of laymen.

In this case, however, even considering the expert testimony, the record at best only supports an inference [that] plaintiff suffered an extremely rare injury in anterior approach cervical fusion surgery which may occur even when due care is exercised. Rarity of the occurrence is not a sufficient predicate for application of res ipsa loquitur. . . . There is no basis in the present case, in expert testimony or otherwise, for saying plaintiff's injury is more likely the result of negligence than some cause for which the defendant is not responsible

. . . .

We do not believe there was any basis in this case for submission of res ipsa loquitur. Trial court did not err in refusing to submit it.

III. *Express warranty.* [The court dismisses this count, saying that the evidence supporting her argument that the physician guaranteed a good result was equivocal in nature: "There comes a point when a question of fact may be generated as to whether the doctor has warranted a cure or a specific result. However, in the present case the evidence does not rise to that level."]

IV. *Battery or trespass.* Plaintiff contends there was also sufficient evidence to submit the case to the jury on the theory of battery or trespass. In effect, she alleges she consented to fusion of two vertebrae (removal of only one protruded disc) thinking there would be a separate operation if additional vertebrae had to be fused. She asserts the fact four vertebrae were fused combined with defendant's assurances and failure to warn her of specific hazards vitiated her consent and makes the paralyzed vocal chord the result of battery or trespass for which defendant is liable even without negligence. There was no evidence or contention by her in the trial court nor is there any assertion here that she would not have consented to the surgery had she known those things she says were withheld from her prior to surgery.

Defendant testified plaintiff was fully advised as to the nature of her problem and the scope of corrective surgery. He acknowledges he did not advise her of the hazard of vocal chord paralysis. He believed the possibility of such occurrence was negligible and outweighed by the danger of undue apprehension if warning of the risk was given.

[The court next begins a discussion of the distinction between *consent* and *informed consent*, quoting with approval from its own landmark California case of *Cobbs v. Grant*:]

Where a doctor obtains consent of the patient to perform one type of treatment and subsequently performs a substantially different treatment for which consent was not obtained, there is a clear case of battery.

However, when an undisclosed potential complication results, the occurrence of which was not an integral part of the treatment procedure but merely a known risk, the courts are divided on the issue of whether this should be deemed to be a battery or negligence.

. . . .

We agree with the majority trend. The battery theory should be reserved for those circumstances when a doctor performs an operation to which the patient has not consented. When the patient gives permission to perform one type of treatment and the doctor performs another, the requisite element of deliberate intent to deviate from the consent given is present. However, when the patient consents to certain treatment and the doctor performs that treatment but an undisclosed inherent complication with a low probability occurs, no intentional deviation from the consent given appears; rather, the doctor in obtaining consent may have failed to meet his due care duty to disclose pertinent information. In that situation the action should be pleaded in negligence.

From our approval of this analysis it should be clear we believe the battery or trespass theory pleaded by plaintiff in this case is limited in its applicability to surgery to which the patient has not consented. There must be a substantial difference between the surgery consented to and the surgery which is done. Plaintiff asserts she consented to only one fusion rather than two. Assuming this is true, the most that could be argued is [that] the second fusion was a battery or trespass. But she does not claim damages for a second fusion. She asks damages because of injury to the laryngeal nerve during surgery. The evidence is undisputed that whether one or two fusions were to be done the path to the axial column had to be cleared by retraction of the visceral column. Hence, any injury caused by such retraction occurred during a procedure to which consent had been given. Retraction of the visceral column during the surgery was not a battery or trespass.

We have no occasion to reach the question whether failure to advise plaintiff of the risk of laryngeal nerve injury would in the circumstances of this case have generated a jury issue on negligence, but we do point out that recovery on such basis is precluded unless a plaintiff also establishes he would not have submitted to the procedure if he had been advised of the risk. . . . There is no evidence plaintiff would have withheld her consent in this case.

. . . .

Affirmed.

Discussion Questions

1. Has due care been shown? Need it be?

2. What is the "second foundation fact" and how does "common experience" matter in relation to it?

3. In a deleted portion of the opinion, the court points out the consequences of the decision to consider the plaintiff's fourth theory negligence rather than battery: (1) expert opinion is not required in a battery case; (2) punitive damages are possible for battery; and (3) the patient has a longer statute of limitations under a negligence theory. Can you think of other consequences? In your opinion, do these factors augur in favor of the decision reached in this case on that point?

4. The opinion states, "There must be a substantial difference between the surgery consented to and the surgery which is done [for a battery case to be made]." What

would amount to a "substantial difference" in your mind? What if during this surgery a throat cancer had been discovered and cleanly removed with no after effects; would that constitute a substantial difference justifying damages for battery even though no other injury (in fact a benefit) had resulted?

5. Why did the court "have no occasion" to decide whether failure to advise the plaintiff of the risk of nerve injury raised a negligence issue?

Shorter v. Drury
103 Wash. 2d 645, 695 P.2d 116 (1985)

Dolliver, J.

This is an appeal from a wrongful death medical malpractice action arising out of the bleeding death of a hospital patient who, for religious reasons, refused a blood transfusion. Plaintiff, the deceased's husband and personal representative, appeals the trial court's judgment on the verdict in which the jury reduced plaintiff's wrongful death damages by 75 percent based on an assumption of risk by the Shorters that Mrs. Shorter would die from bleeding. The defendant doctor appeals the judgment alleging that a plaintiff-signed hospital release form completely barred the wrongful death action. Alternatively, defendant asks that we affirm the trial court's judgment on the verdict. Defendant does not appeal the special verdict in which the jury found the defendant negligent.

The deceased, Doreen Shorter, was a Jehovah's Witness, as is her surviving husband, Elmer Shorter. Jehovah's Witnesses are prohibited by their religious doctrine from receiving blood transfusions.

Doreen Shorter became pregnant late in the summer of 1979. In October of 1979, she consulted with the defendant, Dr. Robert E. Drury, a family practitioner. Dr. Drury diagnosed Mrs. Shorter as having had a "missed abortion". A missed abortion occurs when the fetus dies and the uterus fails to discharge it.

When a fetus dies, it is medically prudent to evacuate the uterus in order to guard against infection. To cleanse the uterus, Dr. Shorter [sic] recommended a "dilation [sic] and curettage" (D and C). There are three alternative ways to perform this operation. The first is with a curette, a metal instrument which has a sharp-edged hoop on the end of it. The second, commonly used in an abortion, involves the use of a suction device. The third alternative is by use of vaginal suppositories containing prostaglandin, a chemical that causes artificial labor contractions. Dr. Drury chose to use curettes.

Although the D and C is a routine medical procedure, there is a risk of bleeding. Each of the three principal methods for performing the D and C presented, to a varying degree, the risk of bleeding. The record below reflects that the curette method which Dr. Drury selected posed the highest degree of puncture-caused bleeding risk due to the sharpness of the instrument. The record also reflects, however, that no matter how the D and C is performed, there is always the possibility of blood loss.

Dr. Drury described the D and C procedure to Mr. and Mrs. Shorter. He advised her there was a possibility of bleeding and perforation of the uterus. Dr. Drury did not discuss any alternate methods in which the D and C may be performed. Examination of Mr. Shorter at trial revealed he was aware that the D and C posed the possibility, albeit remote, of internal bleeding.

The day before she was scheduled to receive the D and C from Dr. Drury, Mrs. Shorter sought a second opinion from Dr. Alan Ott. Mrs. Shorter advised Dr. Ott of Dr. Drury's intention to perform the D and C. She told Dr. Ott she was a Jehovah's Witness. Although he confirmed the D and C was the appropriate treatment, Dr. Ott did not discuss with Mrs. Shorter the particular method which should be used to perform it. He did, however, advise Mrs. Shorter that "she could certainly bleed during the procedure" and at trial confirmed she was aware of that possibility. Dr. Ott testified [that] Mrs. Shorter responded to his warning by saying "she had faith in the Lord and that things would work out . . ."

At approximately 6 a.m. on November 30, Mrs. Shorter was accompanied by her husband to Everett General Hospital. At the hospital the Shorters signed the following form (underlining after heading indicates blanks in form which were completed in handwriting):

GENERAL HOSPITAL OF EVERETT
REFUSAL TO PERMIT BLOOD TRANSFUSION

Date November 30, 1979   Hour 6:15 a.m.

I request that no blood or blood derivatives be administered to Doreen V. Shorter during this hospitalization. I hereby release the hospital, its personnel, and the attending physician from any responsibility whatever for unfavorable reactions or any untoward results due to my refusal to permit the use of blood or its derivatives and I fully understand the possible consequences of such refusal on my part.

[/s/ Doreen Shorter]
Patient

[/s/ Elmer Shorter]
Patient's Husband or Wife

The operation did not go smoothly. Approximately 1 hour after surgery, Mrs. Shorter began to bleed internally and go into shock. Emergency exploratory surgery conducted by other surgeons revealed Dr. Drury had severely lacerated Mrs. Shorter's uterus when he was probing with the curette.

Mrs. Shorter began to bleed profusely. She continued to refuse to authorize a transfusion despite repeated warnings by the doctors she would likely die due to blood loss. Mrs. Shorter was coherent at the time she refused to accept blood. While the surgeons repaired Mrs. Shorter's perforated uterus and abdomen, Dr. Drury and several other doctors pleaded with Mr. Shorter to permit them to transfuse blood into Mrs. Shorter. He likewise refused. Mrs. Shorter bled to death. Doctors for both parties agreed a transfusion in substantial probability would have saved Doreen Shorter's life.

Mr. Shorter thereafter brought this wrongful death action alleging Dr. Drury's negligence proximately caused Mrs. Shorter's death . . . .

The jury found Dr. Drury negligent and that his negligence was "a proximate cause of the death of Doreen Shorter". Damages were found to be $412,000. The jury determined, however, that Mr. and/or Mrs. Shorter "knowingly and voluntarily" assumed the risk of bleeding to death and attributed 75 percent of the fault for her death to her and her husband's refusal to authorize or accept a blood transfusion. Plaintiff was awarded judgment of $103,000. Both parties moved for judgment notwithstanding the verdict. The trial court denied both motions. Plaintiff appealed and defendant cross-appealed to the Court of Appeals, which certified the case [to this court].

The three issues before us concern the admissibility of the "Refusal to Permit Blood Transfusion" (refusal); whether assumption of the risk is a valid defense and if so, whether there is sufficient evidence for the jury to have found the risk was assumed by the Shorters; and whether the submission of the issue of assumption of the risk to the jury violated the free exercise clause of the First Amendment. The finding of negligence by Dr. Drury is not appealed by defendant.

I

Plaintiff argues the purpose of the refusal was only to release the defendant doctor from liability for not transfusing blood into Mrs. Shorter had she required blood during the course of a nonnegligently performed operation. He further asserts the refusal as it applies to the present case violates public policy since it would release Dr. Drury from the consequences of his negligence.

Defendant concedes a survival action filed on behalf of Mrs. Shorter for her negligently inflicted injuries would not be barred by the refusal since enforcement would violate public policy. Defendant argues, however, the refusal does not release the doctor for his negligence but only for the consequences arising out of Mrs. Shorter's voluntary refusal to accept blood, which in this case was death.

While the rule announced by this court is that contracts against liability for negligence are valid except in those cases where the public interest is involved, the refusal does not address the negligence of Dr. Drury. This being so it cannot be considered as a release from liability for negligence.

Plaintiff categorizes the refusal as an all or nothing instrument. He claims that if it is a release of liability for negligence it is void as against public policy and if it is a release of liability where a transfusion is required because of non-negligent treatment then it is irrelevant. We have already stated the document cannot be considered as a release from liability for negligence. The document is more, however, than a simple declaration that the signer would refuse blood only if there was no negligence by Dr. Drury. It is a specific request that no blood or blood derivatives be administered to Mrs. Shorter. The attending physician is released from "any responsibility whatever for unfavorable reactions or any untoward results due to my refusal to permit the use of blood or its derivatives." The release signed by the Shorters further stated: "I fully understand the possible consequences of such refusal on my part."

We find the refusal to be valid. There was sufficient evidence for the jury to find it was not signed unwittingly but rather voluntarily. The record shows Dr. Ott advised Mrs. Shorter that her refusal to accept a transfusion could place her life in jeopardy if she bled from a D and C. Dr. Ott further testified there was a risk of bleeding with a routine D and C and that if she then refused a transfusion she might die. Specifically, Dr. Ott stated he advised Mrs. Shorter that if a perforation occurred at the time of the D and C she would be in grave jeopardy. He also stated Mrs. Shorter said she knew this but remained firm in her conviction to refuse a blood transfusion. Knowing this, and in response to their religious beliefs, the Shorters signed the refusal. In refusing a blood transfusion, the Shorters were acting under the compulsion of circumstances. The compulsion, however, was created by the religious convictions of the Shorters not by the tortious conduct of defendant.

We also hold the release was not against public policy. We emphasize again the release did not exculpate Dr. Drury from his negligence in performing the surgery. Rather, it was an agreement that Mrs. Shorter should receive no blood or blood derivatives. The cases cited by defendant all refer to exculpatory clauses which release a physician or hospital from all liability for negligence. The Shorters specifically accepted the risk which might flow from a refusal to accept blood. Given the particular problems faced when a patient on religious grounds refuses to permit necessary or advisable blood tranfusions, we believe the use of a release such as signed here is appropriate. Requiring physicians or hospitals to obtain a court order would be cumbersome and impractical. Furthermore, it might subject the hospital or physician to an action under [the U.S. civil rights laws]. The alternative of physicians or hospitals refusing to care for Jehovah's Witnesses is repugnant in a society which attempts to make medical care available to all its members.

We believe the procedure used here, the voluntary execution of a document protecting the physician and hospital and the patient is an appropriate alternative and not contrary to the public interest.

If the refusal is held valid, defendant asserts it acts as a complete bar to plaintiff's wrongful death claim. We disagree. While Mrs. Shorter accepted the consequences resulting from a refusal to receive a blood transfusion, she did not accept the consequences of Dr. Drury's negligence which was, as the jury found, a proximate cause of Mrs. Shorter's death. Defendant was not released from his negligence. We next consider the impact of the doctrine of assumption of the risk on this negligence.

II

Plaintiff argues [that] the trial court erred in admitting jury instructions [on the "assumption of risk" theory]. . . .

. . . .

. . . We confine our analysis to the validity of express assumption of risk and the extent to which it applies in the circumstances of this case.

Express assumption of the risk is a defense when:

[T]he plaintiff, in advance, has given his express consent to relieve the defendant of an obligation oft conduct toward him, and to take his chances of injury from a known risk arising from what the defendant is to do or leave undone.

Jurisdictions with comparative negligence statutes have generally held that the defense of express assumption of the risk survives the enactment of these statutes.

. . . .

The next question is whether the Shorters could be found by the jury to have expressly assumed the risk that Dr. Drury's performance of the D and C could be negligent, thereby increasing Mrs. Shorter's chances of bleeding to death. The test is a subjective one: Whether the plaintiff in fact understood the risk; not whether the reasonable person of ordinary prudence would comprehend the risk.

The general rule is that for persons to assume a risk, they must be aware of more than just the generalized risk of their activities; there must be proof they knew of and appreciated the specific hazard which caused the injury. From this rule, plaintiff argues that while he and his wife were aware of the generalized risk of bleeding to death, they did not understand Mrs. Shorter's chances of bleeding to death would be greatly increased by Dr. Drury's negligence. The Shorters, however, did not merely assume a "generalized risk". They assumed the specific risk that Mrs. Shorter might die from bleeding if she refused to permit a blood transfusion.

The Shorters signed the refusal which stated that they waived professional liability for "unfavorable reactions" or "untoward results" due to Mrs. Shorter's refusal to permit the use of blood. Mrs. Shorter consulted with Drs. Drury and Ott, both of whom advised her that the D and C, even if nonnegligently performed, could result in fatal bleeding.

Furthermore, the Shorters were repeatedly advised Mrs. Shorter was bleeding and that without a transfusion her death was imminent.

Plaintiff calls our attention to the common law principle that a person cannot assume the risk of another's negligence. While we do not question the rule, we disagree with plaintiff's assertion that it applies in this case.

. . . Defendant argues, however, and we agree, that the Shorters could be found by the jury to have assumed the risk of death from an operation which had to be performed without blood transfusions and where blood could not be administered under any circumstances including where the doctor made what would otherwise have been correctable surgical mistake. The risk of death from a failure to receive a transfusion to which the Shorters exposed themselves was created by, and must be allocated to, the Shorters themselves.

. . . .

III

Finally, plaintiff asserts the submission of the issue of assumption of the risk to the jury violated the free exercise clause of the First Amendment. Plaintiff concedes he has found no cases involving the effect of a patient's refusal of blood in a malpractice action. Nevertheless, plaintiff claims error in the refusal of the trial court to give his proposed instruction . . . which would have told the jury compensation could not be denied because of a refusal of blood for religious reasons. While the Supreme Court has stated the free exercise clause of the First Amendment forbids the "state condition[ing] receipt of an important benefit upon conduct proscribed by a religious faith", a prerequisite for First Amendment cases is that there be some state action or interference. There is none here. This is a dispute between private individuals; plaintiff is denied no rights under the First Amendment.

. . . .

Affirmed.

Discussion Questions

1. What does *assumption of risk* mean? What does it mean that "a person cannot assume the risk of another's negligence"? How does assumption of risk, in effect, negate the existence of the defendant's negligence?

2. On what grounds does the court allow the partial release to stand? What other methods might medical providers use to protect against the risk of lawsuits from patients who refuse necessary medical treatments?

3. Jehovah's Witnesses' refusal to accept blood transfusions is based on their religious interpretation of the Bible. For example, "A human is not to sustain life with the blood of another creature" (Genesis 9:3–4). Would this religious basis for the refusal augur for a different constitutional result if a state hospital had been involved? (See also discussions of consent in Chapter 10 of this book and the Southwick text.)

Helling v. Carey
83 Wash. 2d 514, 519 P.2d 981 (1974)

Hunter, J.

[This is a malpractice case involving failure to diagnose Barbara Helling's primary open angle glaucoma. The defendants are ophthalmologists who saw Mrs. Helling 11 times for vision exams and contact lenses from 1959 to 1968. Not until October 1968, when she was 32 years old, did the defendants test Mrs. Helling's intraocular pressure. This test indicated that she had glaucoma, that she had lost essentially all peripheral vision, and that her central vision was much reduced. The case turns on the standard of care for ophthalmologists under these circumstances. Expert witnesses on both sides testified that professional standards did not require routine pressure tests for patients under 40 years of age unless "the patients complaints and symptoms reveal to the physician that glaucoma should be suspected." The jury returned a verdict for the defense, the intermediate appellate court affirmed, and the plaintiffs appealed to the supreme court.]

We find this to be a unique case. The testimony of the medical experts is undisputed concerning the standards of the profession for the specialty of ophthalmology. It is not a question in this case of the defendants having any greater special ability, knowledge and information than other ophthalmologists which would require the defendants to comply with a higher duty of care than that "degree of care and skill which is expected of the average practitioner in the class to which he belongs, acting in the same or similar circumstances." The issue is whether the defendants' compliance with the standard of the profession of ophthalmology, which does not require the giving of a routine pressure test to persons under 40 years of age, should insulate them from liability under the facts of this case . . . .

[The court points out evidence that the incidence of glaucoma in persons under the age of 40 is about 1 in 25,000.] However, that one person, the plaintiff in this instance, is entitled to the same protection, as afforded persons over 40, essential for timely detection of the evidence of glaucoma where it can be arrested to avoid the grave and devastating result of this disease. The test is a simple pressure test, relatively inexpensive. There is no judgment factor involved, and there is no doubt that by giving the test the evidence of glaucoma can be detected. . . .

Justice Holmes stated in *Texas & Pac. Ry. v. Behymer*:

What usually is done may be evidence of what ought to be done, but what ought to be done is fixed by a standard of reasonable prudence, whether it usually is complied with or not.

In [another case,] Justice [Learned] Hand stated:

[I]n most cases reasonable prudence is in fact common prudence; but strictly it is never its measure; a whole calling may have unduly lagged in the adoption of new and available devices. It never may set its own tests, however persuasive be its usages. *Courts must in the end say which is required; there are precautions so imperative that even their universal disregard will not excuse their omission.* [Italics added by the court.]

Under the facts of this case reasonable prudence required the timely giving of the pressure test to this plaintiff. The precaution of giving this test to detect the incidence of glaucoma to patients under 40 years of age is so imperative that irrespective of its disregard by the standards of the ophthalmology profession, it is the duty of the courts to say what is required to protect patients under 40 from the damaging results of glaucoma.

We therefore hold, as a matter of law, that the reasonable standard that should have been followed under the undisputed facts of this case was the timely giving of this simple, harmless pressure test to this plaintiff and that, in failing to do so, the defendants were negligent, which proximately resulted in the blindness sustained by the plaintiff for which the defendants are liable.

. . . .

The judgment of the trial court and the decision of the Court of Appeals [are] reversed, and the case is remanded for a new trial on the issue of damages only.

HALE, C.J., and ROSELLINI, STAFFORD, WRIGHT and BRACHTENBACH, JJ, concur.

UTTER, Associate Justice (concurring).

I concur in the result reached by the majority. . . .

The difficulty with this approach is that we, as judges, by using a negligence analysis, seem to be imposing a stigma of moral blame upon the doctors who, in this case, used all the precautions commonly prescribed by their profession in diagnosis and treatment. Lacking their training in this highly sophisticated profession, it seems illogical for this court to say they failed to exercise a reasonable standard of care. It seems to me we are, in reality, imposing liability because, in choosing between an innocent plaintiff and a doctor who acted reasonably according to his specialty but who could have prevented the full effects of this disease by administering a simple, harmless test and treatment, the plaintiff should not have to bear the risk of loss. As such, imposition of liability approaches that of strict liability.

[The opinion explains that strict liability is appropriate "where there is blame on neither side" and it seems appropriate to ask who can best bear the loss. Thus, according to Justice Utter, "strict liability serves a compensatory function in situations where the defendant is, through the use of insurance, the financially more responsible person."]

FINLEY and HAMILTON, JJ, concur.

Discussion Questions

1. Do you agree with the way the court has stated the issue in this case? What does the way it is stated tell you about what the decision is going to be?

2. Do you agree with the concurring opinion? In what other circumstances would strict liability be appropriate?

3. Is this an example of judge-made law? Should this decision have been left to the legislature? Or to the medical profession?

4. What do you suppose was the aftermath of this decision in the medical profession?

5. Note that the Washington legislature attempted, apparently without success, to reverse the effects of this decision (see page 59 in Southwick text). Do you agree, from a policy standpoint, that the courts should be able to dictate what members of a profession ought to do?

Tunkl v. Regents of the Univ. of Calif.
60 Cal. 2d 92, 383 P.2d 441, 32 Cal. Rptr. 33 (1963)

Tobriner, J.

This case concerns the validity of a release from liability for future negligence imposed as a condition for admission to a charitable research hospital. For the reasons we hereinafter specify, we have concluded that an agreement between a hospital and an entering patient affects the public interest and that, in consequence, the exculpatory provision included within it must be invalid under Civil Code section 1668.

Hugo Tunkl brought this action to recover damages for personal injuries alleged to have resulted from the negligence of two physicians in the employ of the University of California Los Angeles Medical Center, a hospital operated and maintained by the Regents of the University of California as a nonprofit charitable institution. Mr. Tunkl died after suit was brought, and his surviving wife, as executrix, was substituted as plaintiff.

The University of California at Los Angeles Medical Center admitted Tunkl as a patient on June 11, 1956. The Regents maintain the hospital for the primary purpose of aiding and developing a program of research and education in the field of medicine; patients are selected and admitted if the study and treatment of their condition would tend to achieve these purposes. Upon his entry to the hospital, Tunkl signed a document setting forth certain "Conditions of Admission." The crucial condition number six reads as follows: "RELEASE: The hospital is a nonprofit, charitable institution. In consideration of the hospital and allied services to be rendered and the rates charged therefor, the patient or his legal representative agrees to and hereby releases The Regents of the University of California, and the hospital from any and all liability for the negligent or wrongful acts or omissions of its employees, if the hospital has used due care in selecting its employees."

Plaintiff stipulated that the hospital had selected its employees with due care. The trial court ordered that the issue of the validity of the exculpatory clause be first submitted to the jury and that, if the jury found that the provision did not bind plaintiff, a second jury try the issue of alleged malpractice. When, on the preliminary issue, the jury returned a verdict sustaining the validity of the executed release, the court entered judgment in favor of the Regents. Plaintiff appeals from the judgment.

We shall first set out the basis for our prime ruling that the exculpatory provision of the hospital's contract fell under the proscription of Civil Code section 1668; we then dispose of two answering arguments of defendant.

We begin with the dictate of the relevant Civil Code section 1668. The section states: "All contracts which have for their object, directly or indirectly, to exempt anyone from responsibility for his own fraud, or willful injury to the person or property of another, or violation of law, whether willful or negligent, are against the policy of the law."

The course of section 1668, however, has been a troubled one. Although, as we shall explain, the decisions uniformly uphold its prohibitory impact in one circumstance, the courts' interpretations of it have been diverse. Some of the cases have applied the statute strictly, invalidating any contract for exemption from liability for negligence. . . . Other cases hold that the statute prohibits the exculpation of gross negligence only; still another case states that the section forbids exemption from active as contrasted with passive negligence.

In one respect, as we have said, the decisions are uniform. The cases have consistently held that the exculpatory provision may stand only if it does not involve "the public interest." . . .

. . . .

If, then, [an] exculpatory clause which affects the public interest cannot stand, we must ascertain those factors or characteristics which constitute the public interest. The social forces that have led to such characterization are volatile and dynamic. No definition of the concept of public interest can be contained within the four corners of a formula. The concept, always the subject of great debate, has ranged over the whole course of the common law; rather than attempt to pre-

scribe its nature, we can only designate the situations in which it has been applied. We can determine whether the instant contract does or does not manifest the characteristics which have been held to stamp a contract as one affected with a public interest.

In placing particular contracts within or without the category of those affected with a public interest, the courts have revealed a rough outline of that type of transaction in which exculpatory provisions will be held invalid. Thus the attempted but invalid exemption involves a transaction which exhibits some or all of the following characteristics. It concerns a business of a type generally thought suitable for public regulation. The party seeking exculpation is engaged in performing a service of great importance to the public, which is often a matter of practical necessity for some members of the public. The party holds himself out as willing to perform this service for any member of the public who seeks it, or at least for any member coming within certain established standards. As a result of the essential nature of the service, in the economic setting of the transaction, the party invoking exculpation possesses a decisive advantage of bargaining strength against any member of the public who seeks his services. In exercising a superior bargaining power the party confronts the public with a standardized adhesion contract of exculpation, and makes no provision whereby a purchaser may pay additional reasonable fees and obtain protection against negligence. Finally, as a result of the transaction, the person or property of the purchaser is placed under the control of the seller, subject to the risk of carelessness by the seller or his agents.

While obviously no public policy opposes private, voluntary transactions in which one party, for a consideration, agrees to shoulder a risk which the law would otherwise have placed upon the other party, the above circumstances pose a different situation. In this situation the releasing party does not really acquiesce voluntarily in the contractual shifting of the risk, nor can we be reasonably certain that he receives an adequate consideration for the transfer. Since the service is one which each member of the public, presently or potentially, may find essential to him, he faces, despite his economic inability to do so, the prospect of a compulsory assumption of the risk of another's negligence. The public policy of this state has been, in substance, to posit the risk of negligence upon the actor; in instances in which this policy has been abandoned, it has generally been to allow or require that the risk shift to another party better or equally able to bear it, not to shift the risk to the weak bargainer.

In the light of the decisions, we think that the hospital-patient contract clearly falls within the category of agreements affecting the public interest. To meet that test, the agreement need only fulfill some of the characteristics above outlined; here, the relationship fulfills all of them. Thus the contract of exculpation involves an institution suitable for, and a subject of, public regulation. That the services of the hospital to those members of the public who are in special need of the particular skill of its staff and facilities constitute a practical and crucial necessity is hardly open to question.

The hospital, likewise, holds itself out as willing to perform its services for those members of the public who qualify for its research and training facilities. While it is true that the hospital is selective as to the patients it will accept, such selectivity does not negate its public aspect or the public interest in it. The hospital is selective only in the sense that it accepts from the public at large certain types of cases which qualify for the research and training in which it specializes. But the hospital does hold itself out to the public as an institution which performs such services for those members of the public who can qualify for them.

In insisting that the patient accept the provision of waiver in the contract, the hospital certainly exercises a decisive advantage in bargaining. The would-be patient is in no position to reject the proffered agreement, to bargain with the hospital, or in lieu of agreement to find another hospital. The admission room of a hospital contains no bargaining table where, as in a private business transaction, the parties can debate the terms of their contract. As a result, we cannot but conclude that the instant agreement manifested the characteristics of the so-called adhesion contract. Finally, when the patient signed the contract, he completely placed himself in the control of the hospital; he subjected himself to the risk of its carelessness.

In brief, the patient here sought the services which the hospital offered to a selective portion of the public; the patient, as the price of admission and as a result of his inferior bargaining position, accepted a clause in a contract of adhesion waiving the hospital's negligence; the patient thereby subjected himself to control of the hospital and the possible infliction of the negligence which he had thus been compelled to waive. The hospital, under such circumstances, occupied a status different than a mere private party; its contract with the patient affected the public interest. We see no cogent current reason for according to the patron of the inn a greater protection than the patient of the hospital; we cannot hold the innkeeper's performance affords a greater public service than that of the hospital.

We turn to a consideration of the two arguments urged by defendant to save the exemptive clause. Defendant first contends that while the public interest may possibly invalidate the exculpatory provision as to the paying patient, it certainly cannot do so as to the charitable one. Defendant secondly argues that even if the hospital cannot obtain exemption as to its "own" negligence it should be in a position to do so as to that of its employees. We have found neither proposition persuasive.

As to the first, we see no distinction in the hospital's duty of due care between the paying and nonpaying patient. The duty, emanating not merely from contract but also tort,

imports no discrimination based upon economic status. . . . To immunize the hospital from negligence as to the charitable patient because he does not pay would be as abhorrent to medical ethics as it is to legal principle.

Defendant's second attempted distinction, the differentiation between its own and vicarious liability, strikes a similar discordant note. In form defendant is a corporation. In everything it does, including the selection of its employees, it necessarily acts through agents. A legion of decisions involving contracts between common carriers and their customers, public utilities and their customers, bailees and bailors, and the like, have drawn no distinction between the corporation's "own" liability and vicarious liability resulting from negligence of agents. We see no reason to initiate so far-reaching a distinction now. If, as defendant argues, a right of action against the negligent agent is in fact a sufficient remedy, then defendant by paying a judgment against it may be subrogated to the right of the patient against the negligent agent, and thus may exercise that remedy.

In substance defendant here asks us to modify our decision in [an earlier case] which removed the charitable immunity; defendant urges that otherwise the funds of the research hospital may be deflected from the real objective of the extension of medical knowledge to the payment of claims for alleged negligence. Since a research hospital necessarily entails surgery and treatment in which fixed standards of care may not yet be evolved, defendant says the hospital should in this situation be excused from such care. But the answer lies in the fact that possible plaintiffs must prove negligence; the standards of care will themselves reflect the research nature of the treatment; the hospital will not become an insurer or guarantor of the patient's recovery. To exempt the hospital completely from any standard of due care is to grant it immunity by the side-door method of a contractual clause exacted of the patient. We cannot reconcile that technique with the teaching of [the earlier case].

We must note, finally, that the integrated and specialized society of today, structured upon mutual dependency, cannot rigidly narrow the concept of the public interest. From the observance of simple standards of due care in the driving of a car to the performance of the high standards of hospital practice, the individual citizen must be completely dependent upon the responsibility of others. The fabric of this pattern is so closely woven that the snarling of a single thread affects the whole. We cannot lightly accept a sought immunity from careless failure to provide the hospital service upon which many must depend. Even if the hospital's doors are open only to those in a specialized category, the hospital cannot claim isolated immunity in the interdependent community of our time. It, too, is part of the social fabric, and prearranged exculpation from its negligence must partly rend the pattern and necessarily affect the public interest.

The judgment is reversed.

Discussion Questions

1. Why is the concept of public interest important to this decision?

2. Do you agree with the factors that the court uses in determining what amounts to matters "affected with a public interest"?

3. Many kinds of organizations other than hospitals have tried to limit their own liability by the use of exculpatory contracts. Some examples include school districts (for children's field trips); the Boy Scouts and Girl Scouts (for various functions); churches (likewise, for activities); and small businesses (disclaiming liability for hat check stands and valet parking). Under what circumstances would you argue that exculpatory contracts should be valid? Where would you draw the line, and how would you define that line?

4. Do you agree that hospitals should not be able to limit their liability through the use of exculpatory contracts? Would such agreements ever be valid in a hospital setting?

Marshall v. Yale Podiatry Group
5 Conn. App. 5, 496 A.2d 529 (1985)

Dupont, C.J.

This case presents the question of whether an orthopedic surgeon is qualified to testify as an expert as to the standard of care required in connection with the performance of foot surgery by a licensed podiatrist certified in the field of surgery.

This is a medical malpractice action arising out of surgery performed by the defendant Jeffrey Yale, a licensed podiatrist in Connecticut, on the plaintiff's right and left feet. Yale is an agent and employee of the defendant Yale Podiatry Group, P.C. His examination of the plaintiff disclosed a hallux limitus of the right foot (restricted, painful range of big toe motion) and a tailor's bunion of the left foot. To alleviate the plaintiff's condition, Yale operated on the plaintiff implanting an artificial joint in the plaintiff's right, big toe and removing a portion of the plaintiff's left small toe.

At trial, the plaintiff called Urelich Weil, an orthopedic surgeon, to testify to the applicable standard of care for such surgery. The defendants objected to Weil's testifying, claiming that he was not qualified to testify as to the applicable standard of care. The trial court sustained the defendants' objection and the plaintiff excepted. Weil was the plaintiff's only expert witness and therefore the plaintiff rested since without his testimony the plaintiff could not prevail. The defendants moved for a directed verdict, which the trial court

granted. The plaintiff moved to set aside the verdict, which the trial court denied and the plaintiff appealed.

The standard of care to which physicians and surgeons are held is "that which physicians and surgeons in the same general neighborhood and in the same general line of practice ordinarily have and exercise in like cases." When the court formulated that test, the "same general neighborhood" was interpreted as a territorial limitation restricted to the confines of the community in which the doctor practiced. In [a 1932 case], the "general neighborhood" was considered the state of Connecticut. It has now been broadened to include the entire nation. These cases reveal a trend towards the liberalization of the rules involving the qualifications of medical experts.

Although the issue of this case does not involve the geographical limitation on medical expert testimony, but rather the "general line of practice" limitation on expert medical testimony offered in a medical malpractice action, the liberalization of the evidentiary rules regarding the former limitation are relevant in analyzing the latter limitation.

Our analysis of cases starts with [a 1975 decision] where the court found that the trial court erred in excluding the plaintiff's expert, a practicing surgeon specializing in breast cancer surgery, from testifying as to the proper medical standards of practice among obstetrician-gynecologists pertaining to breast examinations. In that case, the testimony was "that breast lump examinations are performed in exactly the same manner by obstetrician-gynecologists and surgeons; and that these two specialties are identical with respect to breast lump examination and diagnosis." The threshold question of admissibility is governed by the scope of the witness' knowledge and not the artificial classification of the witness by title.

Our appellate courts have had occasion to address this issue since that case. . . . The common thread tying these decisions together is that where the evidence indicates that the specialties overlap and the applicable standard of care is common to each, a medical expert from either of the overlapping groups who is familiar with that common standard is competent to testify as to the standard of care.

Connecticut has not previously considered whether an orthopedic surgeon can testify as an expert against a podiatrist in a malpractice action. Other jurisdictions, however, have addressed this issue, reaching varying decisional results. The Ohio Supreme Court, citing a Connecticut case, held that the plaintiff's medical expert, a podiatrist, was competent to testify as to the alleged malpractice, applying and failing to remove a cast which was too tight, by the defendant orthopedic surgeon. The record disclosed that the application and removal of casts is an area where these fields of medicine overlap. The court, therefore, concluded that the podiatrist was qualified to testify as an expert. The Georgia Court of Appeals addressed this issue, holding that where the evidence indicates the fields overlap and the methods of treatment are the same for the schools involved, an orthopedic surgeon can testify as an expert as to the standard of care which must be exercised by a podiatrist. The California Court of Appeals has addressed the analogous issue of whether a podiatrist can testify as to the applicable standard of care of an orthopedic surgeon performing foot surgery, holding that he can. The record revealed a familiarity with the surgery and contained testimony that the fields overlapped.

There is, however, a line of authority excluding such testimony. The South Carolina Court of Appeals has held that an orthopedic surgeon was not competent to testify as to the applicable standard of care in a malpractice action against a podiatrist. The record there revealed that the orthopedic surgeon had never performed ambulatory foot surgery nor was he familiar with the surgical procedure performed. Likewise, the North Carolina Court of Appeals has excluded the testimony of an orthopedic surgeon on the applicable standard of care in a malpractice action against a podiatrist. The record also revealed an unfamiliarity with the field of practice. The Illinois Supreme Court has considered whether "a plaintiff may establish the standard of care a podiatrist owes a patient by offering the testimony of a physician or surgeon, or another expert other than a podiatrist." The court held that "in order to testify as an expert on the standard of care in a given school of medicine, the witness must be licensed therein." The dissent casts this as a mechanical and formalistic resolution of the issue.

The decisions allowing and excluding expert testimony in this area generally focus on the expert's familiarity with the school of medicine and the procedures involved. To resolve this issue in the context of this case requires an examination of the testimony proffered to qualify Weil as an expert, in order to determine whether he possessed a sufficient familiarity with the school of medicine and the procedures involved.

In the absence of the jury, Weil was extensively examined regarding his qualifications to testify as an expert. He testified that he has performed hundreds of operations on the feet, that he was familiar with the surgical procedure performed on the plaintiff's feet, and that he was familiar with the treatment, both conservatively and surgically, of keratosis and calluses upon the feet. Further, he testified that he had worked with almost all of the podiatrists in the New Haven area. They had referred patients to him for treatment and he had referred patients to them, generally for conservative treatment, but occasionally for surgical procedures performed in a hospital. He had observed and performed operations where more than one head and neck of a metatarsal was removed for neurological disorders of the feet. Here, the defendant podiatrist removed the fifth metatarsal of the plaintiff's left foot. In addition, the doctor testified that he had performed implant operations and was familiar with implants into the foot and toes, but had never performed an implant operation on the toes. He stated that he was familiar with the standard of care applicable to the treatment of keratosis and bunions and that the standard of care did not change simply because a podiatrist rather than an orthopedic surgeon treated the patient.

The defendant podiatrist testified that, in terms of foot surgery, orthopedic surgeons and podiatric surgeons generally performed the same procedures. He admitted that a certain medical text on surgery on the feet was authoritative. Weil expressed a familiarity with that text insofar as it pertains to the plaintiff's preoperative condition and the surgical and conservative nonsurgical techniques for the treatment of the plaintiff's condition. Although Weil had never performed or assisted in the surgical procedures involved in the treatment of the plaintiff's malady, this was so because he questioned the use of such procedures. The extensive offer of proof discloses that the plaintiff's expert had the requisite familiarity with the particular school of medicine and the procedure involved to substantiate that he had the necessary qualifications to give his opinion as to the standard of care.

There is error, the judgment is set aside and a new trial is ordered.

Discussion Questions

1. What might have been the practical effect for the practice of podiatry if the decision in *Marshall* had been the opposite?

2. Do you believe it is fair to allied health professionals that they be judged by the standards of MDs? Is it fair to MDs that others, with different training, be permitted to practice in the profession? Which viewpoint is better from a public policy perspective?

Morris v. Metriyakool
Jackson v. Detroit Memorial Hosp.
418 Mich. 423, 344 N.W.2d 736 (1984)

Kavanagh, J.

These cases concern arbitration of medical malpractice claims. The most significant issue presented is whether the [Michigan] malpractice arbitration act of 1975 deprives plaintiffs of constitutional rights to an impartial decisionmaker. We hold that it does not.

Plaintiff Diane Jackson was treated in November, 1977, at defendant Detroit Memorial Hospital by defendant Dr. William J. Bloom for a dental malady. At that time, plaintiff agreed to submit to arbitration "any claims or disputes (except for disputes over charges for services rendered) which may arise in the future out of or in connection with the health care rendered to me by this hospital, its employees and those of its independent staff doctors and consultants who have agreed to arbitrate". In August, 1979, plaintiff brought action for malpractice against defendants in the Wayne Circuit Court. Defendants moved for accelerated judgment, on the basis of the agreement to arbitrate. After a hearing, the court found the act constitutional and, finding no duress, mistake, or incompetency in the execution of the agreement, granted defendants' motion. The Court of Appeals reversed, holding that [the arbitration statute] violates the constitutional guarantee of due process by " 'forcing the litigant to submit his or her claim to a tribunal which is composed in such a way that a high probability exists that such tribunal will be biased against the claimant without mandating the use of an arbitration form explicitly detailing the nature of the panel's makeup' ". The Court also held that the arbitration agreement is not a contract of adhesion and that, on the present facts, it is not unconscionable. Defendants applied for leave to appeal, and plaintiffs sought leave to cross-appeal, which we granted.

In the second case before us, plaintiff Delores M. Morris was admitted to defendant South Macomb Hospital on November 9, 1976. At the time of her admission, plaintiff executed an agreement similar to the one executed by plaintiff Jackson to arbitrate any claims against defendant hospital and defendant Dr. S. Metriyakool arising out of her treatment for a hysterectomy. Subsequently, plaintiff brought suit against defendants alleging negligence in the surgical procedure, which caused her to develop peritonitis, and negligence in failing to promptly diagnose and treat the condition. Defendants each moved to submit plaintiff's claims to arbitration in accordance with the agreement. The trial court dismissed plaintiff's complaint with prejudice, but without prejudice to her right to file a claim for arbitration.

The Court of Appeals rejected plaintiff's argument that the composition of the arbitration panel was unconstitutionally biased. It also held that the act does not unconstitutionally or unconscionably deprive a patient of a meaningful opportunity to decide whether to relinquish access to a court and a jury trial. The Court further held that the agreement was not a contract of adhesion. Judge Bronson dissented from the holding of constitutionality. We granted plaintiff's application for leave to appeal.

The malpractice arbitration act provides that a patient "may, if offered, execute an agreement to arbitrate a dispute, controversy, or issue arising out of health care or treatment by a health care provider" or by a hospital. A patient executing such an agreement with a health-care provider may revoke it within 60 days after execution, or, in the case of a hospital, within 60 days after discharge, options which must be stated in the agreement. All such agreements must provide in 12-point boldface type immediately above the space for the parties' signatures that agreement to arbitrate is not a prerequisite to the receipt of health care.

For those who have elected arbitration, the act requires a three-member panel composed of an attorney, who shall be chairperson, a physician, preferably from the respondent's medical specialty, and a person who is not a licensee of the health-care profession involved, a lawyer, or a representative of a hospital or an insurance company. Where the claim is against a hospital only, a hospital administrator may be substituted for the physician. If the claim is against a health-care provider other than a physician, a licensee of the health-care profession involved shall be substituted.

Defendants Detroit Memorial Hospital and Dr. Bloom appeal from the holding that the presence of the medical member unconstitutionally created a biased panel. First, they argue that because the state does not compel arbitration, but only regulates it, state action is not involved.

A basic requirement of due process is a "fair trial in a fair tribunal". Essential to this notion is a fair and impartial decisionmaker. Private conduct abridging individual rights does not implicate the Due Process Clause unless to some significant extent the state, in any of its manifestations, has been found to have become involved in it. . . .

We find it unnecessary, however, to determine here whether the state has significantly involved itself in the challenged action because, even if we were to find so, we have concluded that the composition of the arbitration panel does not offend guarantees of due process.

In the present case . . . it has not been demonstrated that the medical members of these panels have a direct pecuniary interest or that their decision may have any substantial effect on the availability of insurance or insurance premiums. We have been shown no grounds sufficient for us to conclude that these decisionmakers will not act with honesty and integrity. . . .

Plaintiff Jackson also argues that as a class physicians and hospital administrators possess a subliminal bias against patients who claim medical malpractice.

. . . .

We do not believe that the medical members of these panels are so identified and aligned with respondents in malpractice cases that they may be expected to favor the respondents. Physicians and other health care professionals are trained in the medical arts and are oath-bound to treat the ill. Hospital administrators are trained in the proper functioning of hospitals. Neither physicians nor hospital administrators have professional interests that are adverse to patients or even malpractice claimants on a consistent, daily basis. Any identity of interest with respondents is not so strong as to create a subliminal bias for one side and against the other.

Plaintiffs next argue that the arbitration agreement waives constitutional rights to a jury trial and access to a court. Because these fundamental rights are waived, they say, the burden should rest with the defendants to show a valid contract, which they can only do by showing that the waiver was made voluntarily, knowingly, and intelligently. The burden of showing a voluntary waiver is not an easy one, argue plaintiffs, because the arbitration agreement was offered at the time of admission to the hospital in an atmosphere infected with implicit coercion. Additionally, plaintiffs argue that a knowing and intelligent waiver will not be easily shown because the defendants are chargeable with constructive fraud. Constructive fraud is said to arise out of the agreement's failure to highlight the fact of waiver, failure to disclose the composition of the arbitration panel (even though this information is contained in an informational booklet accompanying the agreement), and failure to disclose the attitudes of physicians in general, that they and hospital administrators may be biased and the reasonable probability that insurance rates are affected by awards.

Contracts of adhesion are characterized by standardized forms prepared by one party which are offered for rejection or acceptance without opportunity for bargaining and under the circumstances that the second party cannot obtain the desired product or service except by acquiescing in the form agreement. Regardless of any possible perception among patients that the provision of optimal medical care is conditioned on their signing the arbitration agreement, we believe that the sixty-day rescission period, of which patients must be informed, fully protects those who sign the agreement. The patients' ability to rescind the agreement after leaving the hospital allows them to obtain the desired service without binding them to its terms. As a result, the agreement cannot be considered a contract of adhesion.

We also reject plaintiff's claim that the arbitration agreement is unconscionable. According to the record before us, the arbitration agreement signed by plaintiff Jackson is six paragraphs long. The first sentence of the first paragraph begins, "I understand that this hospital and I by signing this document agree to arbitrate any claims or disputes". The first two sentences of the second paragraph state:

"I understand that Michigan Law gives me the choice of trial by judge or jury or of arbitration. I understand that arbitration is a procedure by which a panel that is either mutually agreed upon or appointed decides the dispute rather than a judge or jury."

This was not a long contract covering different terms, only one of which, obscured among many paragraphs, concerned arbitration. Arbitration was the essential and singular nature of the agreement. We do not believe that an ordinary person signing this agreement to arbitrate would reasonably expect a jury trial. We also reject plaintiffs' argument that the agreement is unconscionable for failure to highlight these terms.

Finally, both plaintiffs ask that we find constructive fraud and hold that the agreements are unconscionable because of failure of the contracts to disclose the composition of the panel, the attitudes of physicians, the fact that the medical member of the panel may be intrinsically biased against plaintiffs, and the reasonable probability that malpractice rates are affected by awards in medical malpractice cases.

We decline. We do not believe that the agreements are unconscionable for failing to include plaintiffs' recommendations. Nor do we believe that defendants have breached a legal or equitable duty which has had the effect of deceiving plaintiffs, nor have defendants received an unmerited benefit.

In *Jackson*, we reverse the finding of unconstitutionality and reinstate the order of the trial court submitting the matter to arbitration.

In *Morris*, we affirm.

Discussion Questions

1. Why are there two cases decided at once here? Do you understand the procedural situation involved?

2. In the *Morris* case, the provider and the patient stipulated the method of resolving a claim for medical injury. How does the health care provider respond to the claim of negotiating from a position of superior power and information or the claim that the plaintiff was coerced into participating in the contract?

3. What do these cases say about alternative methods of resolving medical liability disputes?

4

The Organization and Management of a Corporate Health Care Institution

"Most hospitals and other institutional providers of health care are corporations, and therefore all their personnel should understand the fundamental nature of the corporate form of organization." Thus begins Southwick's chapter on health care organizations, and truer, more straightforward words on the subject would be hard to write.

The corporate form is pervasive in health care because of its many advantages. It is flexible and easy to create, has perpetual existence, allows free transfer of ownership interests, enables the raising of outside capital, creates a career path for talented employees, is taxed lower than individuals (or not at all!), and protects its owners from tort liability. It is even considered a "person" in the eyes of the law for most purposes; it therefore has many of the same constitutional rights that natural persons have under our system of government.

On the other hand, the corporation has certain limitations, the most significant of which is that it possesses only those powers that the law and the corporation's organizing documents permit it to have. And its operation is constrained by certain procedural requirements that can entangle a careless or unsuspecting manager. It is therefore essential for health care executives to know the fundamentals of corporate law. This chapter and the following cases provide that necessary background.

Charlotte Hungerford Hosp. v. Attorney Gen.
26 Conn. Supp. 394, 225 A.2d 495 (1966)

MacDonald, J.

The plaintiff in this action for a declaratory judgment is a nonstock corporation which for many years has owned and operated a voluntary general hospital in a complex of buildings located on a 120-acre tract of wooded land about one mile from the center of the city of Torrington. The land was acquired under a deed of trust providing that the premises thus conveyed "are to be held and used by said grantee for the purpose of maintaining and carrying on a general hospital and, if a majority of corporators so elect, a training school for nurses in connection therewith may be established, and for no other purpose whatsoever." The deed of trust in question, executed in 1917, specifically provided that "if the land herein granted shall cease to be used for the purposes aforesaid * * * title * * * shall thereupon pass to and vest in said town of Torrington * * * to be used forever as a public park." The special act of the General Assembly of Connecticut under which plaintiff was organized in 1917 provides, inter alia, that it shall receive said tract of land "to hold the same subject to all the terms, conditions, restrictions and provisions of said deed and for the purpose of carrying out the trust created by said deed, namely, maintaining and supporting a hospital to be known as The Charlotte Hungerford Hospital."

Plaintiff, the largest general hospital in Litchfield County, has an active medical staff of about forty practicing physicians and surgeons, including specialists as well as general practitioners, and much of their working time is spent on the hospital premises. Because of the size of the hospital grounds and the rather remote location of the main hospital buildings, the establishment of a medical office building on the hospital grounds would be of great convenience and advantage both to the individual doctors and to the hospital, enabling the doctors to spend their office hours in close proximity to the hospital, with its readily available facilities, and providing the hospital with an ever-present staff, almost instantly available when needed.

Although most of the doctors involved heartily support such an undertaking and plaintiff is desirous of constructing and operating a medical office building through the medium of a subsidiary corporation wholly owned and controlled by plaintiff, various questions have arisen with respect to the right, power and authority of plaintiff, under the terms of said deed of trust and special act, to proceed with such a project . . . . The specific questions which the court is requested to answer . . . are (a) whether plaintiff is authorized and empowered . . . to construct and operate, as an integral part of its general hospital complex, a medical office building for members of its medical staff; (b) whether such a medical office building may, under the terms of the aforesaid deed of trust, be located on a portion of the land held by plaintiff thereunder; (c) whether . . . the plaintiff is authorized and empowered to lease . . . a portion of the land included in the aforesaid deed of trust [to a subsidiary corporation that will operate the medical office building]; [and] (d) whether, in addition to offices and office suites for members of plaintiff's medical staff, said building may contain facilities related to or supporting such offices and suites, such as medical laboratories, pharmacies and dispensaries.

The court, after hearing the evidence and the arguments of counsel with full participation by counsel representing the only interested parties, namely, the attorney general of the state of Connecticut, as representative of the public interest in the protection of trusts for charitable uses and purposes pursuant to . . . the General Statutes, and the city of Torrington, contingent beneficiary, has no hesitation in answering all four of the questions posed in the affirmative. It is clear . . . that the proposed project would materially aid the plaintiff in more efficiently carrying out the stated purposes of the trust deed under which it was founded . . . . It is equally clear from the extremely impressive testimony of [the president of the American Hospital Association (AHA) and another witness] that the modern trend is almost universally toward the practice of having nonprofit hospitals provide physicians' private offices for rental to staff members, either in the hospital buildings themselves or on the hospital grounds. . . .

The language of the deed of trust is to be construed in light of the settlor's purpose. And reasonable deviations and expanded interpretations must be made from time to time in order to keep pace with changes in recognized concepts of the proper sphere of general hospital operations. . . . Such deviations are recognized by our Connecticut courts even though the elements for applying cy pres principles are not present.

A decree may enter advising plaintiff of its rights, powers and authority herein by answering the four questions propounded in the affirmative . . . .

Discussion Questions

1. What do the following terms mean: *nonstock corporation, deed of trust, contingent beneficiary, settlor,* and *cy pres*?

2. Who did what to whom? Why is there a lawsuit, and why is the state attorney general the defendant?

3. What does the case tell you about the organization and management of a corporate health care institution?

4. Why is the doctrine of *ultra vires* less important today than formerly?

Woodyard v. Arkansas Diversified Ins. Co.
268 Ark. 90, 594 S.W.2d 13 (1980)

Hickman, J.

The appellant is Arkansas Insurance Commissioner W. H. L. Woodyard, III. The appellee is Arkansas Diversified Insurance Company (ADIC).

ADIC sought a certificate of authority from Woodyard to sell group life insurance to Blue Cross and Blue Shield . . . subscriber groups. Woodyard denied the application. On appeal, his decision was reversed by the Pulaski County Circuit Court as being arbitrary and not supported by substantial evidence. We find on appeal [that] the circuit court was wrong and [we] reverse the judgment. We affirm the commissioner.

The only evidence before the commissioner was presented by ADIC. The appellee candidly admitted it was a wholly owned subsidiary of a corporation named Arkansas Diversified Services, Inc. (ADS) which is a wholly owned subsidiary of Blue Cross and Blue Shield, Inc.

. . . .

ADIC candidly admitted it was created solely to serve Blue Cross customers. It would provide services that could not otherwise be provided by law. While ADS, the parent . . . of ADIC and child of Blue Cross, did offer life insurance in conjunction with Blue Cross and Blue Shield plans, the life policies offered were not ADS's. Some were American Foundation Life; the rest were with a Mississippi company. ADS wanted its own life company to better compete in the market place.

Blue Cross owns all the stock of ADS, which in turn owns all the stock of ADIC. The president of Blue Cross is the president of both ADS and ADIC. Other Blue Cross officials hold positions in ADS and ADIC. The companies use the same location and similar stationery. ADIC will use Blue Cross employees to sell insurance. Underwriting for ADIC will be done by a division of ADS.

There was no real controversy over the commissioner's findings of fact. He concluded that:

(2) . . . [Arkansas law] would apparently authorize a hospital and medical service corporation [of which Blue Cross is one] to invest in a wholly owned subsidiary insurance corporation with the Commissioner's consent.

(3) That Blue Cross is limited by [law] to transact business as a non-profit hospital and medical service corporation.

(4) That ADIC is not a separate corporate entity from Blue Cross since Blue Cross through ADS owns all the capital stock of ADIC. ADIC has common Officers and Directors with Blue Cross, Blue Cross pays the salary for the Officers and employees of ADIC, ADIC will sell its products only to Blue Cross subscriber groups and the record indicates that ADIC is to be treated as a division of Blue Cross. The evidence indicates that ADIC's management will not act independently but will conduct the affairs of ADIC in a manner calculated primarily to further the interest of Blue Cross.

. . . .

The commissioner found that since Blue Cross could not sell life insurance itself, it should not be able to do so through corporate subsidiaries. We find that decision neither arbitrary nor unsupported by substantial evidence.

. . . .

We agree with the commissioner's finding that [Arkansas law] limits the power of medical corporations to providing medical service. If it did not, they could not only sell life insurance, but automobiles or anything else. Clearly, [an] insurance company organized under a charter or statute empowering it to sell one kind of insurance lacks authority to sell another.

The appellees argue that even if the commissioner was right in ruling Blue Cross could not market its own life insurance policies, Blue Cross could . . . invest in a wholly owned subsidiary which would [have that power]. The statutes, however, provide that such an investment can be made only with the commissioner's consent. . . .

Blue Cross is a tax exempt, non-profit corporation enjoying a financial advantage over conventional insurers. Allowing it to sell, through subsidiaries, its own life insurance policies, could be unfair to competitors. While the commissioner did allow Blue Cross to invest in ADS, we can see why he disapproved of ADIC. ADS unlike ADIC, could sell only policies written by insurance companies which lacked the competitive advantages of Blue Cross.

The appellee argues the commissioner arbitrarily pierced the corporate veil of these subsidiaries. . . . [C]ourts will ignore the corporate form of a subsidiary where fairness demands it. Usually, this will be where it is necessary to prevent wrongdoing and where the subsidiary is a mere tool of the parent. We believe both criteria were met here. . . .

Blue Cross, through its president and other officials, candidly admitted why they wanted ADIC to sell insurance. Blue Cross can, through its total control of both subsidiaries by stock, officers and directors, direct all efforts and endeavors of ADIC, and collect all profits.

We cannot say the commissioner was wrong in piercing the corporate veil or in denying the application. The facts are clearly there to support his findings. This order is not contrary to law.

Reversed.

Discussion Questions

1. How does one go about determining what are the powers and authority of a corporation?

2. What does it mean to "pierce the corporate veil"?

3. What difference would it have made if Blue Cross were a for-profit corporation?

Stern v. Lucy Webb Hayes Nat'l. Training School for Deaconesses and Missionaries
381 F. Supp. 1003 (D. D.C. 1974)

Gesell, J.

[This case is a class action in which patients of Sibley Memorial Hospital, known corporately by the name shown in the caption above, challenged various aspects of the hospital's management. The defendants were certain members of the hospital's board of trustees and the hospital itself.]

The two principal contentions in the complaint are that the defendant trustees conspired to enrich themselves and certain financial institutions with which they were affiliated by favoring those institutions in financial dealings with the Hospital, and that they breached their fiduciary duties of care and loyalty in the management of Sibley's funds. . . .

[The court explains the history of the hospital, which was begun by the Methodist Church–related Lucy Webb Hayes School in 1895 and eventually became the school's main activity.]

In 1960 . . . the Sibley Board of Trustees revised the corporate by-laws . . . . Under the new by-laws, the Board was to consist of from 25 to 35 trustees, who were to meet at least twice each year. Between such meetings, an Executive Committee was to represent the Board [and in effect had full power to run the hospital]. . . .

In fact, management of the Hospital from the early 1950's until 1968 was handled almost exclusively by two trustee officers: Dr. Orem, the Hospital Administrator, and Mr. Ernst, the Treasurer. Unlike most of their fellow trustees, to whom membership on the Sibley Board was a charitable service incidental to their principal vocations, Orem and Ernst were continuously involved on almost a daily basis in the affairs of Sibley. They dominated that Board and its Executive Committee, which routinely accepted their recommendations and ratified their actions. Even more significantly, neither the Finance Committee nor the Investment Committee ever met or conducted business from the date of their creation until 1971, three years after the death of Dr. Orem. As a result, budgetary and investment decisions during this period, like most other management decisions affecting the Hospital's finances, were handled by Orem and Ernst, receiving only cursory supervision from the Executive Committee and the full Board.

[It was only after the deaths of Dr. Orem and Mr. Ernst (in 1968 and 1972, respectively) that other trustees began to assert themselves and exercise supervision over the financial affairs of the hospital. At that point, it became known that over the years "unnecessarily large amounts of [Sibley's] money" had been deposited in accounts bearing little or no interest at banks in which trustees had a financial interest. At the same time, the hospital bought certificates of deposit that paid lower-than-market rates and took out loans with interest rates higher than the interest rates being paid on funds deposited.

Since there was no evidence that the trustees, other than Orem and Ernst, had ever actually agreed to engage in or profit from these activities, the court found insufficient evidence to prove a conspiracy among them. The court then proceeds to discuss the allegations of breach of fiduciary duty.]

III. *Breach of Duty.*

Plaintiffs' second contention is that, even if the facts do not establish a conspiracy, they do reveal serious breaches of duty on the part of the defendant trustees and the knowing acceptance of benefits from those breaches by the defendant banks and savings and loan associations.

A. *The Trustees.*

Basically, the trustees are charged with mismanagement, nonmanagement and self-dealing. The applicable law is unsettled.... [H]owever, the modern trend is to apply corporate rather than trust principles in determining the liability of the directors of charitable corporations, because their functions are virtually indistinguishable from those of their "pure" corporate counterparts.

1. *Mismanagement.*

Both trustees and corporate directors are liable for losses occasioned by their negligent mismanagement of investments. However, the degree of care required appears to differ in many jurisdictions. A trustee is uniformly held to a high standard of care and will be held liable for simple negligence, while a director must often have committed "gross negligence" or otherwise be guilty of more than mere mistakes of judgment.

. . . Since the board members of most large charitable corporations fall within the corporate rather than the trust model, being charged with the operation of ongoing businesses, it has been said that they should only be held to the less stringent corporate standard of care. More specifically, directors of charitable corporations are required to exercise ordinary and reasonable care in the performance of their duties, exhibiting honesty and good faith.

2. *Nonmanagement.*

. . . Trustees are particularly vulnerable to such a charge [of failing to supervise investments] because they not only have an affirmative duty to "maximize the trust income by prudent investment," but they may not delegate that duty, even to a committee of their fellow trustees. A corporate director, on the other hand, may delegate his investment responsibility to fellow directors, corporate officers, or even outsiders, but he [*sic*] must continue to exercise general supervision over the activities of his delegates. Once again, the rule for charitable corporations is closer to the traditional corporate rule: directors should at least be permitted to delegate investment decisions to a committee of board members, so long as *all* directors assume the responsibility for supervising such committees by periodically scrutinizing their work.

Total abdication of the supervisory role, however, is improper even under traditional corporate principles. A director who fails to acquire the information necessary to supervise investment policy or consistently fails even to attend the meetings at which such policies are considered has violated his fiduciary duty to the corporation. While a director is, of course, permitted to rely upon the expertise of those to whom he has delegated investment responsibility, such reliance is a tool for interpreting the delegate's reports, not an excuse for dispensing with or ignoring such reports. . . .

3. *Self-dealing.*

Under District of Columbia Law, neither trustees nor corporate directors are absolutely barred from placing funds under their control into a bank having an interlocking directorship with their own institution. In both cases, however, such transactions will be subjected to the closest scrutiny to determine whether or not the duty of loyalty has been violated.

. . . .

. . . Trustees may be found guilty of a breach of trust even for mere negligence in the maintenance of accounts in banks with which they are associated while corporate directors are generally only required to show "entire fairness" to the corporation and "full disclosure" of the potential conflict of interest to the Board.

Most courts apply the less stringent corporate rule to charitable corporations in this area as well. It is, however, occasionally added that a director should not only disclose his interlocking responsibilities but also refrain from voting on or otherwise influencing a corporate decision to transact business with a company in which he has a significant interest or control.

[The court goes on to point out that the hospital board had recently adopted AHA policy guidelines that essentially imposed the standards described above: (1) a duality or conflict of interests should be disclosed to other members of the board, (2) board members should not vote on such matters, and (3) the disclosure and abstention from voting should be recorded in the minutes.]

. . . [T]he Court holds that a director or so-called trustee of a charitable hospital . . . is in default of his fiduciary duty to manage the fiscal and investment affairs of the hospital if it has been shown by a preponderance of the evidence that:

(1) . . . he has failed to use due diligence in supervising the actions of those officers, employees or outside experts to whom the responsibility for making day-to-day financial or investment decisions has been delegated; or

(2) he knowingly permitted the hospital to enter into a business transaction with himself or with any [business entity] in which he then had a substantial interest or held a position as trustee, director, general manager or principal officer [without disclosing that fact]; or

(3) except [with disclosure], he actively participated in or voted in favor of a decision . . . to transact business with himself or with any [business entity] in which he then had a substantial interest or held a position as trustee, director, general manager or principal officer; or

(4) he otherwise failed to perform his duties honestly, in good faith, and with a reasonable amount of diligence and care.

Applying these standards to the facts in the record, the Court finds that each of the defendant trustees has breached his fiduciary duty to supervise the management of Sibley's investments. . . .

. . . .

It is clear that all of the defendant trustees have, at one time or another, affirmatively approved self-dealing transactions. Most of these incidents were of relatively minor significance: one interested trustee would join a dozen disinterested fellow members of the Executive Committee in unanimously approving the opening of a bank account; two or three interested trustees would support a similarly large group in voting to give or renew the mortgage. Others cannot be so easily disregarded. [For example,] defendant Ferris' advice and vote in the relatively small Investment Committee to recommend approval of the investment contract with Ferris & Co. may have been crucial to that transaction. Defendant Reed assumed principal responsibility for account levels between 1969 and 1971, during which period the . . . checking account [at the bank where Reed was a board member and stockholder] grew to more than a million dollars. And defendant Smith, in his capacity as President of Jefferson Federal, personally negotiated the interest rates on a $230,000 certificate account with the Hospital.

That the Hospital has suffered no measurable injury from many of these transactions . . . and that the excessive deposits which were the real source of harm were caused primarily by the uniform failure to supervise rather than the occasional self-dealing vote are both facts that the Court must take into account in fashioning relief, but they do not alter the principle that the trustee of a charitable hospital should al-ways avoid active participation in a transaction in which he or a corporation with which he is associated has a significant interest.

B. *The Financial Institutions.*

While it is thus established that the named trustees acted in breach of fiduciary duty, the institutional defendants are not liable simply because they benefitted from those breaches. Under the prevailing rule of law, a bank or other financial institution is only liable for losses sustained by a trust by reason of its dealings with a trustee if the institution had actual or constructive knowledge that the transaction was in breach of the trustee's fiduciary duty. . . .

Under those principles, the Court finds that the institutional defendants are not liable for any loss of income that may have been suffered by the Hospital. . . .

IV. *Relief.*

[The court notes that the plaintiffs pushed for strict sanctions against the various defendants: the removal of certain board members, the cessation of all business transactions with their related firms, an accounting of all hospital funds, and awards of money damages against the individual defendants. But the court declines to adopt these rather severe measures:]

The function of equity is not to punish but merely to take such action as the Court in its discretion deems necessary to prevent the recurrence of improper conduct. . . . Where voluntary action has been taken in good faith to minimize such recurrence, even though under the pressure of litigation, this is a factor which the Court can take into account in formulating relief.

[The court points out the factors that it considers significant: (1) the defendant trustees are a small minority of the board, whereas all board members were in some way guilty of nonmanagement; (2) the defective practices have been corrected, and those who were most responsible for them have either died or been dismissed; (3) the defendants did not profit personally from the transactions; (4) the defendants will soon leave the board due to age, illness, or the completion of a normal term; and (5) this is essentially the first case in the District of Columbia to discuss these issues comprehensively, thus no clear legal standards previously existed.

For these reasons, the court declines to remove the defendants from the board, to assess money damages, or to take other more severe actions. Instead, it requires new policies and procedures to make certain that all present and future trustees are aware of the requirements of the law and that they fully disclose all hospital transactions with any financial institutions in which they have an interest or position. "Moreover, all such dealings shall be summarized by the Hospital's auditors in their annual audit and a copy of the annual audit shall be made available on request for inspection by any patient of the Hospital at the Hospital's offices during business hours. Such arrangements should continue for a period of five years."

Discussion Questions

1. The late Judge Gerhardt Gesell was a prominent member of the federal bench. Are you aware of other cases he has decided?

2. *Stern* is a landmark decision and two decades later continues to set the standard for hospital board members' fiduciary responsibilities. What exactly is a *fiduciary* duty? What is the difference in that duty between *trust* principles and *corporate* principles?

3. Can you explain the differences in the standard of care for (a) a trustee of a trust, (b) a director for a for-profit corporation, and (c) a director or trustee of a not-for-profit corporation?

4. Based on this opinion, which responsibilities do you believe a hospital governing board can delegate and which can it not? How much supervision must a board exercise over board committees, the medical staff organization, and hospital administration?

5. Do you agree with the court's decisions regarding relief? Do you believe the court, sitting as a court of equity, actually achieved equity in the final result?

Komanetsky v. Missouri State Medical Ass'n.
516 S.W.2d 545 (Mo. Ct. App. 1974)

Kelly, J.

The issue in this case, simply stated, is whether an association of physicians and surgeons of the school of allopathy incorporated under [Missouri Statutes] CH. 352 [relating to religious, scientific, and other charitable associations] may join with an association of physicians and surgeons of the school of osteopathy incorporated as a [general] not-for-profit corporation under [Missouri Statutes] CH. 355 and incorporate a third corporation under CH. 355 for the purpose of affording a review of quality and costs of services rendered by members of the third corporation who are also members of either of the aforesaid parent corporations. We hold that they may.

[This lawsuit was brought by ten physician-members of MSMA to challenge the association's decision to join with MAOPS to create the peer review organization known as HCF. The gist of their complaint was that MSMA members had not been permitted to vote on whether to approve this action, that neither the charitable corporation laws nor MSMA's articles and bylaws gave MSMA the authority to form the new corporation, and that the activities of HCF

would cause plaintiffs irreparable injury. They argued that injury would occur because they would be forced to belong to HCF and this amounted to involuntary servitude; they would have to violate professional ethics by releasing medical records; lay persons would be among those reviewing their professional conduct; and MSMA had appropriated their dues money to set up the new corporation. The plaintiffs sought restitution and injunctive relief.

The trial court found for the defendants, and the plaintiffs appealed, arguing (1) that there was no statutory authority to form HCF, (2) that the decision was not ordinary business and thus should have been voted on by the MSMA members, and (3) that funds were misappropriated and should be repaid.

The court recites at length the corporate structure of MSMA. In summary, that structure includes a legislative body, known as the House of Delegates, which meets annually and consists of delegates elected by the membership; an executive committee, known as the Council, which exercises corporate powers between meetings of the House of Delegates; various standing committees, special committees, and commissions; and various officers of the corporation.

The purposes of the MSMA are "[the] promotion of the science and art of medicine, the protection of public health, the betterment of the medical profession, and, by uniting with similar organizations in other states and territories of the United States, to form the American Medical Association."

The court next describes the purpose and structure of HCF.]

HCF was incorporated by the Presidents of MSMA and MAOPS on August 31, 1970, under authority of the General Not for Profit Corporation Laws of the State of Missouri. Its purpose, according to its Articles of Incorporation, was to promote, develop, define and encourage the distribution of medical services and care by its members to the general public, at a cost reasonable to both patient and physician; to preserve to both the patient and the physician freedom of choice to guard and preserve the physician and patient relationship; to protect public health; to work and study in cooperation with prepaid insurance plans to provide for budgeting for medical care and health services; to provide information and assistance to named agencies, the public, and others as to the fair and reasonable cost of adequate medical care; to work with other associations to promote the development and promotion of the art and science of medical care and health services, the protection of the public health and the betterment of the medical profession; to foster, encourage and coordinate the establishment of uniform, acceptably high standards of medical care and health services by its members with fair and reasonable remuneration for the provision of such medical care and health services; and other stated purposes consistent with aforesaid. The Articles also gave the corporation authority to act alone or in conjunction with any person, firm, association or corporations for the purpose of attaining or furthering any of its objects or purposes provided that same are not inconsistent with the laws of the State of Missouri.

Among the functions HCF was to perform was the review of cases as to quality and cost of medical care upon submission of an inquiry or complaint by patients, physicians and intermediaries. "Intermediaries" was defined to include those who pay the bills, i.e., the federal or state governments, insurance carriers, labor unions, welfare organizations, etc. Peer review, another function of the corporation, was performed by panels consisting of 5 allopathic physicians and 2 doctors of osteopathy; said panels to consist of representatives of members who practice in both rural and urban areas of the state. Since its formation HCF has conducted investigations in some 200 cases involving 300 patient situations.

. . . .

After incorporation of HCF the officers of MSMA at the direction of the Council, appropriated $5,000.00 for HCF. Additional contributions to the corporation were made by MAOPS in the amount of $2,000.00 by Blue Shield of Kansas City in the amount of $15,000.00 and St. Louis Blue Shield in the amount of $25,000.00.

At the April, 1971, annual meeting of the House of Delegates of MSMA, petitioners submitted resolutions seeking a referendum on the action of the defendants with respect to HCF but these motions were rejected by the House of Delegates. Subsequently, the petitioners advised the defendants by letter that they intended to seek a judicial review of their actions if these activities with HCF were not brought to an end. When this notice went unheeded this litigation was initiated.

. . . .

Petitioners . . . argue that there is no power to join with a second corporation to form a third corporation expressly authorized under CH. 352. In further support of this argument they cite [an 1899 case] for the proposition that incorporated associations or societies of the class to which fraternal or benevolent associations belong are creatures of statute, incapable of exercising any power which is not therein either expressly or clearly implied. They also call attention to the powers conferred in § 352.140 [of Missouri Statutes] for the merger or consolidation of one or more corporations organized under this act, and argue from this delegation of powers by express legislative authority the conclusion must follow that in the absence of a specific grant of power to join with another corporation, no such power exists. Defendants state that they have no quarrel with the authorities cited by the petitioners. It is their interpretation of these authorities with which they take issue.

This is a case of first impression in this state and neither petitioners nor defendants have cited any authority directly in point. Each relies on general principles although all agree there is no specific statutory authority for what defendants did here. The critical issue upon which we conclude the case must be decided is whether defendants had the implied power to join with MAOPS and form HCF. In deciding this question we believe that we must first examine the purpose of CH. 352 under which MSMA was incorporated, then consider the purposes for which MSMA was incorporated, and ultimately consider whether formation of HCF in conjunction with MAOPS was within its implied powers.

The thrust of the Chapter is the purpose for which the associations authorized to enjoy the benefits of corporate status devote themselves. The single thread which runs through the entire chapter is "benevolence," i.e., "the disposition to do good," whether it be religious, scientific, fraternal or educational. For this reason, the statute, § 352.010 requires that "the purpose and scope of the association be clearly and fully set forth" so that anyone examining the Articles of Agreement can determine the avowed reason for its incorporation. The "do-good" nature of the associations which may incorporate under the Chapter are more fully detailed in § 352.020 to include "any purely charitable society, hospital, asylum house of refuge, reformatory and eleemosynary institution, fraternal-beneficial associations, or any association whose object is to promote temperance or other virtue conducive to the well-being of the community, and generally, any association formed to provide for some good in the order of benevolence, that is useful to the public, * * *; any association, congregation, society or church organization formed for religious purposes, and any association formed to provide or maintain a cemetery; any school, college, institute, academy or other association founded for educational or scientific purposes, including therein *any association formed to promote* literature, history, *science, information or skill among the learned professions*, intellectual culture in any branch or department, or the establishing of a museum, library, art gallery, or the erection of a public monument, *and, in general, any association, society, company or organization which tends to the public advantage in relation to any or several of the objects above enumerated, and whatever is incident to such objects, . . .*" (Emphasis supplied). We hold that in addition to those powers specifically enumerated in the Chapter, corporations organized under this Chapter have those implied powers which will aid them in achieving the purposes for which they were organized unless said powers are expressly forbidden to them by other statutory enactments, of either the United States or the State of Missouri, and the Constitutions thereof.

In his book "NON-PROFIT CORPORATIONS, ORGANIZATIONS AND ASSOCIATIONS" (2d ed. 1965), Professor Howard L. Oleck, makes no distinction between the powers of a not-for-profit corporation and a corporation incorporated for the purpose of realizing a profit. He says, § 47, l.c. 113:

"Formerly, corporations were viewed as possessing only such powers as were specifically granted to them by the state. This grant of powers was found in the certificate of incorporation . . . or in the special statute granting a charter to the corporation . . . Today, in all the states, a corporation is deemed to possess all the powers of a natural person except those powers which are specifically forbidden to corporations by the law. The old concept of a corporation as a bundle of only a few, specifically granted powers, has been replaced by the concept of a corporation as an artificial person, lacking only those powers which the law specifically denies to it."

And, in § 48, l.c. 116, he continues:

"In the modern view, a corporation possesses all those powers reasonably necessary for the accomplishment of its proper purposes.

What these proper purposes are is stated in the charter of the corporation . . . . When the state accepts the corporate charter for filing, it thereby approves the purposes stated in that charter.

Therefore, the corporation has all those powers reasonably necessary for the accomplishment of its stated purposes, except insofar as specific rules of law, or specific statutes, limit such implied powers." (Emphasis supplied.)

The leading case in this state on the implied powers of a corporation incorporated under this law is [a 1914 case in which the Missouri Supreme Court] said:

"They [implied powers] are defined to be those possessed by a corporation, not indispensably necessary to carry into effect others expressly granted, and [they] comprise all that are *appropriate, convenient, and suitable* for that purpose, including as an incidental right a reasonable choice of the means to be employed in putting into practical effect this class of powers." (Emphasis supplied).

. . . .

Bearing in mind the purposes of MSMA enunciated in Article II of its Constitution we decide that the corporation possessed those powers necessary or proper for the accomplishment and furtherance of those purposes which had been approved by the court in approving the Amended Charter of the association. In view of the broad purposes of MSMA and the powers necessary to achieve its aims and in light of the similar medical and scientific purposes for which HCF was incorporated, we hold that the defendants were acting within the implied powers of MSMA in joining with MAOPS in the incorporation of HCF for the purpose of "the promotion of the science and art of medicine, the protection of public health, the betterment of the medical profession" by reviewing the quality and cost of medical care within the state of Missouri and affording peer review of the professional practices of those members of MSMA and MAOPS who voluntarily made application for membership in HCF.

Petitioners' argument that the decision to join with HCF was one which was not ordinary business and should have been put to a vote of the membership, is likewise without merit.

Petitioners argue that unlike the statutory authority granted to a board of directors for the control and management of the property and business of a corporation organized

under Ch. 351 V.A.M.S., The General Business Corporation Law of Missouri, there is no comparable body authorized to conduct the business of a Ch. 352 corporation; that, by statute, the rights, duties, authority and power of these latter corporations must be found in their by-laws, § 352.110, and that nowhere in the articles of agreement or the by-laws of MSMA is there authority given to the officers, the Councilors or the House of Delegates to go outside the corporate structure and join with another corporate body to form a third corporate entity. Defendants respond to this argument saying that the constitution and by-laws of the corporation establish the House of Delegates as the representatives of the membership, having been elected thereby for that purpose, and that the House of Delegates was authorized to act as defendants did, by an amemdment to a resolutions committee's report of April 3, 1970, directing the Council to "implement the *proposed* peer review procedure with expediency." (Emphasis supplied). The petitioners further contend that the change effected was a fundamental change in MSMA which would require a vote of the membership to be valid. Defendants counter by denying that a fundamental change in the corporation or its purposes was involved.

We have already held that the defendants' acts were not ultra vires the purposes of the corporation or specifically prohibited by statute. We further hold that they are not contrary to public policy. We proceed to consider whether they are ultra vires the authority conferred on the officers, Councilors and House of Delegates.

With respect to the report of the resolutions committee, our study of that report and supporting documents causes us to conclude that the peer review referred to there was concerned with the Missouri Medicare Program and not with peer review of all types of medical care and services included in the HCF program, and that report did not authorize the peer review program subsequently approved by officers and Councilors in the formation of HCF.

Nevertheless, subsequent to the actions of the defendants here under attack, the record is clear that the House of Delegates fully ratified that action. The question then becomes what is the effect of ratification by the House of Delegates?

It is fundamental that ratification by stockholders will not validate ultra vires acts exceeding the express or implied powers of a corporation where estoppel is not applicable or as to those acts which are contrary to public policy or statutorily barred. However, an act merely in excess of the authority conferred on the directors or officers of a corporation may be subsequently ratified by the stockholders. . . .

. . . .

The evidence in this case is that the resolutions passed at the April '71 Annual Session, and the April '72 Annual Session, the publication of the Council minutes of October 3–4, 1970, reflecting the approval of a $5,000.00 appropriation for HCF, and the subsequent approval of those minutes by the House of Delegates lends support to a finding that the House of Delegates was in possession of full knowledge of all material facts when it approved the action of the defendants with respect to the formation of HCF, and it is that body which is charged with the conduct of the business of the corporation when it is in session.

We hold therefore, that the acts of the defendants were ratified by the duly elected representatives of the membership, and, if ultra vires, were thus validated.

We next consider whether the authorization of the incorporation of HCF was an "extraordinary matter" on which the entire membership was entitled to vote. "Extraordinary matters," which would require a vote of the membership, include (1) a radical change of fundamental policy or purposes, (2) dissolution and (3) merger. . . . We are not here confronted with an attempt at merger, consolidation or dissolution. Peer review has been employed in the Practice of medicine in one form or another for many years in the interest of the profession and for the protection of the public; nor was it foreign to MSMA prior to the incorporation of HCF. From our point of vantage, the formation of HCF is an effort on the part of two associations whose membership consists of physicians and surgeons from different schools of medicine, viz, allopathy and osteopathy, to continue to maintain separate but parallel professional associations, and simultaneously afford a public service through a voluntary association via a third corporation "[to] foster, encourage and coordinate the establishment of uniform, acceptably high standards of medical care and health services by the members with fair and reasonable remuneration for the provision of such medical care and health services." This goal is, we think, [consistent] with the action of the General Assembly of this state in 1959 whereby it . . . enacted . . . a number of statutes whose purpose was to establish a common set of laws applicable to both schools of medicine. . . . We also conclude that this action is not in conflict with the purposes of MSMA, nor does it constitute, as petitioners contend, an "extraordinary matter" which is a radical change of fundamental policy.

On two prior occasions the Council of MSMA has formulated other not-for-profit corporations, the Missouri State Medical Foundation in 1961 and the Missouri Medical Service in 1944–45. Although the Council did not join with another association to form these not-for-profit corporations, on both occasions the House of Delegates approved the action of the Council without a vote of the general membership.

There was testimony by Dr. Jost, one of the petitioners, that he could not remember the general membership voting on anything since 1937. Furthermore, the petitioners at the April '71 Annual Meeting of the House of Delegates presented a number of resolutions seeking a referendum of the action of the defendants in establishing HCF which were referred to committee and when called to the floor were defeated by adoption of the committee reports recommending rejection of said resolutions.

We therefore rule [this argument] against petitioners.

With respect to the question of restitution . . . [t]here is in this case no evidence of self-dealing or bad faith on the part of the defendants, nor is there any evidence that any one of them has financially benefitted by the appropriation of the funds to HCF out of the treasury of MSMA. We rule this [argument] against the petitioners also.

[Affirmed.]

Discussion Questions

1. Why do you suppose the dissident members of MSMA who filed this suit were so upset by the prospect of peer review?

2. Why does the court go to some length in explaining the structure of the MSMA, its house of delegates, etc.? Do you understand that structure and how it operated?

3. Do you agree with the court's approach of finding "implied powers" to do all things which are consistent with the corporation's purposes and not otherwise prohibited by law? Could you argue that there should be a more restrictive interpretation for charitable organizations?

4. Why was the vote of the members of MSMA not required?

5. Explain why the officers of MSMA had authority to negotiate this transaction.

6. Why was there no breach of fiduciary duties?

Note

This case should also be considered in relation to the peer review cases discussed in Chapter 15 of Southwick's text and this book.

5

Taxation of Health Care Institutions

As discussed in Chapter 4, most health care organizations are (and until the late 1970s virtually all health care organizations were) not-for-profit corporations, and they are incorporated under certain laws other than those relating to general business corporations.

But being incorporated under not-for-profit corporation laws does not mean that the organization must operate unprofitably: there is no legal barrier to a not-for-profit corporation having revenues that exceed its expenses. The distinction lies in what can be done with those excess revenues.

Given that not-for-profit corporations are permitted to (and, if they expect to survive, must) have some excess of revenues over expenses, a logical question becomes whether those profits are taxable in the same way as are business corporations' profits. The answer to that question lies not in the corporation statutes but, at least in part, in federal and state tax laws.

We say "at least in part" because the answer more and more often depends as much on politics as law. The recent emergence of an antihospital sentiment into the public consciousness has led to the taxation of health care organizations becoming a topic of political discourse and demagoguery. The implications of hospital taxation are therefore not merely legal but practical and operational as well.

The cases discussed in this chapter illustrate various issues relating to the taxation of health care organizations. In particular, the major case, *Utah County v. Intermountain Health Care, Inc.,* sent shock waves through the hospital industry in the mid-1980s. Hospital corporations' exemptions from sales and incomes taxes and various other revenue enhancers are still issues in various states even as this is written.

In addition to the corporation's basic tax status, there are many state law cases involving property taxes on hospital property, and there is little apparent consistency among them. Each case turns on its own specific facts in relation to

the language of the state's exemption statute. (The statutes are similar but not identical.) Challenges to the tax-exempt status of medical office buildings are a good example of the variety of approaches among the states. Cases relating to this topic are also included in the following materials.

Utah County v. Intermountain Health Care, Inc.
709 P.2d 265 (Utah 1985)

Durham, J.

Utah County seeks review of a decision of the Utah State Tax Commission [exempting certain Intermountain Health Care (IHC) hospitals] from *ad valorem* property taxes. At issue is whether such a tax exemption is constitutionally permissible. We hold that, on the facts in this record, it is not, and we reverse.

[IHC is a not-for-profit hospital system that at the time of the case had 21 hospitals in the West. IHC had no stock, no dividends, and none of its revenues or assets inured to the benefit of any private individual.]

Utah County seeks the resolution of two issues: (1) whether [certain statutes] which exempt from taxation hospitals meeting certain requirements, constitute an unconstitutional expansion of the charitable exemption in . . . the Utah Constitution; and (2) whether [the IHC hospitals] are exempt from taxation under . . . the Utah Constitution.[1]

---

1. One of the statutes provides that property dedicated to religious worship or charitable purposes is exempt from taxation if (1) the user is a not-for-profit organization, (2) earnings do not inure to private individuals, (3) the property is not used in a way that profits or compensation benefit any private

Utah County does not seriously dispute that the two hospitals in this case comply with [the statutes in question] but contends instead that these statutes unlawfully expand the charitable exemption granted by . . . the Utah Constitution, which provides in pertinent part:

The property of the state, cities, counties, towns, school districts, municipal corporations and public libraries, lots with the buildings thereon used exclusively for either religious worship or charitable purposes, . . . shall be exempt from taxation. [Ellipsis in the original opinion.]

. . . "[This provision] grants a charitable exemption and our statutes cannot *expand* or *limit* the scope of the exemption or *defeat it*. To the extend the statutes have that effect, they are not valid."

. . . These exemptions confer an indirect subsidy and are usually justified as the *quid pro quo* for charitable entities undertaking functions and services that the state would otherwise be required to perform. A concurrent rationale, used by some courts, is the assertion that the exemptions are granted not only because charitable entities relieve government of a burden, but also because their activities enhance beneficial community values or goals. Under this theory, the benefits received by the community are believed to offset the revenue lost by reason of the exemption.

[In considering the standards under which these rationales are to be applied, however, the court affirms that "the clause exempting property 'used exclusively for . . . charitable purposes' is to be strictly construed." Thus, it holds that an entity qualifies for the exemption only if it meets the definition of a "charity": "the *contribution* or *dedication* of something of value . . . to the common good."]

. . . [T]here are a number of factors which must be weighed in determining whether a particular institution is in fact using its property "exclusively for . . . charitable purposes." These factors are: (1) whether the stated purpose of the entity is to provide a significant service to others without immediate expectation of material reward; (2) whether the entity is supported . . . by donations and gifts; (3) whether the recipients of the "charity" are required to pay for the assistance received, in whole or in part; (4) whether the income received from all sources . . . produces a "profit" to the entity . . . ; (5) whether the beneficiaries of the "charity" are restricted or unrestricted and, if restricted, whether the restriction bears a reasonable relationship to the entity's charitable

objectives; and (6) whether dividends or some other form of financial benefit, or assets upon dissolution, are available to private interests . . . . These factors provide, we believe, useful guidelines for our analysis of whether a charitable purpose or gift exists in any particular case. We emphasize that each case must be decided on its own facts, and the foregoing factors are not all of equal significance, nor must an institution always qualify under all six before it will be eligible for an exemption.

Because the "care of the sick" has traditionally been an activity regarded as charitable in American law, and because the dissenting opinions rely upon decisions from other jurisdictions that in turn incorporate unexamined assumptions about the fundamental nature of hospital-based medical care, we deem it important to scrutinize the contemporary social and economic context of such care. We are convinced that the traditional assumptions bear little relationship to the economics of the medical-industrial complex of the 1980's. Nonprofit hospitals were traditionally treated as tax-exempt charitable institutions because, until late in the 19th century, they were true charities providing custodial care for those who were both sick and poor. The hospitals' income was derived largely or entirely from voluntary charitable donations, not government subsidies, taxes, or patient fees. The function and status of hospitals began to change in the late 19th century; the transformation was substantially completed by the 1920's. "From charities, dependent on voluntary gifts, [hospitals] developed into market institutions financed increasingly out of payments from patients." The transformation was multidimensional: hospitals were redefined from social welfare to medical treatment institutions; their charitable foundation was replaced by a business basis; and their orientation shifted to "professionals, and their patients," away from "patrons and the poor."

[The court next summarizes six factors from Paul Starr's *The Social Transformation of American Medicine* to suggest that by about 1925 hospitals had changed significantly: (1) hospital patients began to reflect the population at large; (2) the percentage of revenue from patient fees increased dramatically; (3) doctors were allowed to charge private patients for hospital-based services; (4) virtually all doctors had hospital privileges; (5) the number of hospitals increased from 178 to over 4,000; and (6) there was a substantial growth in for-profit hospitals. The court summarizes its argument by saying, "All of the above factors indicate a substantial change in the nature of the hospital; a part of that change was the gradual disappearance of the traditional charitable hospital for the poor."]

. . . [T]he revolution in health care . . . has transformed a "healing profession" into an enormous and complex industry, employing millions of people and accounting for a substantial proportion of our gross national product. Dramatic advances in medical knowledge and technology have resulted in an equally dramatic rise in the cost of medical ser-

---

person, and (4) upon dissolution of the organization, the property will not be distributed to any private person.

The second statute provides, "Property used exclusively for religious, hospital, educational, employee representation, or welfare purposes [and that complies with the statute summarized above] shall be deemed to be used for charitable purposes within the exemption provided for in [the Utah Constitution]."

vices. At the same time, elaborate and comprehensive organizations of third-party payers have evolved. Most recently, perhaps as a further evolutionary response to the unceasing rise in the cost of medical services, the provision of such services has become a highly competitive business. . . .

[The court next examines the facts of the case in relation to the six factors articulated earlier for determining whether an activity is a charity. The court finds that the statement of "corporate purposes" in IHC's articles of incorporation meet the first criterion.]

The second factor we examine is whether the hospitals are supported, and to what extent, by donations and gifts. . . . The finding [of the Tax Commission on this point] reads: "The sources of revenue of IHC are derived primarily from patient charges, third parties (Blue Cross, Blue Shield, Medicare, Medicaid), and gifts (wills, endowments and contributions)." [The extent of the gifts was not specified.] The evidence was that both hospitals charge rates for their services comparable to rates being charged by other similar entities, and no showing was made that the donations identified resulted in charges to patients below prevailing market rates. Presumably such differentials, if they exist, could be quantified and introduced into evidence. The defendants have failed to provide such evidence, and it is they who bear the burden of showing their eligibility for exemption.

. . . .

One of the most significant of the factors to be considered in review of a claimed exemption is the third we identified: whether the recipients of the services of an entity are required to pay for that assistance, in whole or in part. The Tax Commission in this case found as follows:

The policy of [IHC's hospitals] is to collect hospital charges from patients whenever it is reasonable and possible to do so; however, no person in need of medical attention is denied care solely on the basis of a lack of funds.

. . . The record shows that the vast majority of the services provided by these two hospitals are [*sic*] paid for by government programs, private insurance companies, or the individuals receiving care. . . . Furthermore, the record also shows that such free service as did exist was deliberately not advertised out of fear of a "deluge of people" trying to take advantage of it. Instead, every effort was made to recover payment for services rendered. . . .

The defendants argue that the great expense of modern hospital care and the universal availability of insurance and government health care subsidies make the idea of a hospital solely supported by philanthropy an anachronism. We believe this argument itself exposes the weakness in the defendants' position. It is precisely because such a vast system of third-party payers has developed to meet the expense of modern hospital care that the historical distinction between for-profit and non-profit hospitals has eroded. . . .

The fourth question we consider is whether the income received from all sources by these IHC hospitals is in excess of their operating and maintenance expenses. Because the vast majority of their services are paid for, the nonprofit hospitals in this case accumulate capital as do their profit-seeking counterparts. . . . [T]here is no showing on the record that surplus funds generated by one hospital in the system will not be utilized for the benefit of facilities in other counties, outside the state of Utah, or purely for administrative costs of the system itself.

Indeed, it is difficult to see a significant difference between the *operation* (as opposed to the form of corporate structure) of defendants' facilities and the operation of [a] for-profit hospital . . . . The significant difference between for-profit and nonprofit hospital corporations is, in effect, the method of distribution of assets upon dissolution of the corporation, which is itself a rare occurrence.

. . . .

The final two factors we address are whether the beneficiaries of the services of the defendants are "restricted" in any way and whether private interests are benefited by the organization or operation of the defendants. Although the policy of IHC is to impose no restrictions, there were some incidents recounted in the testimony which suggested that these institutions do not see themselves as being in the business of providing hospital care "for the poor," an activity which was certainly at the heart of the original rationale for tax exemptions for charitable hospitals. Otherwise, it appears that they meet [the fifth] criterion. On the question of benefits to private interests, certainly it appears that no individuals who are employed by or administer the defendants receive any distribution of assets or income, and some, such as IHC's board of trustees members, volunteer their services. We have noted, however, that IHC owns a for-profit entity, as well as nonprofit subsidiaries, and there is in addition the consideration that numerous forms of private commercial enterprise, such as pharmacies, laboratories, and contracts for medical services, are conducted as a necessary part of the defendants' hospital operations. The burden being on the taxpayer to demonstrate eligibility for the exemption, the inadequacies in the record on these questions cannot be remedied by speculation in the defendants' favor.

In summary, . . . we believe that the defendants in this case confuse the element of gift to the community, which an entity must demonstrate in order to qualify as a charity under our Constitution, with the concept of community benefit, which any of countless private enterprises might provide. . . .

. . . .

Neither can we find on this record that the burdens of government are substantially lessened as a result of the defendants' provision of services. . . . In fact, government is already carrying a substantial share of the operating expenses of defendants, in the form of third-party payments pursuant to "entitlement" programs such as Medicare and Medicaid.

... A hospital, whether nonprofit or for-profit, that provides its services to paying patients relieves no public burden because, in its absence, the government would not (or would have no duty to) provide free health care to patients able to pay for treatment. . . . [And] all hospitals use tax-supported public services, including road construction and maintenance, police protection, fire protection, water and sewer maintenance, and waste removal, to name a few. Exempt hospitals use those services at the expense of nonexempt health care providers and other taxpayers, commercial and individual. . . .

We cannot find, on this record, the essential element of gift to the community, either through the nonreciprocal provision of services or through the alleviation of a government burden, and consequently we hold that the defendants have not demonstrated that their property is being used exclusively for charitable purposes under the Utah Constitution.

. . . Property used exclusively for hospital purposes is not *automatically* being used for charitable purposes, even where the hospital is nonprofit.

We reverse the Tax Commission's grant of an *ad valorem* property tax exemption to defendants as being unconstitutional. We emphasize, contrary to the assertions of the dissents, that this opinion is no more than an extension of the principles of strict construction set forth in [previous cases]. This is a "record" case, and we make no judgment as to the ability of these hospitals or any others to demonstrate their eligibility for constitutionally permissible tax exemptions in the future. We note, however, that reliance on automatic exemptions granted heretofore, and on the kind of minimal efforts to show charity reflected in this record, will no longer suffice.

[The court concludes by saying that this opinion has prospective effect only and that with changes in their operations defendants might be able to qualify for the exemption in the future if they meet the criteria set forth in this decision.]

HALL, C. J., and DAVID SAM, District Judge, concur.

[Two sharp dissenting opinions were filed. One contains the following language: "The majority's suggestions that a nonprofit hospital must have a deficit in its current accounts to qualify for charitable status is both anachronistic and a prescription for lesser quality hospital care, if not bankruptcy. . . . The majority's assertion that 'traditional assumptions bear little relationship to the economics of the medical-industrial complex of the 1980's' is based upon the majority's refusal to acknowledge the development of case law that has occurred over at least the past 45 years."

The other dissenting justice wrote, "Courts long ago fully considered and firmly rejected the notion now advanced by the majority that the charitable character of a hospital is determined by the quantity of its almsgiving." Then, referring to the majority's favorable quotation of student law review articles, the dissenting opinion continues, "In a reck-

less attempt to find support for what appears to be its novel personal ideas, buttressed by references to 'literature' by writers whose credentials are not established, the majority indulges in totally irrelevant arguments." The first dissenter had described those arguments as a "flight of fantasy."]

Discussion Questions

1. This is a lengthy and complicated decision. Do you agree with the outcome?

2. How would you attempt to define the meaning of a *charity*? By what criteria would you judge it?

3. What is the difference between being a not-for-profit corporation and being a tax-exempt corporation? What are the standards?

4. If you were the chief executive officer of one of the IHC hospitals, what would you do differently to try to requalify for the tax exemption?

5. Justice Oliver Wendell Holmes, Jr. once wrote, "It is one of the misfortunes of the law that ideas become encysted in phrases and thereafter for a long time cease to provoke further analysis." Holmes, J. (dissenting) in *Hyde v. United States,* 225 U.S. 347, 384 at 391 (1912). How does this comment relate to the IHC decision?

Greater Anchorage Area Borough v. Sisters of Charity
553 P.2d 467 (Alaska 1976)

Burke, J.

The central issue in this appeal is the tax-exempt status of a building owned by the Sisters of Charity of the House of Providence, under the provisions of Art. IX, Sec. 4, of the Constitution of Alaska[2] and AS 29.53.020.[3]

The Sisters of Charity, a long time health care provider in Alaska, erected the building in question, the Providence Professional Building, adjacent to their hospital on land

---

2. Art. IX, Sec. 4, provides in part:
Exemptions: * * * All, or any portion, of property used exclusively for nonprofit religious, charitable, cemetery or educational purposes, as defined by law, shall be exempt from taxation. Other exemptions of like or different kind may be granted by general law.

3. AS 29.53.020 provides in part:
Required exemptions. (a) The following property is exempt from general taxation:
* * * *
(3) property used exclusively for nonprofit religious, charitable, cemetery, hospital or educational purposes;
* * * *

deeded to them in 1959 by the United States for "hospital site, school and recreational purposes only". The construction of the Professional Building began in 1970; its first full year of operation was 1972.

The Professional Building has four floors, including a basement, and is connected by an underground tunnel to nearby Providence Hospital. Three floors are the subject of this appeal, since the parties agree that the basement and tunnel are used exclusively for hospital purposes and are, therefore, exempt from taxation.

The first, second and third floors are rented to doctors having hospital staff privileges at Providence Hospital, for use as their private office space. Approximately thirty-five doctors rent such space. These doctors, although enjoying staff privileges, are not employed by Providence Hospital, and their patients are not necessarily patients of the hospital. Thus, the actual use made of the first, second and third floors is for office space by doctors engaged in the private practice of medicine.

The doctor-tenants rent space on a square foot basis. Upon leasing, each tenant represents that he enjoys staff privileges, and the Sisters may cancel the lease as to any tenant who ceases to enjoy such privileges. At the time of the hearings below, space was leased to enjoy such privileges. At the time of the hearings below, space was leased for $1.10 per square foot per month, a commercially competitive rate for the Anchorage area. The lease agreement provides that the Sisters shall pay any real property taxes which become payable on the Professional Building and associated lands provided, however, that the rents shall be adjusted annually for any increase in taxes. The agreement also provides that rentals shall be subject to a rental adjustment every two years for whatever reason the Sisters determine necessary. Nothing in the lease agreement restricts the doctor-tenants in the control of their office space.

In 1973, the tax assessor for the Greater Anchorage Area Borough assessed the Providence Professional Building at a value of $2,134,200.00. The tax on this assessment was $43,416.02, which the Sisters of Charity paid under protest.

The assessor determined that the first, second and third floors, and a proportionate share of the land upon which the building is situated, did not qualify for exemption from *ad valorem* taxation, as property being "used exclusively for nonprofit hospital . . . purposes," under AS 29.53.020(a)(3). The Sisters appealed the assessment to the Greater Anchorage Area Borough Assembly, sitting as a board of equalization. The argument on appeal was that the entire property was sufficiently related to hospital purposes to allow total exemption. Upon hearing the evidence and arguments of the parties, the board denied the appeal. The Sisters then appealed to the superior court.

Again, the only issue on appeal was whether the property being assessed was entitled to exemption. No questions were raised regarding the sufficiency of the assessor's ap-

praisal and proration methods or the assessed value of the property.

The superior court initially remanded the matter to the board for a finding of the percentage of the disputed office space which was "reasonably necessary for the fulfillment of the generally recognized functions of a completely modern hospital." When the board did not submit such a finding within the period specified, the court ruled that all of the office space was exempt; upon further consideration of the board's later finding that no part of the board's later finding that no part of the [*sic*] office space was necessary, the court reaffirmed its own ruling. This appeal by the borough followed.

A taxpayer claiming a tax exemption has the burden of showing that the property is eligible for the exemption. Furthermore, the courts must narrowly construe statutes granting such exemptions. The policy behind these rules was expressed in *Animal Rescue League of Boston v. Assessors of Bourne*, [a 1914 Massachusetts case]:

All property is benefited by the security and protection furnished by the State, and it is only just and equitable that expenses incurred in the operation and maintenance of government should be fairly apportioned upon the property of all. An exemption from taxation releases property from this obligation to bear its share of the cost of government and serves to disturb to some extent, that equality in the distribution of this common burden upon all property which is the object and aim of every just system of taxation. While reasonable exemptions based upon various grounds of public policy are permissible, yet taxation is the general rule. * * * It is for this reason that statutes granting exemptions from taxation are strictly construed. A taxpayer is not entitled to an exemption unless he shows that he comes within either the express words or the necessary implication of some statute conferring this privilege upon him.

In this case, therefore, the burden is on the Sisters to show that the office space is exempt. Under AS 29.53.020, this is a two-step process. They must first show . . . that the property is "used exclusively for nonprofit . . . hospital . . . purposes." Then, since income is derived from the property, they must show that it meets the requirements that Sec. 020(c)[4] imposes on property exempt under Sec. 020(a)(3). It is the Sisters' argument that the office space must be considered "reasonably necessary for the fulfillment of the generally recognized functions of a completely modern hospital" and that it therefore can be characterized as used exclusively for hospital purposes. This formulation of the "exclusive use" test derives from *Cedars of Lebanon Hospital v. Los Angeles County* ([Calif.] 1950). We declined to adopt that part of the *Cedars of Lebanon* opinion in *Harmon v. North*

---

4. AS 29.53.020(c) provides:

Property described in (a) or (b) of this section from which income is derived is exempt only if that income is solely from use of the property by nonprofit religious, charitable, hospital, or educational groups for classroom space.

Pac. Union Conference Ass'n of Seventh Day Adventists (Alaska 1969) because of factual differences; we reject it here for the same reason. The California court granted an exemption upon the finding that provision of living quarters for resident doctors and hospital employees was institutionally necessary. Those living quarters were not used for the private practice of medicine; the office space in the Providence Professional Building is. While it is clear from the record before us that the use of the office space by the doctor-tenants in conducting their private practices does provide incidental benefits to the hospital, it is equally clear, and we find as a matter of law, that the office space is not used exclusively for hospital purposes.

The Sisters urge that the owner's use, rather than the actual use, should be considered in making this determination. That analysis, however, would extend the tax exemption to everything owned and used in some way by an exempt institution. If only the uses of the office space by the Sisters are considered, by definition the Sisters' use is exclusive. Nothing in the exemption statute indicates that such a limited reading is justified.

To support their contention that the owner's use alone should be considered in determining exclusive use, the Sisters cite *Matanuska-Sustina Borough v. King's Lake Camp*, (Alaska 1968), where the borough sought to tax a non-profit camp which collected a small user fee from the groups which brought campers there. However, exclusive use was not an issue in that appeal, which concerned the effect of the income from user fees on the exemption, and the establishment of recreation as a charitable use. Thus, *King's Lake* can lend no support to the Sister's position. Similarly, in *Harmon v. North Pac. Union Conference Ass'n of Seventh Day Adventists*, also cited by the Sisters to support their theory of use, this court did not have reason to consider the issue, since the question on appeal involved a specific statutory exemption for the residences of clergy, and not a question of use. We find nothing in these cases inconsistent with analyzing actual use rather than owner's use in determining elibility for an exemption.

A better analogy than *King's Lake* or *Harmon* would be to compare the issue in this case with that decided in *Evangelical Covenant Church of America v. City of Nome* (Alaska 1964). The Church, an exempt institution like the Sisters, ran a radio station, which was used to broadcast religious material. Some of the air time was sold for commercial use, the proceeds going to support the church's work. This court held that the radio station was not used exclusively for religious purposes. While the exempt and the commercial uses of the Professional Building are not as clearly separable as were the uses in *Evangelical*, the lesson of that case is applicable here: when the property in question is used even in part by non-exempt parties for their private business purposes, there can be no exemption.

Following *Cedars of Lebanon Hospital v. Los Angeles County*, and its companion cases, courts in many jurisdic-

tions held exempt such hospital facilities as nurses' and residents' housing, recreational facilities for hospital staff, and parking lots. None of these cases considered office space rented to doctors; where commercial activity of any sort, such as a thrift shop operated by a charity, was considered, the exemption was withdrawn. Of the cases on point, the Sisters, and the superior court, rely on *Philips v. Southern Baptist Hospital*, (Fla. 1969), to support the exemption. In that case, the Florida Supreme Court in a brief per curiam opinion, without analysis, held that office space rented to doctors by the hospital was exempt. We find several decisions of other jurisdictions, which more fully treat the issues and policy consideration involved, to be more persuasive.

In *Gifford Memorial Hospital v. Town of Randolph*, ([Vt.] 1955), the Vermont Supreme Court held not exempt a doctors' office building which brought together, in proximity to the hospital, doctors who had been scattered at distant locations; which allowed the hospital to have full-time emergency coverage; and which improved nurse training and use of laboratory and testing facilities. In applying the Vermont exemption statute, which requires only "primary use" for a charitable purpose, the court looked to the doctors' use of the building in the practice of their profession as the primary use, and held that the benefits to the hospital were insufficient to shift the use to one for the benefit of the hospital.

In *Milton Hospital and Convalescent Home v. Board of Assessors*, ([Mass.] 1971), the hospital claimed an exemption for a professional building in circumstances virtually identical to those here. The Supreme Judicial Court denied the exemption, under a statute not requiring exclusive use,

because the premises leased by [the doctor-tenants] are not being used by them for the purposes for which the hospital is organized. The physicians occupy their offices to conduct their private professional practices for their own personal income. The hospital is not incorporated for the purpose of engaging in the practice of medicine for profit, * * *

Nor is office space a hospital leases to doctors exempt in New York, under *Genesee Hospital v. Wagner* (1975). The doctor's office building at issue there provided all the benefits the Professional Building does, and in addition served to improve the educational function of the hospital. The New York exemption statute requires exclusive use, like the Alaska statute; the court held that the use by the doctors was not exclusively for hospital purposes.

While it is argued that the hospital and the physicians serve the same purpose in the community, that is, to improve the health care of its citizens, . . . for purposes of a tax exemption statute this is too broad a definition in that it fails to take into account the commercial and private practice nature of the physician's operations in the subject office building. The private practice of medicine by a hospital's attending physicians is primarily a commercial enterprise only incidentally related to the hospital's function of providing health care to the community.

The record indicates that the Sisters have performed a service to doctors and patients alike in constructing the Professional Building, and that health care at Providence has been benefited. In order to qualify for an exemption, however, the taxpayer must show, not benefits, but exclusive use. The use of the Professional Building for nonprofit hospital purposes is not exclusive. Therefore, we reverse and remand to the superior court for the entry of an order affirming the Board of Equalization's decision denying the Sisters' appeal.

REVERSED and REMANDED

Barnes Hosp. v. Collector of Revenue
589 S.W.2d 241 (Mo. 1979)

Donnelly, J.

This is an appeal by the Collector of Revenue and the Assessor of the City of St. Louis from a judgment entered by the Circuit Court of the City of St. Louis on August 24, 1978, in favor of respondent, Barnes Hospital, in which the court (1) ordered the Assessor to remove certain property owned by Barnes from the assessment rolls of the City, (2) prohibited the Assessor from placing the property on the tax rolls of the City and (3) prohibited the Collector from levying a tax or compelling payment. Since this case involves a revenue law, we have jurisdiction.

This proceeding involves Queeny Tower, in which full-time and part-time faculty members of Washington University Medical School carry on teaching, research and Barnes Hospital functions, and in which part-time faculty members carry on a private medical practice for individual profit in offices subleased from Barnes Hospital.

On April 28, 1978, Barnes Hospital, a not-for-profit corporation, and owner of Queeny Tower, filed its petition in the Circuit Court seeking to enjoin the Collector, Ronald A. Leggett, from levying a tax or enforcing the collection of same on Queeny Tower for the year 1978 and subsequent years. The petition also sought to enjoin the Assessor, John O'Shaughnessy, from placing Queeny Tower on the tax rolls and from certifying to the Collector any tax bill or list which includes Queeny Tower.

The Barnes Hospital complex consists of eighteen buildings, some of which are owned by Barnes and some by Washington University. Barnes is an important center for teaching medicine and allied fields. Within the complex, teaching programs are conducted by the Washington University Medical School including hospital administration, nursing programs, practical nursing, dietary internships, anesthesia, pharmacy internship programs and radiology technician programs. Barnes and Washington University have jointly developed a world famed reputation, drawing sick and injured from great distances. All patients in Barnes Hospital may be subjects for instruction of the students of the Washington University School of Medicine. The medical staff of the hospital consists solely of the faculty of the school of medicine. Under the hospital bylaws a physician's appointment to the medical staff of the hospital ceases when he ceases to be a member of the faculty of the school of medicine. All the buildings of the Barnes complex are physically connected.

Queeny Tower is a seventeen-story building connected to a building to the east (Rand-Johnson) and has laboratories, patient care rooms, rooms for families, a non-commercial pharmacy, x-ray facilities, hospital offices, a meeting place for the Board, eating facilities, and space for the faculty of Washington University Medical School. Barnes leases 39,989 square feet of space in Queeny Tower to the medical school for which an annual rent is paid constituting less than 0.5% of the total cost of patient care. The medical school in turn subleases a portion to physicians on its part-time faculty to carry on a private practice "in addition to their responsibility to the University for research and teaching."

The trial court made findings of fact, and conclusions of law. It found that the best patient care can be achieved by linking university teaching, research and patient care in the same center. The trial court also found that the location of full-time and part-time members of the faculty in Queeny Tower has improved patient care, research and teaching.

The trial court gave relief to Barnes and enjoined assessment. The Collector and Assessor duly and timely appealed from the judgment of the trial court.

Article X, § 6 of the Constitution of Missouri provides that "all property, real and personal, not held for private or corporate profit and used exclusively . . . for purposes purely charitable . . . may be exempted from taxation by general law."

Section 137.100, RSMo 1978, provides that "All property, real and personal, actually and regularly used exclusively . . . for purposes purely charitable and not held for private or corporate profit . . ." is "exempt from taxation for state, county or local purposes."

There can be no question, under the provisions of [these Missouri laws] that only property which is used exclusively for purposes purely charitable can be held exempt from taxation. The difficulty arises when one poses the question: must the word "property" mean a building or tract in its entirety or may it mean a portion of a building or tract? Historically, this Court has held that the word "property" means a building or tract in its entirety—that buildings or tracts are indivisible for tax purposes.

In *Wyman v. City of St. Louis*, (1852), this Court held that where a building is used in part for a schoolhouse, and in part for other purposes, it is not exempt from taxation; there cannot be a separate assessment for that portion which is used for other than school purposes.

In *State ex rel. Spillers v. Johnston* (1908), this Court diluted the Wyman holding somewhat and said: "The phrase 'exclusively used' has reference to the primary and inherent use as over against a mere secondary and incidental use. * * * If the incidental use * * * does not interrupt the exclusive occupation of the building for school purposes, but dovetails into or rounds out those purposes, then there could fairly be said to be left an exclusive use in the school on which the law lays hold."

However, in *Evangelical Lutheran Synod v. Hoehn* (1946), this Court accurately stated the case law in Missouri to be generally that "where part of a unit tract is used for non-charitable purposes the whole is taxable since it is not used exclusively for charity . . . ."

We have concluded that the holdings in *Wyman, Spillers, Evangelical*, and their progeny, should be overruled and a new sense of direction established.

In [a 1946 legal encyclopedia] it is stated that "[by] the great weight of authority, a statute which in effect exempts from taxation property or buildings used for certain purposes authorizes a partial exemption of a building in case the building is used in part for exempt purposes and in part for nonexempt purposes." Justification for adoption of this position was ably articulated by the Supreme Court of Minnesota in *Christian Business Men's Committee v. State* (1949):

"In the light * * * of modern conditions involving the construction of large buildings, often consisting of many stories, there seems little justification for adhering to an assumed arbitrary rule of thumb that a building is necessarily taxable or nontaxable in its entirety. Big buildings have become the rule in the congested business areas of large cities where ground space is at a premium. The passage of time does not of itself amend the constitution, but it does amend the factual problems, human and physical, to which the constitution applies. If the purpose of tax exemption is to be achieved, we cannot ignore significant changes which have taken place in our physical surroundings. A tax-exempt institution obviously should not be denied the opportunity of acquiring an advantageous location in a congested downtown area simply because it may not be able to occupy for its restricted purpose an entire building consisting of several floors. Although it is a general rule that constitutional provisions exempting property from taxation are to be strictly construed, such provisions, though not subject to extension by construction or implication, are to be given a reasonable, natural, and practical interpretation in the light of modern conditions in order to effectuate the purpose for which the exemption is granted."

We hold that Mo. Const. art. X, § 6 and § 137.100, RSMo 1978, which exempt from taxation property "used exclusively * * * for purposes purely charitable," authorize a partial exemption of a building or tract, where that building, or tract, is used in part for charitable purposes and in part for non-charitable purposes.

Having abandoned the "all-or-nothing" rule of *Wyman* and the "dovetails into or rounds out" rule of *Spillers*, it remains for us to determine the point of departure from precedent. Feeling that justice will best be served by prospective application of the decision announced today, we hold that the new rule shall apply to this case and to all assessments which commence on the first day of January 1980, and thereafter.

In *Franciscan Tertiary Province of Missouri, Inc. v. State Tax Commission* (1978), this Court held that in order for hospital property to be held exempt from taxation under 137.100 *supra*: (1) it must be actually and regularly used exclusively for purposes purely charitable as "charity" is defined in *Salvation Army v. Hoehn*; (2) it must be owned and operated on a not-for-profit basis; and (3) the dominant use of the property must be for the benefit of an indefinite number of people and must directly or indirectly benefit society generally.

The judgment is reversed and the cause remanded for hearing, if necessary, with directions that a judgment be entered enjoining assessment of those portions of Queeny Tower which meet the *Franciscan* test.

Barnes Hosp. v. Collector of Revenue
646 S.W.2d 889 (Mo. Ct. App. 1983)

Pudlowski, J.

This appeal by Barnes Hospital involves taxation of Queeny Tower, a 17-story building connected to, used and owned by Barnes Hospital for the tax exempt purposes of treating patients and providing them with care and services. Washington University Medical School, whose teaching facilities are located within the Barnes Hospital complex and whose faculty members comprise the medical staff of the hospital, leases Queeny Tower from Barnes. The part-time faculty subleases offices in Queeny Tower from Washington University for use in their private practice as well as for use in their teaching, research and Barnes Hospital functions.

The City of St. Louis placed Queeny Tower on its assessment rolls for 1978. Barnes Hospital, a not-for-profit corporation, subsequently filed its petition in the Circuit Court of the City of St. Louis to enjoin the St. Louis City Assessor from placing Queeny Tower on the tax rolls and to enjoin the Collector of Revenue for the City of St. Louis from levying or enforcing tax collection on Queeny Tower for 1978 and subsequent years. After a hearing, the trial court made its findings of facts and conclusions of law in favor of Barnes by decree of August 24, 1978, which enjoined tax assessment or its collection on Queeny Tower. The Collector and Assessor appealed to the Supreme Court which reversed the cause with directions that "a judgment be entered enjoining assessment of those portions of Queeny Tower which meet the *Franciscan* test."

On remand, the trial court conducted three days of hearings, modified its earlier order and entered its judgment in which the trial court permitted the Collector of Revenue and the Assessor of the City of St. Louis:

(1) To assess 16.6% of the buildings of Barnes' property, representing the portion of those buildings occupied by part-time faculty members also engaged in private practice of medicine;

(2) To place those portions of the appellant's property on the assessment rolls of the City of St. Louis for the year 1978 for a total assessment of $315,000; and

(3) To levy a tax for compelled payment on these portions.

We reverse.

The sole question raised is whether property owned by a tax exempt hospital and leased to the medical school for use by its faculty may be taxed where its part-time faculty members, also engaged in limited private practice, maintain their offices therein.

The facts are undisputed. [Here the Court reviews the facts as reported in the Missouri Supreme Court's 1979 decision.]

On remand, in its finding of fact and conclusions of law, the trial court found additionally that the office practice of the part-time faculty members is closely integrated with bedside practice as a role model on patient care. Patient care, instruction of students and the functioning of the clinics for the indigent are materially improved by the presence of part-time doctors in the hospital on a geographically full-time basis. Several highly qualified physician educators testified as expert witnesses that the space-sharing arrangement for the part-time faculty is a necessary concomitant to the hospital's eleemosynary purposes. The heavy load of clinic teaching and patient care falls on the part-time faculty. Without the part-time faculty, Barnes would have to reduce substantially the free clinic work that it does. Its outpatient load exceeds that of St. Louis City Hospital (Starkloff Memorial Hospital), and of both City hospitals before the City closed its Homer G. Phillips Hospital facility. Utilization of the part-time faculty enables the hospital to provide lower cost of care for the indigents within the City. Absent the part-time faculty, Barnes would have to substantially reduce free medical services provided to the City's needy. Equally important is the teaching load of the part-time medical school faculty which is on par with that of the full-time faculty of other departments of the Washington University. In the arrangement where Barnes leases the space to the university, the rent paid to Barnes by the medical school does not yield a corporate profit. Nor does the rent paid by the part-time faculty to the medical school, and, in turn, to Barnes Hospital, generate profit. The hospital sustains a loss.

. . . .

The first prerequisite for exemption is that the property be "used exclusively" for charitable purposes. Nowhere in its decision did the Missouri Supreme Court define the meaning of the statutory words "used exclusively" or "purposes." Thus, the initial proviso of the qualification articulated first in *Franciscan*, the statutory phrase "used exclusively," must be examined. The phrase could mean "solely" or "entirely" in its narrowest sense. We do not construe it in that sense.

Cases analyzing this statutory phrase prior to *Barnes* have not construed it literally, nor do we. In 1974, a building owned by an engineer's club which was used for limited social activities and on occasion was used by private companies, was found to be exempt as a charity from ad valorem taxes. Similarly, residential properties owned by a charitable hospital and occupied by hospital personnel were held to be used exclusively for charitable purposes and hence exempt from taxation. The statutory phrase "used exclusively" has reference to the primary and inherent use as against a mere secondary and incidental use. Our courts since *Barnes* have continued their reliance and acceptance of this definition.

In *Franciscan*, the Missouri Supreme Court held that "the words 'used exclusively * * * for purposes purely charitable' * * * should and do have the same meaning whether applied to property used for a hospital, for training handicapped workers, for operating a YMCA type of program or for providing housing for the aged." Therefore, we are unwilling to deny the exemption to Barnes Hospital on this basis. We reject respondent's contention that the use of the office space in the private practice by the part-time faculty does not meet the [first] prong of the *Franciscan* tri-partite test. We reject the rigid adherence to a literal reading of the statute. We further interpret the Supreme Court in *Barnes* to permit such conclusion.

The policy underlying the statute is to encourage charitable organizations. The meaning we attach to the language of the statute accords with the mandate in *Barnes*. Although it is the general rule that constitutional provisions exempting property are to be strictly construed, such provisions, though not subject to extension by construction or implication, are to be given a reasonable, natural and practical interpretation in light of modern conditions in order to effectuate the purpose for which the exemption is granted.

It is also recognized that each tax exemption case is peculiarly one which must be decided upon its own facts, turning upon the particular record presented. Examining the record against this legal backdrop leads to the conclusion that the office space contingently leased by part-time faculty members also engaged in the private practice of medicine is property actually and regularly used exclusively for purposes purely charitable as required by the *Franciscan* test.

The second prerequisite for charitable exemption is that the property be owned and operated on a not-for-profit basis. No challenge is made that Barnes Hospital is not a charitable or not-for-profit institution. The record satisfies the finding that the rent paid to Barnes Hospital by the Medical School did not yield a profit; on the contrary, the hospital showed a loss. Moreover, even had there been a profit, the exemption would still inure to Barnes Hospital so long as any profit derived from the hospital's operation was achieved incidentally to the primary goal of the organization. The second requirement having been satisfied, we look to the third prerequisite.

The third prong for charitable exemptions is that the dominant use of the property be designed, directly or indirectly, to benefit an indefinite number of people. The evidence adduced at trial clearly satisfies this requirement. The duties conducted by the staff of Barnes Hospital, especially by the part-time faculty, pro tanto benefits the public. The state or municipality generally assumes care of the indigent and helpless. In the City of St. Louis, Barnes Hospital shoulders a segment of this burden, a task more onerous in light of the closing of Homer G. Phillips Hospital. The expert witnesses at trial unanimously agreed that patient care, instruction and functioning of the clinics for the indigent were materially improved by the presence of the part-time doctors in the hospital on a geographically full-time basis. "Part-time" seems a misnomer to describe the contribution made by physicians teaching and monitoring clinics in excess of forty hours per week. The out-patient load at Barnes exceeds that of the City Hospital. Without the part-time faculty, Barnes would have to reduce substantially the free services provided the needy, thereby further encumbering taxpayers, both local and state. We consider the evidence clearly satisfies all three tines of the *Franciscan* test.

For the foregoing reasons, the judgment of the trial court is reversed and the cause remanded with directions that the decree of August 24, 1978, remain in full force and effect and that appellant's questioned property be removed from the tax rolls of St. Louis City and the City Collector be prohibited from levying tax or compelling payment thereon.

All concur.

Discussion Questions

1. How can the Alaska and Missouri courts take two nearly identical tax laws, apply them to similar fact situations, and reach virtually opposite results? For that matter, how can two Missouri courts (one of which is the state's supreme court) do the same?

2. Which of these interpretations do you find more persuasive?

3. After the Missouri Supreme Court's initial decision in *Barnes*—a decision that called for a partial exemption of the property—how can an intermediate appellate court then order that the entire property be removed from the tax rolls?

4. Do you suppose it would matter if the property in question were owned by a for-profit company but leased to a charity for charitable purposes?

5. What if a daily- or hourly-fee parking garage used by employees, patients, families, and visitors was located on a parcel of land owned by and adjacent to a charitable hospital? Is that an exempt use of the property under either Alaska or Missouri law? Does it matter who gets the receipts from the parking garage? Does it matter what fees are charged? Does it change your answer if the garage can also be used by patrons of local businesses that are not connected to the hospital?

6 & 7

Antitrust Law: General Principles and Applications to the Health Care Industry

The word *trust* in the business sense describes a combination of firms or corporations formed by contractual arrangement and usually having the effect of reducing or eliminating competition in the particular industry. Students of U.S. history will recall that the large industrial monopolies of the late 1800s resulted from trust agreements between competing business executives who wished to eliminate their competition, achieve greater efficiency, and maximize their own profits.

The U.S. Congress passed the first antitrust law, the Sherman Antitrust Act, in 1890. The substance of the Sherman Act is simple and broad:

Every contract, combination in the form of trust or otherwise, or conspiracy, in restraint of trade or commerce among the several states, or with foreign nations, is hereby declared to be illegal.

Every person who shall monopolize, or attempt to monopolize, or combine or conspire with any other person or persons, to monopolize any part of the trade or commerce among the several States, or with foreign nations, shall be deemed guilty of a felony. (15 U.S.C. §§ 1–2.)

Armed with this sweeping language, the administrations of Theodore Roosevelt, Taft, and Wilson vigorously enforced the law. As a result, large oil, tobacco, and railroad monopolies (among others) were disassembled and their trusts declared illegal.

Two other statutes, the Clayton Act and the Federal Trade Commission Act, were passed in 1914, and the Robinson-Patman Act was added in 1936. With a few other modifications, these are the basic federal antitrust laws in force today, and it is clear from their history that they were intended to address the economic evils of diminished competition *in industry*. Not until the mid-1970s did it become clear that antitrust law applied to such industries as the learned professions of law, medicine, and health care.

As we have already seen, the character of hospitals has significantly changed in the last 40 years or so. What were essentially small, philanthropic organizations in the immediate post–World War II years are now often regarded as large, complex, "monetarized" corporations (to use Eli Ginzberg's phrase) intent on maximizing revenues and reducing expenditures. In other words, today's hospital is viewed as profit driven.

Ironically, one of hospitals' greatest critics—government—has been largely responsible for this change. Medicare and Medicaid's "cost- or charged-based reimbursement system has undoubtedly given a major impetus to the inflation in the costs of [medical] care" (to quote from page 223 in Southwick's text), and government's reaction has been to encourage the application of business principles to health care management. The pressure to operate more efficiently increased with the advent of the Medicare prospective payment system in the mid-1980s. As a result, the health care sector began in earnest to try to reduce costs, avoid the duplication of services, and increase cooperation.

Paradoxically, even though these trends seemed to meet the government's concerns about rising health care costs, they ran directly contrary to the philosophy of the antitrust laws, which had recently been held to apply to health care for the first time. Therein lies the policy dilemma of the 1990s: until the health care system is reformed, how can the current system be run in a high-quality, cost-efficient manner without violating the antitrust laws' proscription against anti-competitive activities? These issues will be examined in the cases that follow.

Copperweld Corp. v. Independence Tube Corp.
467 U.S. 752 (1984)

Burger, C.J.

We granted certiorari to determine whether a parent corporation and its wholly owned subsidiary are legally capable of conspiring with each other under §1 of the Sherman Act.

I

A

The predecessor to petitioner Regal Tube Co. was established in Chicago in 1955 to manufacture structural steel tubing .... From 1955 to 1968 it remained a wholly owned subsidiary of C. E. Robinson Co. In 1968 Lear Siegler, Inc., purchased Regal Tube Co. and operated it as an unincorporated division. David Grohne, who had previously served as vice president and general manager of Regal, became president of the division after the acquisition.

In 1972 petitioner Copperweld Corp. purchased the Regal division from Lear Siegler; the sale agreement bound Lear Siegler and its subsidiaries not to compete with Regal in the United States for five years. Copperweld then transferred regal's assets to a newly formed, wholly owned Pennsylvania corporation, petitioner Regal Tube Co. The new subsidiary continued to conduct its manufacturing operations in Chicago but shared Copperweld's corporate headquarters in Pittsburgh.

Shortly before Copperweld acquired Regal, David Grohne accepted a job as a corporate officer of Lear Siegler. After the acquisition, while continuing to work for Lear Siegler, Grohne set out to establish his own steel tubing business to compete in the same market as Regal. In May 1972 he formed respondent Independence Tube Corp., which soon secured an offer from the Yoder Co. to supply a tubing mill. In December 1972 respondent gave Yoder a purchase order to have a mill ready by the end of December 1973.

When executives at Regal and Copperweld learned of Grohne's plans, they initially hoped that Lear Siegler's noncompetition agreement would thwart the new competitor. Although their lawyer advised them that Grohne was not bound by the agreement, he did suggest that petitioners might obtain an injunction against Grohne's activities if he made use of any technical information or trade secrets belonging to Regal. The legal opinion was given to Regal and

Copperweld along with a letter to be sent to anyone with whom Grohne attempted to deal. The letter warned that Copperweld would be "greatly concerned if [Grohne] contemplates entering the structural tube market * * * in competition with Regal Tube" and promised to take "any and all steps which are necessary to protect our rights under the terms of our purchase agreement and to protect the know-how, trade secrets, etc., which we purchased from Lear Siegler." ...

When Yoder accepted respondent's order for a tubing mill on February 19, 1973, Copperweld sent Yoder one of these letters; two days later Yoder voided its acceptance. After respondent's efforts to resurrect the deal failed, respondent arranged to have a mill supplied by another company, which performed its agreement even though it too received a warning letter from Copperweld. Respondent began operations on September 13, 1974, nine months later than it could have if Yoder had supplied the mill when originally agreed.

. . . .

B

In 1976 respondent filed this action in the District Court against petitioners and Yoder. The jury found that Copperweld and Regal had conspired to violate [the Sherman Act] but that Yoder was not part of the conspiracy. It also found that Copperweld, but not Regal, had interfered with respondent's contractual relationship with Yoder ... and that Yoder had breached its contract to supply a tubing mill.

... The jury then awarded $2,499,009 against petitioners on the antitrust claim, which was trebled to $7,497,027. It awarded $15,000 against Regal alone on the contractual interference [and a slander count]. The court also awarded attorney's fees and costs after denying petitioners' motions for judgment n.o.v. and for a new trial.

C

The United States Court of Appeals for the Seventh Circuit affirmed. It noted that the exoneration of Yoder from antitrust liability left a parent corporation and its wholly owned subsidiary as the only parties to the § 1 conspiracy. The court questioned the wisdom of subjecting an "intra-enterprise" conspiracy to antitrust liability, when the same conduct by a corporation and an unincorporated division would escape liability for lack of the requisite two legal persons. However, relying on [a previous decision], the Court of Appeals held that liability was appropriate "when there is enough separation between the two entities to make treating them as two independent actors sensible." ...

We granted certiorari to reexamine the intra-enterprise conspiracy doctrine, and we reverse.

II

Review of this case calls directly into question whether the coordinated acts of a parent and its wholly owned subsidiary can, in the legal sense contemplated by § 1 of the Sherman Act, constitute a combination or conspiracy. The so-called "intra-enterprise conspiracy" doctrine provides that § 1 liability is not foreclosed merely because a parent and its subsidiary are subject to common ownership. The doctrine derives from declarations in several of this Court's opinions.

In no case has the Court considered the merits of the intra-enterprise conspiracy doctrine in depth. . . .

The problem began with *United States v. Yellow Cab Co.* [In that case, after acquiring or merging with other taxicab companies, one company controlled taxi operations in four cities. Thus, that opinion stated, the Sherman Act was violated because an unreasonable restraint "may result as readily from a conspiracy among those who are affiliated or integrated under common ownership as from a conspiracy among those who are otherwise independent. . . . The corporate interrelationships of the conspirators, in other words, are not determinative of the applicability of the Sherman Act." Thus, the *Yellow Cab* opinion continues, "the common ownership and control of the various corporate appellees are impotent to liberate the alleged combination and conspiracy from the impact of the Act."]

It is the [above-quoted] language that later breathed life into the intra-enterprise conspiracy doctrine. The passage as a whole, however, more accurately stands for a quite different proposition. It has long been clear that a pattern of acquisitions may itself create a combination illegal under § 1, especially when an original anticompetitive purpose is evident from the affiliated corporations' subsequent conduct. . . . In *Yellow Cab*, the affiliation of the defendants was irrelevant because the original acquisitions were *themselves* illegal. An affiliation "flowing from an illegal conspiracy" would not avert sanctions. Common ownership and control were irrelevant because restraint of trade was "the primary object of the combination," which was created in a "deliberate, calculated" manner. Other language in the opinion is to the same effect.

. . . .

In short, while this Court has previously seemed to acquiesce in the intra-enterprise conspiracy doctrine, it has never explored or analyzed in detail the justifications for such a rule; the doctrine has played only a relatively minor role in the Court's Sherman Act holdings.

III

. . . The central criticism is that the doctrine gives undue significance to the fact that a subsidiary is separately incorporated and thereby treats as the concerted activity of two entities what is really unilateral behavior flowing from decisions of a single enterprise.

We limit our inquiry to the narrow issue squarely presented: whether a parent and its wholly owned subsidiary are capable of conspiring in violation of § 1 of the Sherman Act. We do not consider under what circumstances, if any, a parent may be liable for conspiring with an affiliated corporation it does not completely own.

A

The Sherman Act contains a "basic distinction between concerted and independent action." The conduct of a single firm is governed by § 2 alone and is unlawful only when it threatens [or achieves] actual monopolization. It is not enough that a single firm appears to "restrain trade" unreasonably, for even a vigorous competitor may leave that impression. For instance, an efficient firm may capture unsatisfied customers from an inefficient rival, whose own ability to compete may suffer as a result. This is the rule of the marketplace and is precisely the sort of competition that promotes the consumer interests that the Sherman Act aims to foster. . . . Congress authorized Sherman Act scrutiny of single firms only when they pose a danger of monopolization. . . .

Section 1 of the Sherman Act, in contrast, reaches unreasonable restraints of trade effected by a "contract, combination * * * or conspiracy" between *separate* entities. It does not reach conduct that is "wholly unilateral." Concerted activity subject to § 1 is judged more sternly than unilateral activity under § 2. Certain agreements, such as horizontal price fixing and market allocation, are thought so inherently anticompetitive that each is illegal *per se* without inquiry into the harm [the agreement] has actually caused. Other combinations, such as mergers, joint ventures, and various vertical agreements, hold the promise of increasing a firm's efficiency and enabling it to compete more effectively. Accordingly, such combinations are judged under a rule of reason, an inquiry into market power and market structure designed to assess the combination's actual effect. Whatever form the inquiry takes, however, it is not necessary to prove that concerted activity threatens monopolization.

The reason Congress treated concerted behavior more strictly than unilateral behavior is readily appreciated. Concerted activity inherently is fraught with anticompetitive risk. It deprives the marketplace of the independent centers of decisionmaking that competition assumes and demands. In any conspiracy, two or more entities that previously pursued their own interests separately are combining to act as one for their common benefit. This not only reduces the diverse directions in which economic power is aimed but suddenly increases the economic power moving in one particular direction. Of course, such mergings of resources may well lead to efficiencies that benefit consumers, but their anticompetitive potential is sufficient to warrant scrutiny even in the absence of incipient monopoly.

B

The distinction between unilateral and concerted conduct is necessary for a proper understanding of the terms "contract, combination * * * or conspiracy" in § 1. Nothing in the literal meaning of those terms excludes coordinated conduct among officers or employees of the *same* company. But it is perfectly plain that an internal "agreement" to implement a single, unitary firm's policies does not raise the antitrust dangers that § 1 was designed to police. The officers of a single firm are not separate economic actors pursuing separate economic interests, so agreements among them do not suddenly bring together economic power that was previously pursuing divergent goals. Coordination within a firm is as likely to result from an effort to compete as from an effort to stifle competition. In the marketplace, such coordination may be necessary if a business enterprise is to compete effectively. For these reasons, officers or employees of the same firm do not provide the plurality of actors imperative for a § 1 conspiracy.

There is also general agreement that § 1 is not violated by the internally coordinated conduct of a corporation and one of its unincorporated divisions. . . . [T]here can be little doubt that the operation of a corporate enterprise organized into divisions must be judged as the conduct of a single actor. . . .

Indeed, a rule that punished coordinated conduct simply because a corporation delegated certain responsibilities to autonomous units might well discourage corporations from creating division with their presumed benefits. This would serve no useful antitrust purpose but could well deprive consumers of the efficiencies that decentralized management may bring.

C

For similar reasons, the coordinated activity of a parent and its wholly owned subsidiary must be viewed as that of a single enterprise for purposes of § 1 of the Sherman Act. A parent and its wholly owned subsidiary have a complete unity of interest. Their objectives are common, not disparate; their general corporate actions are guided or determined not by two separate corporate consciousnesses, but one. They are not unlike a multiple team of horses drawing a vehicle under the control of a single driver. . . .

. . . [A] parent and a wholly owned subsidiary *always* have a "unity of purpose or a common design." They share a common purpose whether or not the parent keeps a tight rein over the subsidiary; the parent may assert full control at any moment if the subsidiary fails to act in the parent's best interests.

The intra-enterprise conspiracy doctrine looks to the form of an enterprise's structure and ignores the reality. Antitrust liability should not depend on whether a corporate subunit is organized as an unincorporated division or a wholly owned subsidiary. . . .

If antitrust liability turned on the garb in which a corporate subunit was clothed, parent corporations would be encouraged to convert subsidiaries into unincorporated divisions. . . . Such an incentive serves no valid antitrust goals but merely deprives consumers and producers of the benefits that the subsidiary form may yield.

The error of treating a corporate division differently from a wholly owned subsidiary is readily seen from the facts of this case. Regal was operated as an unincorporated division of Lear Siegler for four years before it became a wholly owned subsidiary of Copperweld. Nothing in this record indicates any meaningful difference between Regal's operations as a division and its later operations as a separate corporation. Certainly nothing suggests that Regal was a greater threat to competition as a subsidiary of Copperweld than as a division of Lear Siegler. . . .

D

[The Court points out that the demise of the "intra-enterprise conspiracy doctrine" leaves a gap in the Sherman Act's treatment of restraints of trade. That is, the anticompetitive effect of the Copperweld-Regal activities is the same whether the companies are thought of as one enterprise or two, yet unreasonable restraint of trade is prohibited by the Sherman Act only if caused by a contract, combination, or conspiracy between separate entities. The Court argues that this omission was intentional for at least two reasons: (1) to continue to scrutinize individual firms' actions for reasonableness "would threaten to discourage the competitive enthusiasm that the antitrust law seeks to promote"; and (2) "whatever the wisdom of the distinction, the Act's plain language leaves no doubt that Congress made a purposeful choice to accord different treatment to unilateral and concerted action."]

The appropriate inquiry in this case, therefore, is not whether the coordinated conduct of a parent and its wholly owned subsidiary may ever have anticompetitive effects, as the dissent suggests. Nor is it whether the term "conspiracy" will bear a literal construction that includes parent corporations and their wholly owned subsidiaries. . . . Rather, the appropriate inquiry requires us to explain the logic underlying Congress' decision to exempt unilateral conduct from § 1 scrutiny, and to assess whether that logic similarly excludes the conduct of a parent and its wholly owned subsidiary. Unless we second-guess the judgment of Congress to limit § 1 to concerted conduct, we can only conclude that the coordinated behavior of a parent and its wholly owned subsidiary falls outside the reach of that provision.

. . . A corporation's initial acquisition of control will always be subject to scrutiny under § 1 of the Sherman Act and § 7 of the Clayton Act. Thereafter, the enterprise is fully subject to § 2 of the Sherman Act and § 5 of the Federal Trade Commission Act. That these statutes are adequate to control dangerous anticompetitive conduct is suggested by the fact that not a single holding of antitrust liability by this Court would today be different in the absence of an intra-enterprise conspiracy doctrine. . . . Elimination of the intra-enterprise conspiracy doctrine with respect to corporations and their wholly owned subsidiaries will therefore not cripple antitrust enforcement. It will simply eliminate treble damages from private state tort suits masquerading as antitrust actions.

IV

We hold that Copperweld and its wholly owned subsidiary Regal are incapable of conspiring with each other for purposes of § 1 of the Sherman Act. To the extent that prior decisions of this Court are to the contrary, they are disapproved and overruled. Accordingly, the judgment of the Court of Appeals is reversed.

It is so ordered.

Discussion Questions

1. In most antitrust cases, facts are everything. Do you clearly understand the facts of this case? Could you coherently explain the factual history to someone else? (It may help to diagram the organizational relationships over time.)

2. What is the basic holding of this case? What changes in the facts would have changed the result?

3. What about Copperweld's rights? It won the case but still has a competitor that it thought it was protected against through the covenant not to compete.

4. Why is the noncompetition covenant *itself* not a violation of the antitrust laws? (Or is it?) Why can Copperweld assert against Independence Tube Corporation the noncompetition agreement it had with Lear-Siegler? (After all, Independence Tube was not a party to that agreement.)

5. The Court makes a strong point that "Congress made a purposeful choice to accord different treatment to unilateral and concerted conduct." Can you think of an area of *criminal* law in which a similar distinction is made? Do you agree that "concerted conduct" (joint action) should be treated differently? Why or why not?

Hospital Building Co. v. Trustees of Rex Hosp.
425 U.S. 738 (1976)

Marshall, J.

This is a suit brought under §§ 1 and 2 of the Sherman Act. Petitioner has alleged that respondents are engaged in an unlawful conspiracy to restrain trade and commerce in the furnishing of medical and surgical hospital services, and that they are attempting to monopolize the hospital business in the Raleigh, N.C., metropolitan area. The District Court dis-

missed petitioner's amended complaint on the pleadings, finding that petitioner had not alleged a sufficient nexus between the alleged violations of the Sherman Act and interstate commerce. The Court of Appeals for the Fourth Circuit, sitting en banc, affirmed the judgment of the District Court, holding that the provision of hospital services is only a "local" activity and that the amended complaint did not adequately allege a "substantial effect" on interstate commerce. We granted certiorari, and now reverse. We hold that the amended complaint, fairly read, adequately alleges a restraint of trade substantially affecting interstate commerce and that dismissal on the pleadings of petitioner's amended complaint was therefore inappropriate.

I

A

Since we are reviewing a dismissal on the pleadings, we must, of course, take as true the material facts alleged in petitioner's amended complaint. Petitioner is a corporation organized for profit under the laws of North Carolina. It operates the Mary Elizabeth Hospital, a 49-bed proprietary hospital in Raleigh, N.C., which offers a general range of medical and surgical services to the public. Respondent Trustees of Rex Hospital (Rex) is a North Carolina corporation which operates Rex Hospital, a private, tax-exempt hospital also located in Raleigh. The other three respondents are the administrator of Rex, one of its individual trustees, and the executive secretary of the local agency responsible for making recommendations to state officials concerning the Raleigh community's need for additional hospital beds. The amended complaint alleges that respondents, along with several co-conspirators not named as defendants in this action, have acted in concert to block the planned relocation of Mary Elizabeth Hospital within the city of Raleigh and its expansion from 49 beds to 140 beds. According to the amended complaint, respondents and their co-conspirators orchestrated a plan to delay and, if possible, prevent the issuance of the state authorization that was a necessary prerequisite to the expansion of Mary Elizabeth. After a delay of some months, the authorization was finally granted, but since then, it is alleged, respondents and their co-conspirators have employed a series of bad-faith tactics, including the bringing of frivolous litigation, to block the implementation of the expansion. The amended complaint also alleges that respondents have maliciously instigated the publication of adverse information about petitioner's expansion plan in order to block the expansion. All these actions, it is contended, have been taken as part of an attempt by Rex to monopolize the business of providing compensated medical and surgical services in the Raleigh area. Petitioner identifies several areas of interstate commerce in which it is involved. According to the amended complaint, petitioner purchases a substantial proportion—up to 80%—of its medicines and supplies from out-of-state sellers. In 1972, it spent $112,000 on these items. A substantial number of the patients at Mary Elizabeth Hospital, it is alleged, come from out of State. Moreover, petitioner claims that a large proportion of its revenue comes from insurance companies outside of North Carolina or from the Federal Government through the Medicaid and Medicare programs. Petitioner also pays a management service fee based on its gross receipts to its parent company, a Delaware corporation based in Georgia. Finally, petitioner has developed plans to finance a large part of the planned $4 million expansion through out-of-state lenders. All these involvements with interstate commerce, the amended complaint claims, have been and are continuing to be adversely affected by respondents' anticompetitive conduct.

. . . .

II

The Sherman Act prohibits every contract, combination, or conspiracy "in restraint of trade or commerce among the several States" and also prohibits monopolizing "any part of the trade or commerce among the several States." It is settled that the Act encompasses far more than restraints on trade that are motivated by a desire to limit interstate commerce or that have their sole impact on interstate commerce. "[W]holly local business restraints can produce the effects condemned by the Sherman Act." As long as the restraint in question "substantially and adversely affects interstate commerce," the interstate commerce nexus required for Sherman Act coverage is established. " 'If it is interstate commerce that feels the pinch, it does not matter how local the operation which applies the squeeze.' "

In this case, the Court of Appeals, while recognizing that Sherman Act coverage requires only that the conduct complained of have a substantial effect on interstate commerce, concluded that the conduct at issue did not meet that standard. We disagree. The complaint, fairly read, alleges that if respondents and their co-conspirators were to succeed in blocking petitioner's planned expansion, petitioner's purchases of out-of-state medicines and supplies as well as its revenues from out-of-state insurance companies would be thousands and perhaps hundreds of thousands of dollars less than they would otherwise be. Similarly, the management fees that petitioner pays to its out-of-state parent corporation would be less if the expansion were blocked. Moreover, the multimillion-dollar financing for the expansion, a large portion of which would be from out of State, would simply not take place if the respondents succeeded in their alleged scheme. This combination of factors is certainly sufficient to establish a "substantial effect" on interstate commerce under the Act.

The Court of Appeals found two considerations crucial in its refusal to find that the complaint alleged a substantial effect on interstate commerce. The Court's reliance on neither was warranted. First, the Court observed: "The effect [on interstate commerce] here seems to us the indirect and fortuitous consequence of the restraint of the intrastate Raleigh area hospital market, rather than the result of activity purposely directed toward interstate commerce." But the fact that an effect on interstate commerce might be termed "indirect" because the conduct producing it is not "purposely directed" toward interstate commerce does not lead to a conclusion that the conduct at issue is outside the scope of the Sherman Act. For instance, in *Burke v. Ford*, Oklahoma liquor retailers brought a Sherman Act action against liquor wholesalers in the State, alleging that the wholesalers had restrained commerce by dividing up the state market into exclusive territories. While the market division was patently not "purposely directed" toward interstate commerce, we held that it nevertheless substantially affected interstate commerce because as a matter of practical economics that division could be expected to reduce significantly the magnitude of purchases made by the wholesalers from out-of-state distillers. "The wholesalers' territorial division * * * almost surely resulted in fewer sales to retailers—hence fewer purchases from out-of-state distillers—than would have occurred had free competition prevailed among the wholesalers." Whether the wholesalers intended their restraint to affect interstate commerce was simply irrelevant to our holding. In the same way, the fact that respondents in the instant case may not have had the purposeful goal of affecting interstate commerce does not lead us to exempt that conduct from coverage under the Sherman Act.

The Court of Appeals further justified its holding of "no substantial effect" by arguing that "no source of supply or insurance company or lending institution can be expected to go under if Mary Elizabeth doesn't expand, and no market price likely will be affected." While this may be true, it is not of great relevance to the issue of whether the "substantial effect" test is satisfied. An effect can be "substantial" under the Sherman Act even if its impact on interstate commerce falls far short of causing enterprises to fold or affecting market price. For instance in *United States v. Employing Plasterers Assn.*, we considered a Sherman Act challenge to an alleged conspiracy between a trade association and union officials to restrain competition among Chicago plastering contractors. As in the instant case, the District Court dismissed the action on the pleadings. It did so on the ground that the complaint amounted to no more than charges of "local restraint and monopoly." The United States appealed directly to this Court . . . , and we reversed. It was sufficient for us that the allegations in the complaint, if proved, could show that the conspiracy resulted in "*unreasonable burdens on the free and uninterrupted flow*" of plastering materials into Illinois. We did not demand allegations, either express or implied, that the conspiracy threaten the demise of out-of-state businesses or that the conspiracy affect market prices. Thus, since in this case the allegations fairly claim that the alleged conspiracy, to the extent it is successful, will place "unreasonable burdens on the free and uninterrupted flow" of interstate commerce, they are wholly adequate to state a claim.

We have held that "a complaint should not be dismissed for failure to state a claim unless it appears beyond doubt that the plaintiff can prove no set of facts in support of his claim which would entitle him to relief." And in antitrust cases, where "the proof is largely in the hands of the alleged conspirators," dismissals prior to giving the plaintiff ample opportunity for discovery should be granted very sparingly. Applying this concededly rigorous standard, we conclude that the instant case is not one in which dismissal should have been granted. Petitioner's complaint states a claim upon which relief can be granted under the Sherman Act. Accordingly, the judgment of the Court of Appeals is reversed, and the case is remanded for further proceedings consistent with this opinion.

Discussion Questions

1. Do you understand why the Sherman Act requires a substantial effect on interstate commerce for conduct to be covered?

2. What if conduct is anticompetitive but does not affect interstate commerce? What would an aggrieved party's remedy be?

3. What does the court mean that "the proof [in antitrust cases] is largely in the hands of the alleged conspirators"?

Arizona v. Maricopa County Medical Soc'y.
457 U.S. 332 (1982)

Stevens, J.

The question presented is whether § 1 of the Sherman Act has been violated by agreements among competing physicians setting, by majority vote, the maximum fees that they may claim in full payment for health services provided to policyholders of specified insurance plans. The United States Court of Appeals for the Ninth Circuit held that the question could not be answered without evaluating the actual purpose and effect of the agreements at a full trial. [The State of Arizona, the plaintiff, filed an interlocutory appeal arguing that the stipulated facts disclosed price-fixing conspiracies that are illegal per se under the Sherman Act and therefore that a full trial to evaluate their anticompetitive effect was not necessary.]

II

The Maricopa Foundation for Medical Care is a nonprofit Arizona corporation composed of licensed doctors of medicine, osteopathy, and podiatry engaged in private practice. Approximately 1,750 doctors, representing about 70% of the practitioners in Maricopa County, are members.

The Maricopa Foundation was organized in 1969 for the purpose of promoting fee-for-service medicine and to provide the community with a competitive alternative to existing health insurance plans. The foundation performs three primary activities. It establishes the schedule of maximum fees that participating doctors agree to accept as payment in full for services performed for patients insured under plans approved by the foundation. It reviews the medical necessity and appropriateness of treatment provided by its members to such insured persons. It is authorized to draw checks on insurance company accounts to pay doctors for services performed for covered patients. . . .

The Pima Foundation for Medical Care, which includes about 400 member doctors, performs similar functions. For the purposes of this litigation, the parties seem to regard the activities of the two foundations as essentially the same. No challenge is made to their peer review or claim administration functions. . . .

At the time this lawsuit was filed, each foundation made use of "relative values" and "conversion factors" in compiling its fee schedule. . . . The relative value was multiplied by the conversion factor to determine the maximum fee. The fee schedule has been revised periodically. The foundation board of trustees would solicit advice from various medical societies about the need for change in either relative values or conversion factors in their respective specialties. The board would then formulate the new fee schedule and submit it to the vote of the entire membership.

The fee schedules limit the amount that the member doctors may recover for services performed for patients insured under plans approved by the foundations. To obtain this approval the insurers . . . agree to pay the doctors' charges up to the scheduled amounts, and in exchange the doctors agree to accept those amounts as payment in full for their services. The doctors are free to charge higher fees to uninsured patients, and they also may charge any patient less than the scheduled maxima. . . .

The impact of the foundation fee schedules on medical fees and on insurance premiums is a matter of dispute. The State of Arizona contends that the periodic upward revisions of the maximum-fee schedules have the effect of stabilizing and enhancing the level of actual charges by physicians, and that the increasing level of their fees in turn increases insurance premiums. The foundations, on the other hand, argue that the schedules impose a meaningful limit on physicians' charges, and that the advance agreement by the doctors to accept the maxima enables the insurance carriers to limit and calculate more efficiently the risks they underwrite and therefore serves as an effective cost-containment mechanism that has saved patients and insurers millions of dollars. . . .

. . . .

III

The respondents recognize that our decisions establish that price-fixing agreements are unlawful on their face. But they argue that the *per se* rule does not govern this case because the agreements at issue are horizontal and fix maximum prices, are among members of a profession, are in an industry with which the judiciary has little antitrust experience, and are alleged to have procompetitive justifications. Before we examine each of these arguments, we pause to consider the history and the meaning of the *per se* rule against price-fixing agreements.

A

[The Court begins this discussion with a recognition that most antitrust cases are considered under a "rule of reason" analysis. That is, Congress could not have meant that "every" agreement "in restraint of trade" is illegal, so in most cases the courts look to the reasonableness of an agreement to determine "whether under all the circumstances of the case the restrictive practice imposes an unreasonable restraint on competition." This is an expensive and time consuming process; therefore, experience has led to the creation of certain categories of per se antitrust violations, of which price fixing is one. If a case involves activities that fit under one of the per se categories, the courts will apply "a conclusive presumption that the restraint is unreasonable." The court recognizes that this may occasionally create an apparent injustice, but it adds, "For the sake of business certainty and litigation efficiency, we have tolerated the invalidation of some agreements that a fullblown inquiry might have proved to be reasonable."

The Court next reviews certain cases involving *uniform* price fixing and then moves to consider *maximum* price fixing, to which it holds that the per se rules apply equally well. The Court quotes with favor an earlier maximum-price-fixing case: "[S]uch agreements, no less than those to fix minimum prices, cripple the freedom of traders and thereby restrain their ability to sell in accordance with their own judgment." This rationale was affirmed in a later case that the Court also quotes with approval: "Maximum and minimum price fixing may have different consequences in many situations. But schemes to fix maximum prices, by substituting the perhaps erroneous judgment of a seller for the forces of the competitive market, may severly intrude upon the ability of buyers to compete and survive in that market. . . . [I]f the actual price charged under a maximum price scheme is nearly always the fixed maximum price, . . . the scheme tends to acquire all the attributes of an arrangement fixing minimum prices."]

B

. . . In this case, the [per se] rule is violated by a price restraint that tends to provide the same economic rewards to all prac-

titioners regardless of their skill, their experience, their training, or their willingness to employ innovative and difficult procedures in individual cases. Such a restraint also may discourage entry into the market and may deter experimentation and new developments by individual entrepreneurs. It may be a masquerade for an agreement to fix uniform prices, or it may in the future take on that character.

Nor does the fact that doctors—rather than nonprofessionals—are the parties to the price-fixing agreements support the respondents' position. . . . [T]he claim that the price restraint will make it easier for customers to pay does not distinguish the medical profession from any other provider of goods or services. [And the Court had recently struck down the "learned professions exception" to the antitrust laws in a case involving the Virginia State Bar association.]

We are equally unpersuaded by the argument that we should not apply the *per se* rule in this case because the judiciary has little antitrust experience in the health care industry. The argument quite obviously is inconsistent with [an earlier case in which the Court held,] "[w]hatever may be its peculiar problems and characteristics, the Sherman Act, so far as price-fixing agreements are concerned, establishes one uniform rule applicable to all industries alike." . . .The respondents' principle argument is that the *per se* rule is inapplicable because their agreements are alleged to have procompetitive justifications. The argument indicates a misunderstanding of the *per se* concept. The anticompetitive potential inherent in all price-fixing agreements justifies their facial invalidation even if procompetitive justifications are offered for some. . . .

. . . .

It is true that a binding assurance of complete insurance coverage—as well as most of the respondents' potential for lower insurance premiums—can be obtained only if the insurer and the doctor agree in advance on the maximum fee that the doctor will accept as full payment for a particular service. Even if a fee schedule is therefore desirable, it is not necessary that the doctors do the price fixing.

. . . .

C

Our adherence to the *per se* rule is grounded not only on economic prediction, judicial convenience, and business certainty, but also on a recognition of the respective roles of the Judiciary and the Congress in regulating the economy. Given its generality, our enforcement of the Sherman Act has required the Court to provide much of its substantive content. By articulating the rules of law with some clarity and by adhering to rules that are justified in their general application, however, we enhance the legislative prerogative to amend the law. The respondents' arguments against application of the *per se* rule in this case therefore are better directed to the Legislature. Congress may consider the exception that we are not free to read into the statute.

IV

. . . .

. . . The agreement under attack is an agreement among hundreds of competing doctors concerning the price at which each will offer his [or her] own services to a substantial number of consumers. It is true that some are surgeons, some anesthesiologists, and some psychiatrists, but the doctors do not sell a package of three kinds of services. If a clinic offered complete medical coverage for a flat fee, the cooperating doctors would have the type of partnership arrangement in which a price-fixing agreement among the doctors would be perfectly proper. But the fee agreements disclosed by the record in this case are among independent competing entrepreneurs. They fit squarely into the horizontal price-fixing mold.

The judgment of the Court of Appeals is reversed.

[The decision was a four-to-three vote in which Justices Stevens, Brennan, White, and Marshall constituted the majority; Chief Justice Burger and Justices Rehnquist and Powell dissented. Justices Blackmun and O'Connor did not participate in the decision.]

Discussion Questions

1. Is this result good policy from a health care standpoint?

2. Why is the kind of price fixing involved here illegal but resource-based relative value scales are not? What about insurance companies' "usual and customary" limits on physician fees? Or diagnosis-related-group prices?

3. Why are "respondents' arguments . . . better directed to the Legislature"?

4. Do you believe the per se rule is generally a good and fair principle?

5. Do you believe health care organizations should be subject to antitrust laws?

United States v. Carilion Health Sys.
707 F. Supp. 840 (W.D. Va. 1989)

Turk, C.J.

This antitrust action, brought by the U.S. Justice Department's Antitrust Division to prevent the merger of two hospitals in Roanoke, Virginia, is before the court for entry of judgment. Based on the findings of fact to follow, the court concludes that the government has failed to prove that the planned merger of the defendants would constitute an unreasonable restraint of trade under the antitrust laws and will enter judgment for the defendants.

The government filed this action in May, 1988, and claimed that defendants' planned affiliation would violate Sherman Act § 1 and Clayton Act § 7. The court dismissed

the government's Clayton Act claim in September,[1] and the remaining claim under Sherman Act § 1 was tried for three weeks . . . between December 12, 1988, and January 17, 1989. . . .

Findings of Fact

Defendant Carilion Health System is a non-stock, nonprofit holding company that owns three nonprofit hospitals in Virginia and manages six others. The company also owns a number of for-profit subsidiaries, including a helicopter ambulance service, an eye, ear, nose and throat clinic, a pharmacy, an insurance company and a health club. Carilion's largest facility is Roanoke Memorial Hospitals in Roanoke, a facility licensed by Virginia health planning authorities for 677 acute inpatient beds, of which the hospital staffs and operates 609. Occupancy averages something less that 500 patients. Roanoke Memorial is a teaching affiliate for the University of Virginia Medical School in Charlottesville.

Carilion also owns Bedford County Memorial Hospital in Bedford, a facility licensed for 75 beds, and Radford Community Hospital in Radford, a facility licensed for 160 beds that staffs and operates about 120 beds. In addition, Carilion manages Franklin Memorial Hospital in Rocky Mount, licensed for 60 beds, Giles Memorial Hospital in Pearisburg, licensed for 60 beds, Wythe County Community Hospital in Wythe County and Tazewell Community Hospital in Tazewell County.

Defendant Community Hospital of Roanoke Valley is a nonstock, non-profit corporation that owns a hospital by the same name in downtown Roanoke. The facility has 400 licensed beds of which 220 are staffed. Occupancy averages about 175 patients. Both Carilion and Community have been organized principally to provide hospital services to the general public, and both provide indigent care to the extent that funds are available. The boards of directors of both institutions are comprised in large part of business leaders from the Roanoke area who have sought to minimize health care costs to employers and patients.

Both Roanoke Memorial and Community draw more than half their patients from the Roanoke metropolitan area, including the cities of Roanoke and Salem and Roanoke County. About 53 percent of Roanoke Memorial's patients come from this area, while Community draws about 74 percent of its patients from there. If defendants' planned affiliation took place, a third facility in the Roanoke area, Lewis-Gale Hospital in Salem, would not be involved in the

---

1. In dismissing the claim, the court noted that § 7 had two clauses, one that prohibited certain stock acquisitions, and a second that barred certain assets acquisitions by persons "subject to the jurisdiction of the Federal Trade Commission." The court found that the clause addressed to stock acquisitions did not apply to defendants because no stock was involved in their transaction. Both defendants are nonstock, nonprofit corporations. The assets clause did not apply either, the court ruled, because the FTC Act did not confer jurisdiction over nonprofit entities on the FTC. . . .

transaction. Owned by Hospital Corporation of America, Lewis-Gale is licensed for 406 beds, of which it operates about 335. The hospital's average occupancy is about 242. Lewis-Gale receives about 70 percent of its patients from the Roanoke area.

All three of these hospitals draw substantial numbers of patients from outside the immediate vicinity of Roanoke. Roanoke Memorial draws 27 percent of its patients from an area that includes Alleghany, Bedford, Botetourt, Craig, Floyd, Franklin, Giles, Montgomery, Pulaski, Rockbridge and Wythe Counties and the cities of Lynchburg and Radford in Virginia, as well as Greenbriar, Mercer and Monroe Counties in West Virginia. The hospital treats at least 100 patients a year from each of these localities and from each of the following: Amherst, Campbell, Patrick, Smyth and Tazewell Counties and Carroll County together with the City of Galax. Roanoke Memorial receives an average of $5,000 in revenue from each patient. Community draws 18 percent of its patients from an area that includes Alleghany, Bedford, Botetourt, Craig, Floyd, Franklin, Montgomery and Rockbridge Counties and the City of Lynchburg, all in Virginia. Twenty percent of the patients who receive treatment at Lewis-Gale come from an area that includes Bedford, Craig, Botetourt, Floyd, Franklin and Montgomery Counties.

Professionals in the hospital industry distinguish among types of care various facilities provide, based on the sophistication of services they render and the seriousness and complexity of the illnesses they treat. Primary care services involve the prevention, early detection and treatment of disease. Such services include obstetrics, gynecology, internal medicine and general surgery. A hospital that limits itself to providing primary care usually has some diagnostic equipment to do X-rays and laboratory analysis. Secondary care involves more sophisticated treatment and may include cardiology, respiratory care and physical therapy. Equipment and laboratory capabilities are more sophisticated. Tertiary care is designed to arrest disease in process. It usually includes heart surgery and such cancer treatments as chemotherapy and requires still more sophisticated equipment than primary or secondary services do. Research hospitals associated with university medical schools also provide state-of-the-art quaternary level care.

All three of the hospitals in Roanoke and Salem provide primary, secondary and some types of tertiary care. Roanoke Memorial provides a significantly greater variety of care at this level and thus tends to treat more serious illnesses than the other two hospitals. Community, while offering some tertiary services, provides the least such care of the three hospitals.

Within its licensed capacity, Lewis-Gale has about 160 unfilled beds. While the hospital would need some time and money to again staff the 70 beds that it no longer operates, it could do so and could then take in at least about 100 more patients before its occupancy would be uncomfortably close to capacity. Hospital administrators testified that they are uncomfortable with occupancy above about 85 percent of capacity.

About 20 other hospitals within the geographic area [that] Roanoke Memorial and, to some extent, Community serve provide primary and, in some cases, secondary level services. . . .

. . . .

These facts show that the Roanoke hospitals compete with the various hospitals in the counties that surround Roanoke to provide primary and secondary level care to patients from those areas. A patient who desires care at a hospital away from home generally must be referred to a doctor who practices near that hospital and has admitting privileges there, but this can be done with little difficulty.

In providing tertiary care, the Roanoke hospitals do not face competition from the hospitals in surrounding counties, but several other large hospitals in Virginia and North Carolina do compete with them. . . .

Various witnesses agreed that some medical needs are treated exclusively on an outpatient basis, while others are treated only in a hospital. Most also agreed, however, that a significant number of problems could be treated either on an in or outpatient basis. Reasonable doctors differ as to when a problem must be treated in a hospital or when outpatient treatment is appropriate. Moreover, various insurance carriers, including Blue Cross and Blue Shield of Virginia, two of whose executives testified at trial, have restructured their reimbursement policies in recent years in order to encourage patients to use outpatient services, which are less expensive than inpatient care. Because patients or their doctors can choose to have problems treated either in a hospital or in an outpatient clinic or doctor's office in a significant number of cases, the court finds that certain clinics and other providers of outpatient services compete with the defendants' hospitals to treat various medical needs.

New entry into the hospital market would be financially difficult. Expansion of an existing hospital, however, would cost substantially less. Expansion beyond licensed capacity would require state approval. Such approval is unlikely until at least July 1, when a state moratorium is scheduled to expire. However, most hospitals now staff substantially fewer beds than their licensed capacity and could expand to their full licensed quotas without obtaining state approval. Moreover, the number of problems treated on an inpatient basis has declined steadily in recent years and can be expected to continue to fall. Defendants' hospitals and their competitors can therefore be expected to have even more beds to fill within their licensed capacity, and competition for patients can therefore be expected to intensify further. . . .

Hospitals have high fixed costs, and their financial health depends on high occupancy. . . .

Because hospitals have high fixed costs, Roanoke Memorial or Community would sustain significant financial harm if either lost a significant number of patients to any of their various competitors: local hospitals in outlying rural areas that compete to provide primary and secondary services to patients who live in those areas; large hospitals in Virginia and North Carolina that compete to provide tertiary level services to patients in western Virginia; outpatient clinics and other facilities that compete to treat medical problems that might otherwise have been treated in a hospital; and Lewis-Gale.

Under defendants' planned affiliation, which defendants approved on July 30, 1987, Carilion would acquire sole membership in and ownership of Community, and Community would gain minority representation on Carilion's board of directors. Defendants want to merge in order to enhance the competitive positions of both Roanoke Memorial and Community. Roanoke Memorial needs more space in which to offer its obstetrics services and for various other clinical and administrative functions. On the other hand, Community's occupancy had declined faster than that of Roanoke's other hospitals. Community has extra space and needs more patients. Defendants plan to consolidate all obstetrics and other clinical services of both hospitals at Community. The merger also can be expected to help the two hospitals strengthen and expand joint operations, which already have begun in the areas of data processing and laundry. Credible testimony at trial satisfies the court the merger will produce capital avoidance and other clinical and administrative efficiencies that will save the two hospitals at least $40 million over the first five years of the affiliation.

. . . .

In conclusion, the court finds that the planned merger would probably improve the quality of health care in western Virginia and reduce its cost and will strengthen competition between the two large hospitals that would remain in the Roanoke area. Defendants' boards of directors could be expected to help insure that savings realized from the affiliation will be passed on to consumers.

Conclusions of Law

The government brings this action under Sherman Act § 1, which provides that "[e]very contract, combination in the form of trust or otherwise, or conspiracy, in restraint of trade or commerce * * * is declared to be illegal. * * *" While "any commercial contract" could be deemed to be a restraint of trade that violates the provision, courts use a " 'rule of reason' analysis for determining whether most business combinations or contracts violate the prohibitions of the Sherman Act." Whether a particular combination is unreasonable depends on such factors as "the facts peculiar to the business in which the restraint is applied, the nature of the restraint and its effects, and the history of the restraint and the reason for its adoption."

. . . .

In analyzing a merger under § 1, the court must evaluate the percentage of business the new merged entity would control, "the strength of remaining competition, whether the action springs from business requirements or purpose to monopolize, the possible development of the industry, consumer demands, and other characteristics of the market."

Relevant Market

The government challenges the effect of defendants' merger on competition to provide acute inpatient hospital serv.:es in the Roanoke Valley. To determine the percentage of business the merged entity would control and the strength of remaining competition, "[i]t is first necessary to delimit the market in which the concerns compete" to provide inpatient services.

Based on the finding above that providers of outpatient services compete with providers of inpatient services for the same patients in a significant number of cases, the court concludes that the relevant service market for this case includes not only other inpatient hospitals but also various outpatient clinics that treat medical problems for which patients might otherwise have sought treatment in an inpatient hospital setting.

Based on the finding above that the Roanoke hospitals compete with hospitals in surrounding counties to provide primary and, in some cases, secondary services to residents of those counties, the court concludes that all those areas are included in the relevant geographic market for this case with respect to primary and secondary services. Specifically, the market includes all the counties and cities from which Roanoke Memorial draws at least 100 patients a year. This area is comprised of 16 counties and three independent cities of Virginia and three counties of West Virginia. Competitors to provide primary and secondary services in the relevant geographic market include not only defendants and Lewis-Gale but nearly 20 hospitals in the counties and cities that surround Roanoke, including a relatively large institution in Lynchburg, as well as relevant outpatient clinics throughout those areas.

Based on the finding above that hospitals in central Virginia and northern North Carolina compete with defendants and Lewis-Gale to provide tertiary level services to the same residents of western Virginia that the three Roanoke hospitals serve, the court concludes that for tertiary level services the relevant geographic market includes hospitals in Charlottesville and Richmond, Virginia, and in Winston-Salem and Durham, North Carolina. . . .

Reasonableness of Restraint

The government argues that defendants' merger would give Roanoke Memorial and Community a market concentration of over 70 percent, based on share of patient occupancy. The court must reject this calculation, however, as it is based on market assumptions that the court cannot accept. The record does not allow the court to produce a concentration figure because the size and occupancy of many of the hospitals in the market were not disclosed at trial. However the market is defined, the merger would doubtless give Carilion a larger market share than it now enjoys. When the various hospitals in the market area surrounding Roanoke are included, however, defendants' market share, even adjusted for the six other hospitals in the market that are owned or managed by Carilion, cannot be expected to approach the estimates advanced by the government. The market share is further reduced by the share of patients drawn away by large research hospitals in central Virginia and northern North Carolina and by various outpatient clinics throughout the geographic market.

In any case, "[t]he relative effect of percentage command of market varies with the setting in which that factor is placed." The court has found that defendants rely for their financial health on filling their beds with various patients who, even after defendants' merger, could turn to one or more other providers for care. These include residents of outlying areas who could go to hospitals near their homes rather than going into Roanoke, patients needing tertiary care who could get it at various hospitals in central Virginia and northern North Carolina and persons who could have their problems treated on an outpatient basis. More importantly, Lewis-Gale, which plans to increase its tertiary service offerings and is considering an affiliation with a major medical school in the region, promises to be a major competitor. The hospital's 160 legally available beds can be expected to put substantial competitive pressure on the merged Carilion hospitals as the number of patients who are hospitalized anywhere continues to decline. The continuing decline in the number of patients in the market increasingly reduces the importance of state legal restraints on hospital expansion, restraints which themselves appear likely to be removed. Financial and legal barriers to expansion by existing hospitals therefore cannot be viewed as prohibitive, and so defendants' various competitors in the geographic market would be able to expand their capacity if necessary in order to compete more vigorously with defendants. The strength of remaining competition and the ease with which remaining competitors can further challenge defendants thus outweighs the increased market share defendants would acquire through their combination.

Also relevant is the fact that defendants seek to merge in order to strengthen, rather than reduce, competition. Based on Roanoke Memorial's serious need to expand and Community's need for more patients, they have found various ways in which more efficient operations can save money and thereby enable them to offer their services more competitively than ever, to patients' benefit. Greater competitiveness—in both prices charged and the quality of services offered—serves to benefit both patients and those who pay for their health care. That business requirements and consumer demand, rather than a monopolistic design, motivate defendants' intention to merge argues strongly in favor of the planned merger's reasonableness.

Defendants' nonprofit status also militates in favor of finding their combination reasonable. Defendants' boards of directors both include business leaders who can be expected to demand that the institutions use the savings achieved through the merger to reduce hospital charges, which are paid in many cases by employers, either directly or through insurance carriers. Defendants concede, of course, that Sherman Act § 1 applies to nonprofit entities. Leading cases on the subject, however, do not address nonprofit entities' charitable activities. . . . Without deciding whether defendants' nonprofit status should exempt their merger from § 1 scrutiny, the court concludes that their nonprofit status weighs in favor of their merger's being reasonable.

The court therefore . . . finds that the merger would not constitute an unreasonable restraint of trade under Sherman Act § 1. The court will therefore enter judgment for the defendants and must deny the injunctive relief the government seeks. The court will enter an appropriate order this day.

United States v. Rockford Memorial Corp.
898 F.2d 1278 (7th Cir 1990)

Posner, J.

The United States brought suit under section 7 of the Clayton Act and section 1 of the Sherman Act . . . to enjoin a merger of the two largest hospitals—both nonprofits—in Rockford, Illinois, a city of 140,000 people. The district judge held that the merger violated section 7, and issued the injunction; he did not reach the section 1 charge.

The defendants appeal, arguing first that section 7 does not apply to a merger between nonprofit enterprises. Surprisingly, this is an issue of first impression at the appellate level, with the exception of an unpublished opinion by the Fourth Circuit, of which more later. Section 7 provides that "[1] no person * * * shall acquire * * * the whole or any part of the *stock or other share capital* and [2] no person *subject to the jurisdiction of the Federal Trade Commission* shall acquire the whole or any part of the assets of another person," where the effect may be substantially to lessen competition, or to tend to create a monopoly. (Emphasis added.) Illinois law forbids a nonprofit corporation to have, and these hospitals do not have, stock or share capital. So the clause we have labeled [1] would seem not to apply. And, the defendants argue, the FTC has no jurisdiction over a nonprofit corporation—so that the merger is not covered by the clause referring to asset acquisitions, clause [2], either—because section 4 of the Federal Trade Commission Act confines the Commission's jurisdiction under the Act to a "company * * * or association, incorporated or unincorporated, which is organized to carry on business for its own profit or that of its members."

The first argument, knocking out clause [1], is strong. The second argument, however, in assuming that the reference in section 7 to "[persons] subject to the jurisdiction of the Federal Trade Commission" is to the Federal Trade Commission Act, overlooks the possibility that the reference is actually to the provision in the Clayton Act itself [that] . . . vests authority to enforce the prohibitions of the Clayton Act in five agencies. These are the Interstate Commerce Commission [ICC], with respect to the common carriers regulated by that Commission; the Federal Communications Commission [FCC], with respect to the common carriers regulated by it; ditto for the Civil Aeronautics Board [CAB] (now defunct); the Federal Reserve Board [FRB], for banks; and, for everyone else, the FTC: "Authority to enforce compliance with sections 2, 3, 7, and 8 of this Act by the persons respectively subject thereto is hereby vested in * * * the Federal Trade Commission where applicable to all other character of commerce." . . . We believe that the force of the assets-acquisition provision in section 7 is, therefore, merely to exempt mergers in the regulated industries enumerated in section 11 [i.e., those regulated by the ICC, FCC, CAB, and FRB]. Those industries do not include the hospital industry. The Clayton Act evinces a purpose of limiting the Federal Trade Commission's jurisdiction vis-à-vis that of other federal agencies charged with enforcing the Act in the industries that they regulate, but it evinces no purpose of exempting nonprofit firms in industries within the domain that the Act bestows on the Commission ("all other character of commerce").

. . . .

. . . [W]e believe (contrary to *United States v. Carilion Health System*) that the merger *is* subject to section 7, once the reference in that section to the jurisdiction of the FTC is understood, as we think it should be understood, to refer to section 11 of the Clayton Act rather than to section 4 of the FTC Act.

The government [also argues that] the merger violates section 1 of the Sherman Act, as charged alternatively in the complaint. Although the district judge did not find it necessary to reach the issue, we can do so, without impropriety, since the subordinate findings that the judge made demonstrate a section 1 violation. . . .

We doubt whether there is a substantive difference today between the standard for judging the lawfulness of a merger challenged under section 1 of the Sherman Act and the standard for judging the same merger challenged under section 7 of the Clayton Act. It is true that the operative language of the two provisions is different and that some of the old decisions (old by antitrust standards anyway) speak as if that should make a difference. A transaction violates section 1 of the Sherman Act if it restrains trade; it violates the Clayton Act if its effect may be substantially to lessen competition. But both statutory formulas require, and have received, judi-

cial interpretation; and the interpretations have, after three quarters of a century, converged.

. . . .

. . . As we noted recently in another (and very similar) hospital-merger case, *Hospital Corporation of America v. FTC*, the current understanding of section 7 is that it forbids mergers that are likely to "hurt consumers, as by making it easier for the firms in the market to collude, expressly or tacitly, and thereby force price above or farther above the competitive level."

A merger with such effects would also violate section 1. The defendants' argument that section 7 prevents probable restraints and section 1 actual ones is word play. Both statutes as currently understood prevent transactions likely to reduce competition substantially. . . .

Even if we are wrong that the standards under section 1 of the Sherman Act and section 7 of the Clayton Act have converged, . . . the defendants are still in deep trouble. The Court in *Columbia Steel* thought that a merger which created a 24 percent firm was not anticompetitive in the unusual conditions of the industry. Here we have a far larger merger and, as we shall see, such unusual conditions as may be present in the hospital industry reinforce rather than undermine the inference naturally to be drawn from the defendants' combined market share.

But all this is provided the district court's market definition is accepted. The "market" is the denominator of the fraction the numerator of which is the output of the defendants or some other select group of firms; the denominator is given by the output of the suppliers to which a group of customers can turn for their requirements of a particular product. Market share is the fraction of that output that is controlled by a particular supplier or particular suppliers whose market power we wish to assess. The higher the aggregate market share of a small number of suppliers, the easier it is for them to increase price above the competitive level without losing so much business to other suppliers as to make the price increase unprofitable; this is the power we call market power.

The district judge estimated the combined market share of the parties to the merger (hospitals of roughly equal size—the two largest in Rockford) at between 64 and 72 percent, depending on whether beds, admissions, or patient days are used as the measure of output. And he estimated the combined market share of the three largest hospitals in Rockford after the merger at 90 percent. Three firms having 90 percent of the market can raise prices with relatively little fear that the fringe of competitors will be able to defeat the attempt by expanding their own output to serve customers of the three large firms. An example will show why. To take away 10 percent of the customers of the three large firms in our hypothetical case, thus reducing those firms' aggregate market share from 90 percent to 81 percent, the fringe firms would have to increase their own output by 90 percent (from 10 to 19 percent of the market). This would take a while, surely, and would force up their costs, perhaps steeply—the fact they are so small suggests that they would incur sharply rising costs in trying almost to double their output, and that it is this prospect which keeps them small. So the three large firms could collude to raise price (within limits of course) above the competitive level without incurring the additional transaction costs and risk of exposure that would result from their trying to coordinate their actions with that of their small competitors.

This analysis, however, collapses if customers can turn to suppliers who (or products that) have been excluded from the market. The market defined by the district judge consists of the provision of inpatient services by acute-care hospitals in Rockford and its hinterland. The defendants point out correctly that a growing number of services provided by acute-care hospitals are also available from nonhospital providers. But the force of the point eludes us. If a firm has a monopoly of product X, the fact that it produces another product, Y, for which the firm faces competition is irrelevant to its monopoly unless the prices of X and Y are linked. For many services provided by acute-care hospitals, there is no competition from other sorts of provider. If you need a kidney transplant, or a mastectomy, or if you have a stroke or a heart attack or a gunshot wound, you will go (or be taken) to an acute-care hospital for inpatient treatment. The fact that for other services you have a choice between inpatient care at such a hospital and outpatient care elsewhere places no check on the prices of the services we have listed, for their prices are not linked to the prices of services that are not substitutes or complements. If you need your hip replaced, you can't decide to have chemotherapy instead because it's available on an outpatient basis at a lower price. Nor are the prices of hip replacement and chemotherapy linked. The defendants' counsel correctly noted that diet soft drinks sold to diabetics are not a relevant product market, but that is because the manufacturers cannot separate their diabetic customers from their other customers and charge the former a higher price. Hospitals can and do distinguish between the patient who wants a coronary bypass and the patient who wants a wart removed from his foot; these services are not in the same product market merely because they have a common provider. The defendants do not argue for the broader market on the basis of substitutability in supply—that is, the ability of a provider of outpatient services to switch to inpatient services should the price of the latter rise as a result of collusive pricing, making such services more profitable.

The more difficult issue is the geographical market. The defendants offered evidence, which the judge accepted, that their service area is a ten-county area of northern Illinois and southern Wisconsin centered on Rockford. Medicare records the address of all hospital patients, so it was possible to determine the zip codes from which the defendants draw their patients. The district judge noticed that 87 percent of the defendants' patients come from an area surrounding Rockford and consisting of the rest of Winnebago County (the county in which Rockford is located) and pieces of several other counties; the remaining patients are widely scattered. The defendants accept the area picked out by the district judge as a reasonable approximation of their service area (though not of the relevant market). There are four other acute-care hospitals in that area. Their output (as measured, we said, by beds, admissions, or patient days, all of which are highly correlated) plus that of the defendants is the market that the judge used to estimate the defendants' market share.

The defendants point out correctly that the hospitals in the defendants' service area may not exhaust the alternatives open to the residents of that area. Maybe a lot of people who live in Rockford, or if not in Rockford then at the edge of the Rockford hospitals' service area at the farthest possible distance from Rockford that is still within that area, use hospitals outside the area. Maybe—but the record shows that the six hospitals in the defendants' service area, plus a hospital in Beloit just north of the service area, account for 83 percent of the hospitalizations of residents of the service area, and that 90 percent of Rockford residents who are hospitalized are hospitalized in Rockford itself. For highly exotic or highly elective hospital treatment, patients will sometimes travel long distances, of course. But for the most part hospital services are local. People want to be hospitalized near their families and homes, in hospitals in which their own—local—doctors have hospital privileges. There are good hospitals in Rockford, and they succeed in attracting most of the hospital patients not only from Rockford itself but from the surrounding area delineated by the district judge. The exclusion of the Beloit hospital from the market was not adequately explained, but apparently does not affect the figures materially.

It is always possible to take pot shots at a market definition (we have just taken one), and the defendants do so with vigor and panache. Their own proposal, however, is ridiculous—a ten-county area in which it is assumed (without any evidence and contrary to common sense) that Rockford residents, or third-party payors, will be searching out small, obscure hospitals in remote rural areas if the prices charged by the hospitals in Rockford rise above competitive levels. Forced to choose between two imperfect market definitions, the defendants' and the district judge's (the latter a considerable expansion of the government's tiny proposed market), and bound to review the judge's determination under the deferential "clearly erroneous" standard, we choose the less imperfect, the district judge's.

The defendants' immense shares in a reasonably defined market create a presumption of illegality. . . .

We [next discuss] the emphasis that the defendants place on their status as nonprofit corporations. This status, they argue, removes any ground for concern that they might seek to maximize profits through avoidance of price or service competition. . . . We are aware of no evidence—and the defendants present none, only argument—that nonprofit suppliers of goods or services are more likely to compete vigorously than profit-making suppliers. Most people do not like to compete, and will seek ways of avoiding competition by agreement tacit or explicit, depending of course on the costs of agreeing. The ideology of nonprofit enterprise is cooperative rather than competitive. If the managers of nonprofit enterprises are less likely to strain after that last penny of profit, they may be less prone to engage in profit-maximizing collusion but by the same token less prone to engage in profit-maximizing competition.

The question cannot be resolved a priori, and once the government showed that the merger would create a firm having a market share approaching, perhaps exceeding, a common threshold of monopoly power—two-thirds—it behooved the defendants to present evidence that the normal inference to be drawn from such a market share would mislead.

It is regrettable that antitrust cases are decided on the basis of theoretical guesses as to what particular market-structure characteristics portend for competition, but to place on the government an insuperable burden of proof is not the answer. We would like to see more effort put into studying the actual effect of concentration on price in the hospital industry as in other industries. If the government is right in these cases, then, other things being equal, hospital prices should be higher in markets with fewer hospitals. This is a studiable hypothesis, by modern methods of multivariate statistical analysis, and some studies have been conducted correlating prices and concentration in the hospital industry. Unfortunately, this literature is at an early and inconclusive stage, and the government is not required to await the maturation of the relevant scholarship in order to establish a prima facie case. The principles of civil procedure do not require that the plaintiff make an airtight case, only that his case satisfy some minimum threshold of persuasiveness and be better than the defendant's case. The government showed large market shares in a plausibly defined market in an industry more prone than many to collusion. The defendants responded with conjectures about the motives of nonprofits, and other will o' the wisps, that the district judge was free to reject, and did. The judge's findings establish a violation of section 1 under the standards of *Columbia Steel*, and the judgment must therefore be affirmed without our needing to decide whether the district judge was correct in holding that section 7 does reach mergers between nonprofit corporations.

The defendants press upon us a recent, not-to-be published (and therefore nonprecedential) opinion by the Fourth Circuit, *United States v. Carilion Health System*, affirming a decision in favor of the defendants in a hospital-merger case much like this one. The discussion in the Fourth Circuit's opinion is brief, indeed perfunctory, consisting as it does very largely of a conclusion that the district court's findings were not clearly erroneous; in any event the court did not want its decision to have a precedential effect. As for the discussion by the district court in *Carilion*, we find it unpersuasive as well as inconsistent with our analysis in *Hospital Corporation of America*—a case cited by neither the district court nor the court of appeals in *Carilion*.

AFFIRMED.

Discussion Questions

1. The facts in the *Carilion* and *Rockford Memorial* cases are remarkably similar, yet the outcomes are virtually opposite. Can you reconcile the results?

2. Which interpretation of the Clayton Act § 7 issue do you find more persuasive?

3. Which approach to defining the relevant service and geographic markets is more reasonable?

4. The two courts show remarkably different philosophies and attitudes regarding not-for-profit corporations. With which do you agree?

8

Admission and Discharge

It is said of most areas of the law that general propositions do not decide concrete cases. Although this is certainly true, it is also true that for analytical purposes we usually begin with general propositions and move to the specifics. But when we do, we often find that there are more exceptions to a rule than applications of it.

This observation is especially true in the area of admission and discharge. The general proposition regarding admission is simple enough to state: persons have no legal right to be admitted to a hospital. The exceptions to this black letter rule, however, would fill many pages of a legal encyclopedia. There might be a right to admission (or at least treatment) in an emergency, at a government hospital, at a Hill-Burton-funded facility, when certain contracts are involved, under nondiscrimination statutes, when universal-access regulations apply, at the request of a police officer, under the terms of a court order, when the facility caused the patient's condition, and so on.

Likewise, the determination of proper discharge from the hospital is not as simple as it may seem. Certainly, as a general proposition, one is discharged when the treating physician writes an order allowing the patient to go home. But patients have been known to leave earlier (against medical advice) or to remain afterwards because they have nowhere else to go (e.g., the alone elderly, crack babies). In addition, when the patient is under some form of legal compulsion (arrest, involuntary psychiatric detention, etc.), the discharge decision may not entirely be the physician's to make. Finally, even when discretion does exist, liability factors may influence the discharge (like in *Tarasoff v. Regents of the Univ. of Calif.*, below).

The following cases exemplify some of the issues surrounding questions of admission and discharge.

Hill v. Ohio County
468 S.W.2d 306 (Ky. 1971)

Smith, Special Commissioner

[This case is a wrongful death action against Ohio County, Kentucky, the owner of Ohio County Hospital. The trial court granted a motion for summary judgment in favor of the defendant, without giving any reasons for that action. The "uncontradicted material facts" are as follows:]

Decedent approached Nurse Hartley [who was "in charge of the 'floor,' " according to the court] at her desk in the hospital before 9 a.m. on May 12, 1967, said that her name was Juanita Monroe, her doctor was in Illinois, she had come to Ohio County to attend a funeral and she was afraid she would not be able to get back to Illinois before she had her baby. Nurse Hartley assumed she wanted to be admitted for obstetrical (herein OB) care.

There were only four doctors admitted to practice in the hospital. Nurse Hartley consulted her list and found that Dr. Beard (according to the doctors' informal agreement among themselves) was "on call" that week. He was at the time in the operating room. Upon Nurse Hartley's inquiry whether to admit decedent, Dr. Beard [required] that he did not handle OB cases. Upon advice from the hospital administrator that another of the four doctors, Dr. Johnson, was making rounds, Nurse Hartley asked him the same question and Dr. Johnson replied that he did not handle "walk-in OBs."

Decedent did not advise that she had been delivered of a child at the Ohio County Hospital in June 1964, admitted by Dr. Charles Price of Hartford (one of the four doctors practicing in the Hospital) and had again consulted Dr. Price within the past year.

Decedent was advised that she could get OB service in Owensboro and Louisville, with doctors on call, and replied she did not want to go to Owensboro or Louisville, but would call a taxi to go home. Nurse Hartley assisted her in making the call. Being advised that decedent was still there more than an hour later, Nurse Hartley consulted with the hospital administrator and was told to call Bill Danks, ambulance driver, who promptly appeared and offered to take decedent wherever she wanted to go. She declined, and a taxi finally took her away.

Her baby was born at home (apparently unattended) during the night. Decedent called Bill Danks who came immediately, and about 6 a.m. called Dr. Johnson, who asked some questions concerning the state of mother and child and advised Danks to take them to Owensboro. Decedent was dead on arrival at the Owensboro Hospital, some 25 miles from Hartford.

Ohio County Hospital is a public hospital, constructed (at least in part) with Hill-Burton funds which are for construction only. It is a one-floor building and the county pays the cost of operation, including an administrator (not a doctor) and at least two registered nurses. There are no salaried doctors, no residents or interns, and only four local doctors are admitted to practice. The hospital rules properly provide that no patient may be admitted without an order from a doctor to do so—[Kentucky law] provides that no one may practice medicine without being licensed to do so.

. . . .

[The court quotes favorably from *American Jurisprudence* (Second):]

With respect to a public hospital, it has been said that since all persons cannot participate in its benefits, no one has, individually, a right to demand admission. The trustees or governing board of a public hospital alone determine the right of admission to the benefits of the institution, and their discretion in this regard will not be reviewed by the courts at the suit of an individual applicant.

. . . .

In the instant case, the decedent was not admitted to the hospital nor was the element of critical emergency apparent. The hospital nurse acted in accordance with valid rules for admission to the facility. The uncontradicted facts demonstrate that no breach of duty by the hospital occurred. The nurse could not force the private physicians to accept decedent as a patient. The nurse did all she could do for the decedent on the occasion in question. Therefore, the hospital and the nurse were entitled to a dismissal as a matter of law.

The judgment is affirmed.

Discussion Questions

1. If you had been the judge, what other facts, if any, would you have wanted to know before you decided the outcome of this case?

2. What other issues could you have raised as plaintiff's lawyer?

3. Would the case be decided differently today than it was over 20 years ago? On what grounds?

4. The party named Hill was the plaintiff. The patient was referred to in an excerpted part of the opinion as "plaintiff's intestate." What does this mean and what is Hill's status to be plaintiff?

5. What is the significance, if any, of the fact that the hospital is a public hospital that received Hill-Burton funds?

6. Explain why Dr. Beard and Dr. Johnson would not have been personally liable for refusal to attend the patient had they been joined as defendants in this action.

Simkins v. Moses H. Cone Memorial Hosp.

323 F.2d 959 (4th Cir. 1963)

Sobeloff, C.J.

The threshold question in this appeal is whether the activities of the two defendants [located in Greensboro, North Carolina] . . . are sufficiently imbued with "state action" to bring them within the Fifth and Fourteenth Amendment prohibitions against racial discrimination. Beyond this initial inquiry lies the question of the constitutionality of a portion of the Hill-Burton Act and a regulation pursuant thereto.

The plaintiffs are Negro physicians, dentists and patients suing on behalf of themselves and other Negro citizens similarly situated. Their complaint seeks declaratory and injunctive relief against the defendant hospitals and their respective administrators and directors. The basis of their complaint is that the defendants have discriminated, and continue to discriminate, against them because of their race . . . . [They] seek an injunction restraining the defendants from continuing to deny Negro physicians and dentists the use of staff facilities on the ground of race; an injunction restraining the defendants from continuing to deny . . . admission of patients on the basis of race . . . ; and a judgment declaring unconstitutional [a portion of the Hill-Burton law and regulations] which authorize the construction of hospital facilities and the promotion of hospital services with funds of the United States on a "separate-but-equal" basis.

. . . . [T]hroughout the proceedings the Government, unusually enough, has joined the plaintiffs in this attack on the congressional Act and the regulation made pursuant thereto.

[The Hill-Burton Act, as passed in 1946, had a general provision prohibiting racial discrimination, but an exception was provided "in cases where separate hospital facilities are provided for separate population groups, if the plan makes equitable provision on the basis of need for facilities and services of like quality for each such group." The implementing regulations, as amended in 1956, had a similar exception.

The Court summarizes the factual background of the case and concludes that the racial discrimination was "clearly established" but that the defendant hospitals, both of which had accepted Hill-Burton grant money, were privately owned and operated. The district court, on that basis, found that no state action existed and therefore that no relief could be granted. However, on this point the appellate court commented, "Participation in the Hill-Burton program subjects hospitals to an elaborate and intricate pattern of governmental regulations, both state and federal . . . ." On this basis, the court proceeds to state the issue and analyze it as follows.]

. . . In our view the initial question is . . . whether the state or the federal government, or both, have become so involved in the conduct of these otherwise private bodies that their activities are also the activities of these governments and performed under their aegis without the private body necessarily becoming either their instrumentality or their agent in a strict sense. As the Supreme Court recently said in *Burton v. Wilmington Parking Authority*, [which was] a case involving racial discrimination by a privately owned restaurant operating on government property,

"The Civil Rights Cases [a set of Supreme Court decisions issued in 1883] 'embedded in our constitutional law' the principle 'that the action inhibited by the [Equal Protection Clause] of the Fourteenth Amendment is only such action as may fairly be said to be that of the States. That Amendment erects no shield against merely private conduct, however discriminatory or wrongful.' . . . It is clear, as it always has been since the Civil Rights Cases, that 'Individual invasion of individual rights is not the subject-matter of the amendment,' and that private conduct abridging individual rights does no violence to the Equal Protection Clause *unless to some significant extent the State in any of its manifestations has been found to have become involved in it. . . .*" [Italics in the original.]

Weighing the circumstances we are of the opinion that this case is controlled by Burton, where the Court held that the "activities, obligations and responsibilities of the [Parking] Authority, the benefits mutually conferred, together with the obvious fact that the restaurant is operated as an integral part of a public building devoted to a public parking service, indicates that degree of state participation and involvement in discriminatory action which it was the design of the Fourteenth Amendment to condemn."

Here the most significant contacts compel the conclusion that the necessary "degree of state [in the broad sense, including federal] participation and involvement" is present as a result of the participation by the defendants in the Hill-Burton program. The massive use of public funds and extensive state-federal sharing in the common plan are all relevant factors. We deal here with the appropriation of millions of dollars of public monies pursuant to comprehensive governmental plans. But we emphasize that this is not merely a controversy over a sum of money. Viewed from the plaintiffs' standpoint it is an effort by a group of citizens to escape the consequences of discrimination in a concern touching health and life itself. As the case affects the defendants it raises the question of whether they may escape constitutional responsibilities for the equal treatment of citizens, arising from participation in a joint federal and state program allocating aid to hospital facilities throughout the state.

Not every subvention by the federal or state government automatically involves the beneficiary in "state action," and it is not necessary or appropriate in this case to undertake a precise delineation of the legal rule as it may operate in circumstances not now before the court. Prudence and established judicial practice counsel against such an attempt at needlessly broad adjudication. Our concern is with the Hill-Burton program, and examination of its functioning leads to the conclusion that we have state action here. Just as the Court in the parking Authority case attached major significance to "the obvious fact that the restaurant is operated as an integral part of a public building devoted to a public parking service," we find it significant here that the defendant hospitals operate as integral parts of comprehensive joint or intermeshing state and federal plans or programs designed to effect a proper allocation of available medical and hospital resources for the best possible promotion and maintenance of public health. Such involvement in discriminatory action "it was the design of the Fourteenth Amendment to condemn."

. . . .

These federal provisions undertaking to authorize segregation by state-connected institutions are unconstitutional. The rest [of the statute], providing for hospital facilities without discrimination, however, remains in effect. . . . The general prohibition against discrimination stands; only the exception tolerating "separate-but-equal" falls. . . .

. . . .

Giving recognition to its responsibilities for public health, the state elected not to build publicly owned hospitals, which concededly could not have avoided a legal requirement against discrimination. Instead it adopted and the defendants participated in a plan for meeting those responsibilities by permitting its share of Hill-Burton funds to go to existing private institutions. The appropriation of such funds to the [defendants] effectively limits Hill-Burton funds available in the future to create non-segregated facilities in the Greensboro area. In these circumstances, the plaintiffs can have no effective remedy unless the constitutional discrimination complained of is forbidden.

The order of the District Court is reversed and the case is remanded for the entry of an order in conformity with the opinion of this court.

Reversed and remanded.

HAYNSWORTH, Circuit Judge, with whom BOREMAN, Circuit Judge, joins [filed a dissenting opinion].

Discussion Questions

1. Do you agree with the way in which the court has stated the issue for decision in this case? If not, how else would you state it?

2. Recalling the legal and political climate of the 1950s and 1960s, why would the U.S. government join the plaintiffs in an attack on one of its own laws? Why should not the government merely have amended the law and changed the regulation involved in this case?

3. The regulation at issue was adopted in 1956. What famous, relevant Supreme Court discrimination decision was handed down not long before that date?

4. Compare this case with *Jackson v. Metropolitan Edison* in Chapter 1, and consider *Burton v. Wilmington Parking Auth.* (referred to in the *Simkins* excerpt). Be prepared to discuss the relationship among them. Can the decisions be reconciled, or are they fundamentally inconsistent? What is the consistent rationale, if there is one, by which the cases can be considered?

5. Judge Haynsworth, who dissented in this case, was front-page news about 20 years ago. Do you know why?

Tarasoff v. Regents of the Univ. of Calif.
17 Cal. 3d 425, 551 P.2d 334, 131 Cal. Rptr. 14 (1976)

Tobriner, J.

On October 27, 1969, Prosenjit Poddar killed Tatiana Tarasoff. Plaintiffs, Tatiana's parents, allege that two months earlier Poddar confided his intention to kill Tatiana to Dr. Lawrence Moore, a psychologist employed by the Cowell Memorial Hospital at the University of California at Berkeley. They allege that on Moore's request, the campus police briefly detained Poddar, but released him when he appeared rational. They further claim that Dr. Harvey Powelson, Moore's superior, then directed that no further action be taken to detain Poddar. No one warned plaintiffs of Tatiana's peril.

Concluding that these facts set forth causes of action against neither therapists and policemen involved, nor against the Regents of the University of California as their employer, the superior court sustained defendants' demurrers to plaintiffs' second amended complaints without leave to amend. This appeal ensued.

Plaintiffs' complaints predicate liability on two grounds: defendants' failure to warn plaintiffs of the impending danger and their failure to bring about Poddar's confinement pursuant to the Lanterman-Petris-Short Act [the California law allowing involuntary, psychiatric admission of persons considered dangerous to themselves or others]. Defendants, in turn, assert that they owed no duty of reasonable care to

Tatiana and that they are immune from suit under the California Tort Claims Act of 1963.

We shall explain that defendant therapists cannot escape liability merely because Tatiana herself was not their patient. When a therapist determines, or pursuant to the standards of his profession should determine, that his patient presents a serious danger of violence to another, he incurs an obligation to use reasonable care to protect the intended victim against such danger. The discharge of this duty may require the therapist to take one or more of various steps, depending upon the nature of the case. Thus it may call for him to warn the intended victim or others likely to apprise the victim of the danger, to notify the police, or to take whatever other steps are reasonably necessary under the circumstances.

In the case at bar, plaintiffs admit that defendant therapists notified the police, but argue on appeal that the therapists failed to exercise reasonable care to protect Tatiana in that they did not confine Poddar and did not warn Tatiana or others likely to apprise her of the danger. Defendant therapists . . . are public employees, consequently, and to the extent that plaintiffs seek to predicate liability upon the therapists' failure to bring about Poddar's confinement, the therapists can not claim immunity under Government Code section 856[1] since no specific statutory provision . . . shields them from liability based upon failure to warn Tatiana or others likely to apprise her of the danger, and Government Code section 820.2[2] does not protect such failure as an exercise of discretion.

Plaintiffs therefore can amend their complaints to allege that, regardless of the therapists' unsuccessful attempt to confine Poddar, since they knew that Poddar was at large and dangerous, their failure to warn Tatiana or others likely to apprise her of the danger constituted a breach of the therapists' duty to exercise reasonable care to protect Tatiana. . . .

1. *Plaintiffs' complaints*

Plaintiffs, Tatiana's mother and father, filed separate but virtually identical second amended complaints. The issue before us on this appeal is whether those complaints now state, or can be amended to state, causes of action against defen-

---

1. Editors' note:

§ 856. Determinations in accordance with applicable enactments

(a) Neither a public entity nor a public employee acting within the scope of his employment is liable for any injury resulting from determining in accordance with any applicable enactment:

(1) Whether to confine a person for mental illness or addiction.

(2) The terms and conditions of confinement for mental illness or addiction.

(3) Whether to parole, grant a leave of absence to, or release a person confined for mental illness or addiction.

(b) A public employee is not liable for carrying out with due care a determination described in subdivision (a).

(c) Nothing in this section exonerates a public employee from liability for injury proximately caused by his negligent or wrongful act or omission in carrying out or failing to carry out:

dants. We therefore begin by setting forth the pertinent allegations of the complaints.

Plaintiffs' first cause of action, entitled "Failure to Detain a Dangerous Patient," alleges that on August 20, 1969, Poddar was a voluntary outpatient receiving therapy at Cowell Memorial Hospital. Poddar informed Moore, his therapist, that he was going to kill an unnamed girl, readily identifiable as Tatiana, when she returned home from spending the summer in Brazil. Moore, with the concurrence of Dr. Gold, who had initially examined Poddar, and Dr. Yandell, assistant to the director of the department of psychiatry, decided that Poddar should be committed for observation in a mental hospital. Moore orally notified Officers Atkinson and Teel of the campus police that he would request commitment. He then sent a letter to Police Chief William Beall requesting the assistance of the police department in securing Poddar's confinement.

Officers Atkinson, Brownrigg, and Halleran took Poddar into custody, but, satisfied that Poddar was rational, released him on his promise to stay away from Tatiana. Powelson, director of the department of psychiatry at Cowell Memorial Hospital, then asked the police to return Moore's letter, directed that all copies of the letter and notes that Moore had taken as therapist be destroyed, and "ordered no action to place Prosenjit Poddar in 72-hour treatment and evaluation facility."

Plaintiffs' second cause of action, entitled "Failure to Warn On a Dangerous Patient," incorporates the allegations of the first cause of action, but adds the assertion that defendants negligently permitted Poddar to be released from police custody without "notifying the parents of Tatiana Tarasoff that their daughter was in grave danger from Posenjit Poddar." Poddar persuaded Tatiana's brother to share an apartment with him near Tatiana's residence; shortly after her return from Brazil, Poddar went to her residence and killed her. . . .

[The court holds that the first cause of action is barred by the principle of governmental immunity. The third and fourth—not summarized in this book—were also held to be invalid.] We direct our attention, therefore, to the issue of whether plaintiffs' second cause of action can be amended to state a basis for recovery.

---

(1) A determination to confine or not to confine a person for mental illness or addiction.

(2) The terms or conditions of confinement of a person for mental illness or addiction.

(3) A determination to parole, grant a leave of absence to, or release a person confined for mental illness or addiction.

2. Editors' note:

§ 820.2. Discretionary acts

Except as otherwise provided by statute, a public employee is not liable for an injury resulting from his act or omission where the act or omission was the result of the exercise of the discretion vested in him, whether or not such discretion be abused.

2. *Plaintiffs can state a cause of action against defendant therapists for negligent failure to protect Tatiana.*

The second cause of action can be amended to allege that Tatiana's death proximately resulted from defendants' negligent failure to warn Tatiana or others likely to apprise her of her danger. Plaintiffs contend that as amended, such allegations of negligence and proximate causation, with resulting damages, establish a cause of action. Defendants, however, contend that in the circumstances of the present case they owed no duty of care to Tatiana or her parents and that, in the absence of such duty, they were free to act in careless disregard of Tatiana's life and safety.

In analyzing this issue, we bear in mind that legal duties are not discoverable facts of nature, but merely conclusory expressions that, in cases of a particular type, liability should be imposed for damage done. As stated in *Dillon v. Legg*: "The assertion that liability must * * * be denied because defendant bears no 'duty' to plaintiff 'begs the essential question—whether the plaintiff's interests are entitled to legal protection against the defendant's conduct. * * * [Duty] is not sacrosanct in itself, but only an expression of the sum total of those considerations of policy which lead the law to say that the particular plaintiff is entitled to protection.' "

In the landmark case of *Rowland v. Christian* (1968), Justice Peters recognized that liability should be imposed "for injury occasioned to another by his want of ordinary care or skill" as expressed in section 1714 of the Civil Code. Thus, Justice Peters, quoting from *Heaven v. Pender* (1883) stated: " 'whenever one person is by circumstances placed in such a position with regard to another * * * that if he did not use ordinary care and skill in his own conduct * * * he would cause danger of injury to the person or property of the other, a duty arises to use ordinary care and skill to avoid such danger.' "

We depart from "this fundamental principle" only upon the "balancing of a number of considerations"; major ones "are the foreseeability of harm to the plaintiff, the degree of certainty that the plaintiff suffered injury, the closeness of the connection between the defendant's conduct and the injury suffered, the moral blame attached to the defendant's conduct, the policy of preventing future harm, the extent of the burden to the defendant and consequences to the community of imposing a duty to exercise care with resulting liability for breach, and the availability, cost and prevalence of insurance for the risk involved."

The most important of these considerations in establishing duty is foreseeability. As a general principle, a "defendant owes a duty of care to all persons who are foreseeably endangered by his conduct, with respect to all risks which make the conduct unreasonably dangerous." As we shall explain, however, when the avoidance of foreseeable harm requires a defendant to control the conduct of another person, or to warn of such conduct, the common law has traditionally imposed liability only if the defendant bears some special relationship to the dangerous person or to the potential victim. Since the relationship between a therapist and his patient satisfies this requirement, we need not here decide whether foreseeability alone is sufficient to create a duty to exercise reasonable care to protect a potential victim of another's conduct.

Although, as we have stated above, under the common law, as a general rule, one person owed no duty to control the conduct of another, nor to warn those endangered by such conduct, the courts have carved out an exception to this rule in cases in which the defendant stands in some special relationship to either the person whose conduct needs to be controlled or in a relationship to the foreseeable victim of that conduct. Applying this exception to the present case, we note that a relationship of defendant therapists to either Tatiana or Poddar will suffice to establish a duty of care; as explained in . . . the Restatement Second of Torts, a duty of care may arise from either "(a) a special relation * * * between the actor and the third person which imposes a duty upon the actor to control the third person's conduct, or (b) a special relation * * * between the actor and the other which gives to the other a right of protection."

Although plaintiffs' pleadings assert no special relation between Tatiana and defendant therapists, they establish as between Poddar and defendant therapists the special relation that arises between a patient and his doctor or psychotherapist. Such a relationship may support affirmative duties for the benefit of third persons. Thus, for example, a hospital must exercise reasonable care to control the behavior of a patient which may endanger other persons. A doctor must also warn a patient if the patient's condition or medication renders certain conduct, such as driving a car, dangerous to others.

Although the California decisions that recognize this duty have involved cases in which the defendant stood in a special relationship both to the victim and to the person whose conduct created the danger, we do not think that the duty should logically be constricted to such situations. Decisions of other jurisdictions hold that the single relationship of a doctor to his patient is sufficient to support the duty to exercise reasonable care to protect others against dangers emanating from the patient's illness. The courts hold that a doctor is liable to persons infected by his patient if he negligently fails to diagnose a contagious disease, or, having diagnosed the illness, fails to warn members of the patient's family.

Since it involved a dangerous mental patient, the decision in *Merchants Nat. Bank & Trust Co. of Fargo v. United States* [1967] comes closer to the issue. The Veterans Administration arranged for the patient to work on a local farm, but did not inform the farmer of the man's background. The farmer consequently permitted the patient to come and go freely during nonworking hours; the patient borrowed a car, drove to his wife's residence and killed her. Notwithstanding the lack of any "special relationship" between the Veterans Administration and the wife, the court found the Veterans Administration liable for the wrongful death of the wife.

In their summary of the relevant rulings [two scholars] conclude that the "case law should dispel any notion that to impose on the therapists a duty to take precautions for the safety of persons threatened by a patient, where due care so requires, is in any way opposed to contemporary ground rules on the duty relationship. On the contrary, there now seems to be sufficient authority to support the conclusion that by entering into a doctor-patient relationship the therapist becomes sufficiently involved to assume some responsibility for the safety, not only of the patient himself, but also of any third person whom the doctor knows to be threatened by the patient."

Defendants contend, however, that imposition of a duty to exercise reasonable care to protect third persons is unworkable because therapists cannot accurately predict whether or not a patient will resort to violence. In support of this argument amicus representing the American Psychiatric Association and other professional societies cites numerous articles which indicate that therapists, in the present state of the art, are unable reliably to predict violent acts; their forecasts, amicus claims, tend consistently to overpredict violence, and indeed are more often wrong than right. Since predictions of violence are often erroneous, amicus concludes, the courts should not render rulings that predicate the liability of therapists upon the validity of such predictions.

The role of the psychiatrist, who is indeed a practitioner of medicine, and that of the psychologist who performs an allied function, are like that of the physician who must conform to the standards of the profession and who must often make diagnoses and predictions based upon such evaluations. Thus the judgment of the therapist in diagnosing emotional disorders and in predicting whether a patient presents a serious danger of violence is comparable to the judgment which doctors and professionals must regularly render under accepted rules of responsibility.

We recognize the difficulty that a therapist encounters in attempting to forecast whether a patient presents a serious danger of violence. Obviously, we do not require that the therapist, in making that determination, render a perfect performance; the therapist need only exercise "that reasonable degree of skill, knowledge, and care ordinarily possessed and exercised by members of [that professional specialty] under similar circumstances." Within the broad range of reasonable practice and treatment in which professional opinion and judgment may differ, the therapist is free to exercise his or her own best judgment without liability; proof, aided by hindsight, that he or she judged wrongly is insufficient to establish negligence.

In the instant case, however, the pleadings do not raise any question as to failure of defendant therapists to predict that Poddar presented a serious danger of violence. On the contrary, the present complaints allege that defendant therapists did in fact predict that Poddar would kill, but were negligent in failing to warn.

Amicus contends, however, that even when a therapist does in fact predict that a patient poses a serious danger of violence to others, the therapist should be absolved of any responsibility for failing to act to protect the potential victim. In our view, however, once a therapist does in fact determine, or under applicable professional standards reasonably should have determined, that a patient poses a serious danger of violence to others, he bears a duty to exercise reasonable care to protect the foreseeable victim of that danger. While the discharge of this duty of due care will necessarily vary with the facts of each case, in each instance the adequacy of the therapist's conduct must be measured against the traditional negligence standard of the rendition of reasonable care under the circumstances. As explained in [the same scholars' article]: " * * * the ultimate question of resolving the tension between the conflicting interests of patient and potential victim is one of social policy, not professional expertise. * * * In sum, the therapist owes a legal duty not only to his patient, but also to his patient's would-be victim and is subject in both respects to scrutiny by judge and jury."

Contrary to the assertion of amicus, this conclusion is not inconsistent with our recent decision in *People v. Burnick*. Taking note of the uncertain character of therapeutic prediction, we held in *Burnick* that a person cannot be committed as a mentally disordered sex offender unless found to be such by proof beyond a reasonable doubt. The issue in the present context, however, is not whether the patient should be incarcerated, but whether the therapist should take any steps at all to protect the threatened victim; some of the alternatives open to the therapist, such as warning the victim, will not result in the drastic consequences of depriving the patient of his liberty. Weighing the uncertain and conjectural character of the alleged damage done the patient by such a warning against the peril to the victim's life, we conclude that professional inaccuracy in predicting violence cannot negate the therapist's duty to protect the threatened victim.

The risk that unnecessary warnings may be given is a reasonable price to pay for the lives of possible victims that may be saved. We would hesitate to hold that the therapist who is aware that his patient expects to attempt to assassinate the President of the United States would not be obligated to warn the authorities because the therapist cannot predict with accuracy that his patient will commit the crime.

Defendants further argue that free and open communication is essential to psychotherapy; that "Unless a patient * * * is assured that * * * information [revealed by him] can and will be held in utmost confidence, he will be reluctant to make the full disclosure upon which diagnosis and treatment * * * depends." The giving of a warning, defendants contend, constitutes a breach of trust which entails the revelation of confidential communications.

We recognize the public interest in supporting effective treatment of mental illness and in protecting the rights of patients to privacy and the consequent public importance of safeguarding the confidential character of psychotherapeutic communication. Against this interest, however, we must weigh the public interest in safety from violent assault. The Legislature has undertaken the difficult task of balancing the countervailing concerns. In Evidence Code section 1014, it established a broad rule of privilege to protect confidential communications between patient and psychotherapist. In Evidence Code section 1024, the Legislature created a specific and limited exception to the psychotherapist-patient privilege: "There is no privilege * * * if the psychotherapist has reasonable cause to believe that the patient is in such mental or emotional condition as to be dangerous to himself or to the person or property of another and that disclosure of the communication is necessary to prevent the threatened danger."

We realize that the open and confidential character of psychotherapeutic dialogue encourages patients to express threats of violence, few of which are ever executed. Certainly a therapist should not be encouraged routinely to reveal such threats; such disclosures could seriously disrupt the patient's relationship with his therapist and with the persons threatened. To the contrary, the therapist's obligations to his patient require that he not disclose a confidence unless such disclosure is necessary to avert danger to others, and even then that he do so discreetly, and in a fashion that would preserve the privacy of his patient to the fullest extent compatible with the prevention of the threatened danger.

The revelation of a communication under the above circumstances is not a breach of trust or a violation of professional ethics; as stated in the Principles of Medical Ethics of the American Medical Association (1957), section 9: "A physician may not reveal the confidence entrusted to him in the course of medical attendance * * * *unless he is required to do so by law or unless it becomes necessary in order to protect the welfare of the individual or of the community.*" [Emphasis added by the court.] We conclude that the public policy favoring protection of the confidential character of patient-psychotherapist communications must yield to the extent to which disclosure is essential to avert danger to others. The protective privilege ends where the public peril begins.

Our current crowded and computerized society compels the interdependence of its members. In this risk-infested society we can hardly tolerate the further exposure to danger that would result from a concealed knowledge of the therapist that his patient was lethal. If the exercise of reasonable care to protect the threatened victim requires the therapist to warn the endangered party or those who can reasonably be expected to notify him, we see no sufficient societal interest that would protect and justify concealment. The containment of such risks lies in the public interest. For the foregoing reasons, we find that plaintiffs' complaints can be amended to state a cause of action against defendants Moore, Powelson,

Gold, and Yandell and against the Regents as their employer, for breach of a duty to exercise reasonable care to protect Tatiana.

Discussion Questions

1. The *Tarasoff* decision is premised on the psychotherapist's duty to determine the dangerousness of a patient. How should that determination be made? Can the reliability of the determination only be determined retrospectively? Are you persuaded by the court's explanation of the reasons for dismissing experts' opinions that such determinations are inherently unreliable?

2. Would the same result have been obtained if the patient had been threatening violence to himself and later committed suicide? Would the same result have been obtained if the patient had been threatening violence to the community in general?

3. How can one rationalize *Tarasoff*'s result with the individual rights of patients to be free of unreasonable restraints on their liberty? Especially where, as here, a state agency is involved, how would a psychotherapist's decision protect the due process of such a patient?

Wickline v. State
192 Cal. App. 3d 1630, 239 Cal. Rptr. 810 (1986)

Rowen, J.

This is an appeal from a judgment for plaintiff entered after a trial by jury. For the reasons discussed below, we reverse the judgment.

Principally, this matter concerns itself with the legal responsibility that a third party payor, in this case, the State of California, has for harm caused to a patient when a cost containment program is applied in a manner which is alleged to have affected the implementation of the treating physician's medical judgment.

The plaintiff, respondent herein, Lois J. Wickline (plaintiff or Wickline) sued defendant, appellant herein, State of California . . . . The essence of the plaintiff's claim is found in paragraph 16 of her second amended complaint which alleges: "Between January 6, 1977, and January 21, 1977, [an unnamed] employee of the State of California, while acting within the scope of employment, negligently discontinued plaintiff's Medi-Cal eligibility, causing plaintiff to be discharged from Van Nuys Community Hospital prematurely and whil[e] in need of continuing hospital care. As a result of said negligent act, plaintiff suffered a complete occlusion of the right infra-renoaorta, necessitating an amputation of plaintiff's right leg."

I

Responding to concerns about the escalating cost of health care, public and private payors have in recent years experimented with a variety of cost containment mechanisms. We deal here with one of those programs: The prospective utilization review process.

At the outset, this court recognizes that this case appears to be the first attempt to tie a health care payor into the medical malpractice causation chain and that it, therefore, deals with issues of profound importance to the health care community and to the general public. For those reasons we have permitted the filing of amicus curiae briefs in support of each of the respective parties in the matter to assure that due consideration is given to the broader issues raised before this court by this case.

Traditionally, quality assurance activities, including utilization review programs, were performed primarily within the hospital setting under the general control of the medical staff. The principal focus of such quality assurance review schema was to prevent overutilization due to the recognized financial incentives to both hospitals and physicians to maximize revenue by increasing the amount of service provided and to insure that patients were not unnecessarily exposed to risks as a result of unnecessary surgery and/or hospitalization.

Early cost-containment programs utilized the retrospective utilization review process. In that system the third party payor reviewed the patient's chart after the fact to determine whether the treatment provided was medically necessary. If, in the judgment of the utilization reviewer, it was not, the health care provider's claim for payment was denied.

In the cost-containment program in issue in this case, prospective utilization review, authority for the rendering of health care services must be obtained before medical care is rendered. Its purpose is to promote the well recognized public interest in controlling health care costs by reducing unnecessary services while still intending to assure that appropriate medical and hospital services are provided to the patient in need. However, such a cost-containment strategy creates new and added pressures on the quality assurance portion of the utilization review mechanism. The stakes, the risks at issue, are much higher when a prospective cost-containment review process is utilized than when a retrospective review process is used.

A mistaken conclusion about medical necessity following retrospective review will result in the wrongful withholding of payment. An erroneous decision in a prospective review process, on the other hand, in practical consequences, results in the withholding of necessary care, potentially leading to a patient's permanent disability or death.

II

Though somewhat in dispute, the facts in this case are not particularly complicated. [The court here embarks on a lengthy recitation of the facts, which can be summarized as follows. Mrs. Wickline was a woman in her mid-40s when she began having circulatory problems in her back and legs due to arteriosclerosis. After receiving prior approval from Medi-Cal (the California Medicaid agency) for a ten-day hospital admission, a vascular surgeon performed an operation to place a synthetic graft onto an artery in one of Mrs. Wickline's legs. Because of complications, two additional surgeries were necessary and her convalescence was delayed. Her physician requested an eight-day extension of her hospital stay. Based on the recommendation of the "on-site nurse" (a Medi-Cal employee who reviews such requests at the hospital), a Medi-Cal consultant (one of a number of physicians employed to make such decisions for the Los Angeles region) approved only a four-day extension. This decision was made on the basis of a phone conversation with the on-site nurse. Noting that her condition was not critical, the attending physicians reluctantly accepted this decision ("while still of the subjective, non-communicated, opinion that Wickline was seriously ill and that the danger to her was not over") and discharged the patient after the four-day extension. For the next few days the patient remained at home, and her condition deteriorated. Eventually, infection set in, she returned to the hospital on an emergency basis, and her right leg had to be amputated below the knee.]

III

From the facts thus presented, appellant takes the position that it was not negligent as a matter of law. Appellant contends that the decision to discharge was made by each of the plaintiff's three doctors, was based upon the prevailing standards of practice, and was justified by her condition at the time of her discharge. It argues that Medi-Cal had no part in the plaintiff's hospital discharge and therefore was not liable even if the decision to do so was erroneously made by her doctors.

Further, appellant raises the defense of the doctrine of discretionary immunity pursuant to Government Code section 820.2, and, finally, argues that the language of Government Code section 818.4 can reasonably be interpreted to apply to provide the State with absolute immunity in this matter.

IV

Civil Code section 1714, derived from the common law, reads in pertinent part as follows: "Every one is responsible, not only for the result of his willful acts, but also for an injury occasioned to another by his want of ordinary care or skill in the management of his property or person, except so far as the latter has, willfully or by want of ordinary care, brought the injury upon himself."

In *Rowland v. Christian* (1968), the court reexamined the negligence liability rules applicable in this state and came

to the conclusion that the principle embodied in this code section . . . serves as the foundation of our negligence law. Rephrased, it establishes the general rule that " 'All persons are required to use ordinary care to prevent others being injured as a result of their conduct.' " And, " 'in the absence of statutory provision declaring an exception to the fundamental principle enunciated by section 1714 of the Civil Code, no such exception should be made unless clearly supported by public policy.' "

The opinion then sets forth broad criteria for determining the applicability of both the principal rule and the exceptions: "A departure from this fundamental principle involves the balancing of a number of considerations; the major ones are the foreseeability of harm to the plaintiff, the degree of certainty that the plaintiff suffered injury, the closeness of the connection between the defendant's conduct and the injury suffered, the moral blame attached to the defendant's conduct, the policy of preventing future harm, the extent of the burden to the defendant and consequences to the community of imposing a duty to exercise care with resulting liability for breach, and the availability, cost, and prevalence of insurance for the risk involved."

Applying those standards to the facts in issue in this matter causes this court to conclude that appellant's contentions are well taken and that it is absolved from liability in this case as a matter of law.

Negligence is not absolute or to be measured in all cases in accordance with some precise standard, but always relates to some circumstance of time, place and person.

Dr. Kaufman, the chief Medi-Cal Consultant for the Los Angeles field office, was called to testify on behalf of the defendant. He testified that in January 1977, the criteria, or standard, which governed a Medi-Cal Consultant in acting on a request to consider an extension of time was founded on title 22 of the California Administrative Code. That standard was "the medical necessity" for the length and level of care requested. That, Dr. Kaufman contended, was determined by the Medi-Cal Consultant from the information provided him [on the case] form. The Medi-Cal Consultant's decision required the exercise of medical judgment and, in doing so, the Medi-Cal Consultant would utilize the skill, knowledge, training and experience he had acquired in the medical field.

Dr. Kaufman supported Dr. Glassman's [the Medi-Cal consultant's] decision. He testified, based upon his examination of the MC-180 form in issue in this matter, that Dr. Glassman's four-day hospital stay extension authorization was ample to meet the plaintiff's medically necessary needs at that point in time. Further, in Dr. Kaufman's opinion, there was no need for Dr. Glassman to seek information beyond that which was contained in Wickline's 180 form.

Dr. Kaufman testified that it was the practice in the Los Angeles Medi-Cal office for Medi-Cal Consultants not to review other information that might be available, such as [other forms], unless called by the patient's physician and requested to do so and, instead, to rely only on the information contained in the MC-180 form. Dr. Kaufman also stated that Medi-Cal Consultants did not initiate telephone calls to patient's [*sic*] treating doctors because of the volume of work they already had in meeting their prescribed responsibilities. Dr. Kaufman testified that any facts relating to the patient's care and treatment that was [*sic*] not shown on the 180 form was [*sic*] of no significance.

As to the principal issue before this court, i.e., who bears responsibility for allowing a patient to be discharged from the hospital, her treating physicians or the health care payor, each side's medical expert witnesses agreed that, in accordance with the standards of medical practice as it existed in January 1977, it was for the patient's treating physician to decide the course of treatment that was medically necessary to treat the ailment. It was also that physician's responsibility to determine whether or not acute care hospitalization was required and for how long. Finally, it was agreed that the patient's physician is in a better position than the Medi-Cal Consultant to determine the number of days medically necessary for any required hospital care. The decision to discharge is, therefore, the responsibility of the patient's own treating doctor.

Dr. Kaufman testified that if, on January 21, the date of the plaintiff's discharge from Van Nuys, any one of her three treating doctors had decided that in his medical judgment it was necessary to keep Wickline in the hospital for a longer period of time, they, or any of them, should have filed another request for extension of stay in the hospital, that Medi-Cal would expect those physicians to make such a request if they felt it was indicated, and upon receipt of such a request further consideration of an additional extension of hospital time would have been given.

Title 22 of the California Administrative Code, section 51110, provided, in pertinent part, at the relevant time in issue here, that: "The determination of need for acute care shall be made in accordance with the usual standards of medical practice in the community."

The patient who requires treatment and who is harmed when care which should have been provided is not provided should recover for the injuries suffered from all those responsible for the deprivation of such care, including, when appropriate, health care payors. Third party payors of health care services can be held legally accountable when medically inappropriate decisions result from defects in the design or implementation of cost-containment mechanisms as, for example, when appeals made on a patient's behalf for medical or hospital care are arbitrarily ignored or unreasonably disregarded or overridden. However, the physician who complies without protest with the limitations imposed by a third party payor, when his medical judgment dictates otherwise, cannot avoid his ultimate responsibility for his patient's care. He cannot point to the health care payor as the liability scape-

goat when the consequences of his own determinative medical decisions go sour.

There is little doubt that Dr. Polonsky [the vascular surgeon] was intimidated by the Medi-Cal program[,] but he was not paralyzed by Dr. Glassman's response nor rendered powerless to act appropriately if other action was required under the circumstances. If, in his medical judgment, it was in his patient's best interest that she remain in the acute care hospital setting for an additional four days beyond the extended time period originally authorized by Medi-Cal, Dr. Polonsky should have made some effort to keep Wickline there. He himself acknowledged that responsibility to his patient. It was his medical judgment, however, that Wickline could be discharged when she was. All the plaintiff's treating physicians concurred[,] and all the doctors who testified at trial, for either plaintiff or defendant, agreed that Dr. Polonsky's medical decision to discharge Wickline met the standard of care applicable at the time. Medi-Cal was not a party to that medical decision and therefore cannot be held to share in the harm resulting if such decision was negligently made.

In addition thereto, while Medi-Cal played a part in the scenario before us in that it was the resource for the funds to pay for the treatment sought, and its input regarding the nature and length of hospital care to be provided was of paramount importance, Medi-Cal did not override the medical judgment of Wickline's treating physicians at the time of her discharge. It was given no opportunity to do so. Therefore, there can be no viable cause of action against it for the consequences of that discharge decision.

The California Legislature's intent, in enacting the Medi-Cal Act, was to provide "mainstream" medical care to the indigent. The Legislature had expressly declared that Medi-Cal recipients should be able "whenever possible and feasible * * *, to the extent practical, * * * to secure health care in the same manner employed by the public generally, and without discrimination or segregation based purely on their economic disability."

Welfare and Institutions Code section 14132 provided, in pertinent part, as follows: "The following is the schedule of benefits under this chapter: [¶](b) In-patient hospital services, * * * are covered subject to utilization controls." Welfare and Institutions Code section 14133 provided, in pertinent part: "Utilization controls that may be applied to the services set forth in section 14132 which are subject to utilization controls shall be limited to: [¶](a) Prior authorization, which is approval by a department [of health] consultant, of a specified service in advance of the rendering of that service based upon a determination of medical necessity."

Title 22 of the California Administrative Code set forth the pertinent regulations applicable to the State's Medi-Cal program. Section 51327 thereof dealt with inpatient hospitalization for other than emergency services and stated, in pertinent part, as follows:

"(a)(2) Nonemergency hospitalization is covered only if prior authorization is obtained from the Medi-Cal Consultant before the hospital admission is effected. The Medi-Cal Consultant's authorization shall be for a specified number of days of hospital care. Continued necessary hospitalization beyond the specified number of days shall be covered after approval by the Medi-Cal Consultant has been obtained by the hospital on or before the last day of the previously approved period of hospitalization."

In the case before us, the Medi-Cal Consultant's decision, vis-a-vis the request to extend Wickline's hospital stay, was in accord with then existing statutory law.

V

This court appreciates that what is at issue here is the effect of cost-containment programs upon the professional judgment of physicians to prescribe hospital treatment for patients requiring the same. While we recognize, realistically, that cost consciousness has become a permanent feature of the health care system, it is essential that cost limitation programs not be permitted to corrupt medical judgment. We have concluded, from the facts in issue here, that in this case it did not.

For the reasons expressed herein, this court finds that appellant is not liable for respondent's injuries as a matter of law. That makes unnecessary any discussion of the other contentions of the parties.

The judgment is reversed

Discussion Questions

1. Critics of prospective review of hospital utilization predicted that the result of those activities would be patients discharged from hospitals "sicker and quicker," as in Mrs. Wickline's case. Clearly, without such a cost-containment mechanism in this case (and assuming ability to pay had not been an issue), Mrs. Wickline would have stayed in the hospital longer and probably would not have lost her leg. Yet the court in this case placed the responsibility on the treating physicians to make the discharge decision and to take the matter up again with the Medi-Cal officials. Do you agree with laying the responsibility on the physicians in this manner? Does this result make good public policy?

2. Why was this case brought against Medi-Cal and not the physicians or the hospital?

3. Under what circumstances might a third-party payer be liable for a medically inappropriate decision resulting from prospective utilization review?

4. Are there other means of reducing health care costs that would avoid the kinds of difficulties this case represents?

Payton v. Weaver
131 Cal. App. 3d 38, 182 Cal. Rptr. 225 (1982)

Grodin, J.

Occasionally a case will challenge the ability of the law, and society, to cope effectively and sensitively with fundamental problems of human existence. This is such a case. Appellant, Brenda Payton, is a 35-year-old black woman who suffers from a permanent and irreversible loss of kidney function, a condition known as chronic end stage renal disease. To stay alive, she must subject herself two or three times a week to hemodialysis (dialysis), a process in which the patient's circulatory system is connected to a machine through which the blood is passed. Using salts and osmotic membranes, artificial kidneys in the machine drain the blood of excess liquids and accumulated impurities. Without such treatment, the volume of liquids in the patient's system will increase dangerously; liquid will begin to fill the lungs, making breathing difficult and possibly leading to heart failure. The resulting toxic waste buildup and chemical imbalances can also threaten the function of the heart and other organs.

Brenda has other difficulties. Unable to care for her children, she lives alone in a low-income housing project in West Oakland, subsisting on a $356 per month Social Security check. She has no family support; one brother is in prison and another is a mental patient. She confesses that she is a drug addict, having been addicted to heroin and barbiturates for over 15 years. She has alcohol problems, weight problems and, not surprisingly, emotional problems as well.

Despite these difficulties Brenda appears from the record to be a marvelously sympathetic and articulate individual who in her lucid moments possesses a great sense of dignity and is intent upon preserving her independence and her integrity as a human being. At times, however, her behavior is such as to make extremely difficult the provision of medical care which she so desperately requires.

The other principal figure in this case is respondent John C. Weaver, Jr., a physician specializing in kidney problems. He conducts his practice through respondent Biomedical Application of Oakland, Inc. (BMA), which operates an outpatient dialysis treatment unit on the premises of respondent Providence Hospital.

Dr. Weaver began treating Brenda in 1975 when, after the birth of Brenda's twin daughters, her system rejected a transplanted kidney. He has been treating her ever since. To her, "Dr. Weaver is and was and still is the man between me and death * * * other than God, I don't think of nobody higher than I do Dr. Weaver."

On December 12, 1978, Dr. Weaver sent Brenda a letter stating he would no longer permit her to be treated at BMA because of her "persistent uncooperative and antisocial behavior over * * * more than * * * three years * * * her persistent refusal to adhere to reasonable constraints of hemodialysis, the dietary schedules and medical prescriptions * * * the use of barbiturates and other illicit drugs and because all this resulted in disruption of our program at BMA."

In the latter part of 1978, Brenda applied for admission to the regular dialysis treatment programs operated by respondents Alta Bates and Herrick Hospitals, and was refused.

For several months Dr. Weaver continued to provide Brenda with necessary dialysis on an emergency basis, through Providence. On April 23, 1979, he again notified her by letter that he would no longer treat her on an outpatient basis. This letter led to Brenda's filing of a petition for mandate to compel Dr. Weaver, BMA, and Providence to continue to provide her with outpatient dialysis services. That litigation was settled by a stipulated order which called for continued treatment provided Brenda met certain conditions: that she keep all appointments at their scheduled time; that she refrain from use of alcohol and drugs; that she maintain prescribed dietary habits; and that she "in all respects cooperate with those providing her care and abide by her physician's prescribed medical regimen." Later, a sixth stipulation was added: that Brenda would "enter into and participate in good faith in a program of regular psychotherapy and/or counselling."

Dr. Weaver and BMA continued treatment of Brenda as an outpatient pursuant to the stipulation, but on March 3, 1980, Dr. Weaver, contending that Brenda had failed to fulfill any part of the bargain, again notified her that treatment would be terminated. He provided her with a list of dialysis providers in San Francisco and the East Bay, and volunteered to work with her counsel to find alternative care.

Brenda then instituted a second proceeding, again in the form of a petition for writ of mandate, this time naming Herrick and Alta Bates Hospitals as respondents, along with Dr. Weaver, BMA and Providence. As pertinent here, the petition alleges that all respondents have "wrongfully failed and refused and continue to fail and refuse to provide Petitioner with regular hemodialysis treatment and medical supervision as required by her chronic end-stage kidney condition"; and, more specifically, that the refusal by Herrick and Alta Bates to admit her as an outpatient to their dialysis treatment programs violated their obligations under Health and Safety Code section 1317 to provide "emergency" treatment. The petition also contained allegations that Herrick and Alta Bates had discriminated against her on grounds of race and indigency, in violation of the Civil Rights Act of 1968 and the Hill-Burton Act, but the trial court found these allegations to be unsupported, and they are not at issue here.

The trial court, after a lengthy evidentiary hearing, found that Brenda had violated each and every condition which she had accepted as part of the stipulated order providing for continued treatment, and that finding is basically undisputed. There was evidence that Brenda continued, after the stipulated order, to buy barbiturates from pushers on the street at least twice a week; that she failed to restrict her diet, gaining as much as 15 kilograms between dialysis treatments; that she continued to be late and/or miss appointments; that due primarily to missed appointments she had 30 emergencies requiring hospitalization in the 11 months preceding trial; that she would appear for treatment in an intoxicated condition; that she discontinued her program of counseling after a brief period; and, as the trial court found, she displayed in general "gross non-cooperation with her treating physician, BMA of Oakland and Providence Hospital." The trial court found that her behavior in these respects was "knowing and intentional."

Brenda's behavior was found to affect not only Dr. Weaver but the other patients and the treating staff as well. Dialysis treatment is typically provided to several patients at a time, all of them connected to a single dialysis machine. There was evidence that Brenda would frequently appear for treatment late or at unscheduled times in a drugged or alcoholic condition, that she used profane and vulgar language, and that she had on occasion engaged in disruptive behavior, such as bothering other patients, cursing staff members with obscenities, screaming and demanding that the dialysis be turned off and that she be disconnected before her treatment was finished, [and] pulling the dialysis needle from the connecting shunt in her leg causing blood to spew, and exposing her genitals in a lewd manner. The trial court found that during the times she has sought treatment "her conduct has been disruptive, abusive, and unreasonable such as to trespass upon the rights of other patients and to endanger their rights to full and adequate treatment," and that her conduct "has been an imposition on the nursing staff." The court determined that, on balance, the rights and privileges of other patients endangered by Brenda's conduct were superior to the rights or equities which Brenda claimed.

The court also found, contrary to Brenda's contentions, that Dr. Weaver had given sufficient notice to Brenda, and that Dr. Weaver was not responsible for Brenda being refused dialysis by any other respondent. It concluded that Dr. Weaver had "discharged all obligations imposed by the patient-physician relationship" with Brenda.

As to Alta Bates and Herrick Hospitals the court found that they had not refused Brenda "emergency" treatment in violation of Health and Safety Code section 1317. In late 1978, after receiving notification from Dr. Weaver that he would no longer treat her, Brenda made application to the regular outpatient dialysis programs at these two hospitals and was refused—for reasons, as the trial court found, that did not include her race, her indigency, or any actions on the part of Dr. Weaver. It concluded, on the basis of reasoning which we shall discuss later in this opinion, that Brenda's chronic kidney disease did not itself constitute an "emergency" within the meaning of that section.

Finally, the trial court found that Brenda "has freedom of several choices available by which she can be kept away from dangerous drugs and alcohol, helped to stay on a proper dietary regimen, and in all other ways caused to cooperate with those attempting to provide her with care," so that she is "not without means to arrange for her own care." It concluded, after a weighing of the equities, that Brenda "has no legal right to compel medical service from any of the Respondents for chronic or regular care of her kidney problems through dialysis," and so denied her petition for writ of mandate. At the same time, however, the court stayed execution of its judgment and continued in effect its temporary order requiring Dr. Weaver, and BMA, to provide hemodialysis to Brenda on a regular basis pending appeal.

Discussion

We begin our analysis by considering the trial court's conclusion that Dr. Weaver and the clinic with which he is associated have no present legal obligation to continue providing Brenda with dialysis treatment. Brenda does not claim that Dr. Weaver has any such obligation on the basis of the stipulated order that was entered in the prior proceeding, nor could she reasonably do so. The trial court found that she was estopped from so claiming by her frequent violations of the conditions contained in that order, and that finding is amply supported by the evidence.

Rather, Brenda relies upon the general proposition that a physician who abandons a patient may do so "only * * * after due notice, and an ample opportunity afforded to secure the presence of other medical attendance."

The trial court found, however, that Dr. Weaver gave sufficient notice to Brenda, and discharged all his obligations in that regard, and that finding, also, is amply supported. Dr. Weaver supplied Brenda with a list of the names and telephone numbers of all dialysis providers in San Francisco and the East Bay, and it is apparent from the record that nothing would have pleased him more than to find an alternative facility for her, but there is no evidence that there is anything further he could have done to achieve that goal under the circumstances.

During the proceedings, the trial court observed that Dr. Weaver "is one of the most sensitive and honest physicians that I have been exposed to either in a courtroom or out of a courtroom," that he was "in fact sensitive to [Brenda's] needs, that he has attempted to assist her to the best of his medical abilities, that he continues to have concern for her as a person and has continued to serve her medical needs," and that "[the] man has the patience of Job." It appears that Dr. Weaver has behaved according to the highest standards of the medical profession, and that there exists no basis in law or in equity to saddle him with a continuing sole obligation for Brenda's welfare. The same is true of the clinic, the BMA.

We turn now to Brenda's contention that Herrick and Alta Bates Hospitals violated their obligations under Health and Safety Code section 1317, the text of which is set forth in the margin,[3] by denying her admission to their regular outpatient dialysis programs in late 1978. The trial court found that at the time Brenda applied for admission to these programs she was not in an "emergency condition," by which the court obviously meant that she was in no imminent physical danger on the day she applied. Brenda contends, however, that her illness is itself "a chronic/acute emergency which requires that she receive medical treatment every third day to avoid death," and that such a condition qualifies for mandated service under section 1317.

The trial court, in response to Brenda's contention, found that a patient with end stage renal disease "will not become a medical emergency if that person obeys medical orders, avoids drug abuse and appears for and has regularly scheduled hemodialysis treatments," and that regular outpatient dialysis treatment requires expertise and equipment not normally found in emergency rooms. It concluded that a chronic requirement for continued dialysis treatment does not constitute a need for "emergency" services or care within the meaning of section 1317. It declared, in that connection, that should Brenda present herself at any emergency department of any of the respondent health care providers claiming a need for emergency care, "a determination shall be made at that time by qualified physicians to see whether her condition constitutes an emergency" and, if so, she would be entitled to medical services under section 1317. Since that was not the situation at the time of Brenda's application to the two hospitals, the court found no liability.

We agree with the trial court's conclusion. While end stage renal disease is an extremely serious and dangerous disease, which can create imminent danger of loss of life if not properly treated, the need for continuous treatment as such cannot reasonably be said to fall within the scope of section 1317. There are any number of diseases or conditions which could be fatal to the patient if not treated on a continuing basis. If a patient suffering from such a disease or condition were to appear in the emergency room of a hospital in need of immediate life-saving treatment, section 1317 would presumably require that such treatment be provided. But it is unlikely that the Legislature intended to impose upon whatever health care facility such a patient chooses the unqualified obligation to provide continuing preventive care for the patient's lifetime.

It does not necessarily follow that a hospital, or other health care facility, is without obligation to patients in need of continuing medical services for their survival. While it has

---

3. Health and Safety Code section 1317 provides in pertinent part: "Emergency services and care shall be provided to any person requesting such services or care, or for whom such services or care is requested, for any condition in which the person is in danger of loss of life, or serious injury or illness, at any health facility licensed under this chapter that maintains and operates an emergency department to provide emergency services to the public when such health facility has appropriate facilities and qualified personnel available to provide such services or care."

been said that "[a] private hospital owes the public no duty to accept any patient not desired by it, and it is not necessary to assign any reason for its refusal to accept a patient for hospital service", it is questionable whether a hospital which receives public funding under the Hill-Burton Act, and perhaps from other sources, can reasonably be said to be "private" in that sense. Rather, where such a hospital contains a unique, or scarce, medical resource needed to preserve life, it is arguably in the nature of a "public service enterprise," and should not be permitted to withhold its services arbitrarily, or without reasonable cause. And, while disruptive conduct on the part of a patient may constitute good cause for an individual hospital to refuse continued treatment, since it would be unfair to impose serious inconvenience upon a hospital simply because such a patient selected it, it may be that there exists a collective responsibility on the part of the providers of scarce health resources in a community, enforceable through equity, to share the burden of difficult patients over time, through an appropriately devised contingency plan.

Whatever the merits of such an approach might be in a different factual context, however—and we recognize that it poses difficult problems of administration and of relationship between hospitals and physicians—it cannot serve as a basis for imposition of responsibility upon these respondents under the circumstances present here. Apart from the fact that the record does not demonstrate to what extent respondent hospitals are the sole providers of dialysis treatment in the area accessible to Brenda, her present behavior, as found by the trial court, is of such a nature as to justify their refusal of dialysis treatment on either an individual or collective basis. Whatever collective responsibility may exist, it is clearly not absolute, or independent of the patient's own responsibility.

What we have said to this point is analytically sufficient to dispose of Brenda's legal arguments, and thus to sustain the trial court's ruling, but the circumstances are such that we cannot responsibly avoid confronting the more fundamental question posed by Brenda's challenge, and considered at some length by the parties in their briefs and at oral argument, namely: what alternatives exist for assuring that Brenda does not die from lack of treatment as a result of her uncooperative and disruptive behavior?

One possibility which has been considered is an involuntary conservatorship under the Lanterman-Petris-Short (LPS) Act. Such a conservatorship is appropriate in the case of persons "gravely disabled as a result of mental disorder or impairment by chronic alcoholism". The County of Alameda has apparently determined, however, that the conditions of that statute cannot be met in Brenda's case.

A second possibility is an involuntary conservatorship under the provisions of Probate Code section 1801 et seq.

Under section 1801, subdivision (a), "[a] conservator * * * may be appointed for a person who is unable properly to provide for his or her personal needs for physical health, food, clothing, or shelter." Such a conservator "may consent to medical treatment to be performed upon the conservatee, and may require the conservatee to receive such medical treatment, in any case which the conservator determines in good faith based upon medical advice that the case is an emergency case in which the medical treatment is required * * * ." This possibility remains a viable alternative.

A third possibility, and the one which appears from recent developments to be the most promising, is a voluntary conservatorship under Probate Code section 1802. While Brenda has heretofore resisted consenting to such a conservatorship, her attorneys advise us in a postargument declaration that they are willing to use their influence to persuade Brenda to consent and that they believe they can arrange for her placement in a private, closed psychiatric facility. They suggest that we remand the matter to the superior court for the institution of appropriate proceedings. Respondents also appear to consider a voluntary conservatorship the best approach.

We have no authority to "remand" for the institution of a voluntary conservatorship, as Brenda's attorneys suggest. The trial court's order requiring Dr. Weaver to provide dialysis treatment to Brenda pending appeal will, however, remain in effect until our decision becomes final. If, during that period, Brenda institutes proceedings for a voluntary conservatorship, and a conservator is appointed, it will be that person's obligation to arrange for continued treatment under statutory authority, and subject to such conditions as the court may impose.

The judgment is affirmed.

Discussion Questions

1. What is a *writ of mandate*, and what does it do?

2. What are your feelings about the plaintiff? About the physician? Was a reasonable effort made to treat Ms. Payton fairly? Should someone be required to continue to treat her? If so, who?

3. Was Ms. Payton's condition an emergency to your mind? If not, what factors persuade you that it was not an emergency? What if Ms. Payton simply shows up at a different emergency room every three to four days in immediate need of dialysis? Would that constitute an emergency each time she did so? These kinds of questions will be considered further in the next chapter.

9

Emergency Care

There is generally no duty to come to another person's aid, even if a danger is obvious, immediate, and easily avoided. Thus, it was sometimes said that "no one has a duty to keep the blind man from walking off a cliff." In fact, under the common law, one who voluntarily came to another's aid and in doing so caused an injury could be held liable if the rescue was held to have been accomplished negligently. Thus, physicians were afraid to render aid at the scene of an accident, and hospitals were reluctant to treat all who appeared at their doors.

For these reasons, as was seen in Chapter 8 and such cases as *Hill v. Ohio County*, there is generally no legal right to be admitted to a hospital. "That is," according to Southwick, "as a general rule the hospital has no common law or statutory duty to admit or even serve all who apply for accommodation or service, except in a medical emergency."

On the other hand, he continues, "It is perfectly evident that the American public expects service from the nation's hospitals and their medical staffs"; therefore the current trend is to find reasons to impose on hospitals a duty at least to stabilize patients who present to an emergency room with conditions requiring immediate medical treatment. Various state and federal statutes as well as some judicial decisions have imposed this duty to provide emergency care.

The following cases exemplify the courts' handling of these situations.

Thompson v. Sun City Community Hosp., Inc.
141 Ariz. 597, 688 P.2d 605 (1984)

Feldman, J.

. . . .

Michael Jessee, plaintiff's son, was injured on the evening of September 4, 1976. Jesse was 13 years old at the

time of this accident. He was rushed by ambulance from the place of the accident . . . to the Boswell Memorial Hospital operated by Sun City Community Hospital, Inc. (Boswell) in Sun City. Among Jessee's injuries was a transected femoral artery. The injury was high in the left thigh and interrupted the flow of blood to the distal portion of the leg. Upon arrival at the emergency room at 8:22 p.m., Jessee was examined and initially treated by Dr. Steven Lipsky, the emergency room physician. Fluids were administered and blood was ordered. The leg injury prompted Dr. Lipsky to summon Dr. Alivina Sabanas, an orthopedic surgeon. She examined Jessee's leg and determined that he needed surgery. Dr. Jon Hillegas, a vascular surgeon, was consulted by phone.

At some time after 9:30 p.m. Jessee's condition "stabilized" and the decision was made to transfer him to County Hospital. There is no clear indication in the record of *who* ordered the transfer. Dr. Lipsky determined that Jessee was "medically transferable" but stated that "Michael Jessee was transferred for economic reasons after we found him to be medically transferable." Dr. Lipsky had no authority to admit patients to Boswell. Dr. Sabanas, who did have such authority and who knew that Jessee needed vascular surgery, claimed that Jessee was transferable from an orthopedic standpoint. Dr. Hillegas told Dr. Lipsky that Jessee could be transferred when "stabilized." A witness for the plaintiff testified that "The doctor at Boswell [apparently Dr. Lipsky] said [to Jessee's mother], 'I have the shitty detail of telling you that Mike will be transferred to County * * * .' " A Boswell administrator testified that emergency "charity" patients are transferred from Boswell to County whenever a physician, in his professional judgment, determines that "a transfer could occur."

Thus at 10:13 Jessee was discharged from the Boswell emergency room, placed in an ambulance, and taken to County. The doctors who attended to him at County began administering fluids and ordered blood. They testified that

Jessee's condition worsened but that he was eventually "stabilized" and taken to surgery at about 1:00 a.m. Jessee underwent abdominal surgery and, immediately thereafter, surgery to repair his torn femoral artery. He survived but has residual impairment of his left leg. His mother . . . brought a malpractice action against Boswell and the physicians.

. . . In any case such as this there are two types of causation questions. The first, relating to the question of breach of duty, pertains to the cause for the transfer to another hospital. Was the patient transferred for medical or other reasons? The second question relates to the cause of injury and is concerned with whether the transfer, with its attendant movement and delay, caused a new or additional injury or aggravated any injury which already existed. The first question was answered by defense counsel in chambers, prior to any testimony being taken in the case:

We admit and stipulate that the plaintiff in this case was transferred from Boswell to County Hospital for financial reasons. There is no question about it.

. . . .

In this state, the duty which a hospital owes a patient in need of emergency care is determined by the statutes and regulations interpreted by this court in *Guerrero v. Copper Queen Hospital*. Construing the statutory and regulatory scheme governing health care and the licensing of hospitals as of 1972, we held [in the *Guerrero* case] that it was the "public policy of this state" that a general "hospital may not deny emergency care to any patient without cause."

. . . .

[In addition to the *Guerrero* rationale, t]he emergency services section of the JCAH states that:

no patient should arbitrarily be transferred if the hospital where he was initially seen has means for adequate care of his problem.

The "Patient Rights" section of the JCAH manual makes it clear that the financial resources of a patient are among the "arbitrary" considerations within the contemplation of the above language:

no person should be denied impartial access to treatment or accommodations that are available and *medically indicated*, on the basis of such considerations as * * * the nature of the source of payment for his care.

. . . .

The [applicable] statute [requiring hospitals to provide facilities for emergency care and requiring the County to pay for emergency treatment of indigents] was in effect in 1975 when we decided *Guerrero* and is still in effect. It provides the answer to a serious problem. Charging hospitals with a legal duty to render emergency care to indigent patients does not ignore the distinctions between private and public hospitals. Imposition of a duty to render emergency care to indigents simply charges private hospitals with the same duty as public hospitals under a statutory plan which permits reimbursement from public funds for the emergency care charges incurred at the private hospital.

This legislative and regulatory history provides no reason to retreat from or modify *Guerrero*. We therefore affirm its holding that, as a matter of public policy, licensed hospitals in this state are required to accept and render emergency care to all patients who present themselves in need of such care. The patient may not be transferred until all medically indicated emergency care has been completed. This standard of care has, in effect, been set by statute and regulation embodying a public policy which requires private hospitals to provide emergency care that is "medically indicated" without consideration of the economic circumstances of the patient in need of such care. Thus, the word "cause" used in the quoted portion of *Guerrero* refers to something other than economic considerations. Interpreting the standard of care in accordance with the public policy defined in *Guerrero*, we hold that reasonable "cause" for transfer before completion of emergency care refers to medical considerations relevant to the welfare of the patient and not economic considerations relevant to the welfare of the hospital. . . .

. . . .

. . . The undisputed evidence established that the patient was transferred for financial reasons while emergency care was medically indicated. As a matter of law this was a breach of the hospital's duty. Thus, the only question before the jury on the issue of the hospital's liability was whether its breach of duty was a cause of some compensable damage.

[The case concludes with a complicated discussion of the question of the causation of damage. The issue turns on the fact that the delay in Jess[e]e's eventual surgery might or might not have made a difference in his eventual degree of disability and that no one can say for sure what the outcome would have been in either event. Expert opinion was that even if Jess[e]e had been admitted at Boswell and surgery had been promptly performed, there was still only a 5 to 10 percent chance that he would have completely recovered. On the other hand, it was agreed that the chance of recovery was better without the delay than with it, and it is the chance of recovery itself that the law should protect.

Arizona tort law had previously required the plaintiff to prove that the defendant's conduct had aggravated the original injury. Jess[e]e wanted that rule changed so that he could prevail even if all he could prove was that the defendant's acts or omissions had "increased the risk of harm." The opinion summarizes the court's holding on this point as follows.]

We . . . adopt the rule of [the] *Restatement (Second) of Torts* . . . [:]

One who undertakes, * * *, to render services to another which he should recognize as necessary for the protection of the other's person or things, is *subject to liability* to the other for physical harm resulting from his failure to exercise reasonable care to perform his undertaking, if (a) his failure to exercise such care increases the risk of such harm, * * * . [Emphasis added by the court.]

. . . That defendant is "subject to liability" means that the issue of causation may go to the jury upon proof of increase in the risk of harm. The jury is left to decide the issue of probability.

. . . .

The judgments in favor of defendants Hillegas and Lipsky are affirmed. The judgment in favor of Boswell is reversed and the case remanded for further proceedings. . . .

Discussion Questions

1. From a medical standpoint, how serious was Jessee's injury? Was it reasonable to transfer him before surgery? Do you have enough information to make a judgment about such questions?

2. In your opinion, does this case establish good public policy? Whose responsibility is it to establish public policy?

3. What would have been the result, from a public policy standpoint, if the case had turned out the other way?

4. If Arizona statutes required counties to reimburse private hospitals for emergency care rendered to indigents, why would Boswell transfer Jessee to County? What difference would it make to Boswell since they would get paid anyway?

5. What kind of reasonable cause for the transfer of a patient can you contemplate?

6. What do you suppose happened when the case against the hospital went back to the trial court?

7. Why were the judgments in favor of Dr. Hillegas and Dr. Lipsky affirmed?

Gragg v. Neurological Assocs.
152 Ga. App. 586, 263 S.E.2d 496 (1979)

Smith, J.

Appellants, Mr. and Mrs. C. A. Gragg, brought this malpractice action for damages allegedly occurring when an angiogram was performed upon Mr. Gragg. We agree with appellants' contention that the trial court erred in concluding the Good Samaritan Statute to be applicable, and we therefore reverse the court's grant of summary judgment to appellee, Dr. William Spenser.

[According to the opinion, Mr. Gragg was undergoing an angiogram when his physician, Dr. Peter Reitt (who had performed hundreds of angiograms previously), "encountered difficulty in . . . maneuver[ing] the catheter from the left to the right carotid artery." This difficulty happens occasionally and is not felt to be due to negligence. Dr. Reitt then called Dr. Spenser, a specialist who was present in the hospital, to assist, and the procedure was completed "with a little difficulty." Fifteen minutes later, Mr. Gragg suffered a stroke that resulted in "permanent total paralysis of the left arm and hip and with permanent partial loss of the use of the left arm and hand."]

Solely on the basis of the Good Samaritan Statute the trial court granted summary judgment to appellee Spenser. That statute provides: "Any person, including those licensed to practice medicine and surgery pursuant to the provisions of this Chapter, and including any person licensed to render service ancillary thereto, who in good faith renders emergency care at the scene of an accident or emergency to the victim or victims thereof without making any charge therefor, shall not be liable for any civil damages as a result of any act or omission by such person in rendering the emergency care or as a result of any act or failure to act to provide or arrange for further medical treatment or care for the injured person." We believe the Good Samaritan Statute is inapplicable to the factual situation before us. [Paragraph break added by the editor.]

Here Mr. Gragg was receiving the care of a qualified, experienced physician, Dr. Reitt, before Dr. Spenser's arrival in surgery. Dr. Reitt had performed the angiogram on three hundred occasions prior to this one and was aware of the possibility that the difficulty which he encountered could occur. The deposition testimony also showed that the discontinuance of the angiogram would not itself have placed Gragg's health in any immediate danger and that Dr. Reitt was fully capable of proceeding on alone in face of the complication and would have chosen to do so, had Dr. Spenser not been available. We hold that, as a matter of law, the hardship encountered here during the process of a diagnostic procedure being conducted by an experienced physician did not constitute such an accident or emergency as would invoke the provisions of the Good Samaritan Statute.

Judgment reversed.

Discussion Questions

1. Virtually all states have enacted Good Samaritan laws similar to Georgia's to protect physicians and other health care personnel who render medical assistance at the scene of an emergency. (Some protect all Good Samaritans, whether medical professionals or not.) What do you suppose was the motivation for such statutes? How effective do you think they have been in achieving their purpose, and in how many cases do you think they have protected a defendant?

2. How much does location matter in determining whether the Good Samaritan statute should apply? What if a hospital visitor has a coronary in the lobby while waiting for an elevator? Or on the sidewalk between the parking garage and the main entrance? Or a heart patient has a coronary in the waiting room of the outpatient clinic?

3. What if there is a slip-and-fall injury outside the hospital? Does it matter, with regard to the Good Samaritan statute, whether the location is a public sidewalk or one maintained by the hospital? What if there is an automobile accident on the public street in front of the hospital, or a block away, or away from a hospital but in front of a physician's office?

4. Is the presence of a woman in labor an emergency for purposes of the Good Samaritan statute? (Cf. *Hill v. Ohio County.*)

Fjerstad v. Knutson
271 N.W.2d 8 (S.D. 1978)

Porter, J. (on reassignment)

CASE SUMMARY

This is an action by the special administrator of the estate of Dezso Csoka for his wrongful death, allegedly caused by negligent medical services rendered to decedent by defendants. The trial court rendered judgment, based on a jury verdict, for defendants. On appeal plaintiff contends: (1) The trial court erred in instructing the jury that it could not find defendant Sioux Valley Hospital liable unless it found defendant Knutson liable . . . .

We conclude that the separate liability of Sioux Valley Hospital was not properly presented to the jury, and we therefore reverse and remand for a new trial against Sioux Valley Hospital. We affirm that part of the judgment which found defendant Knutson not liable.

FACTS

Decedent Dezso Csoka and his family went on vacation in late June, 1973, and were returning to their home near Chicago when they arrived in Rapid City on July 2. Decedent felt ill on his arrival, but did not seek medical attention because he wanted to return to Chicago and see his own doctor. On July 4 the Csoka family traveled across South Dakota, with decedent driving the entire distance. Decedent's condition had deteriorated upon their arrival in Sioux Falls. He and his family rented a motel room and then went to the emergency room at Sioux Valley Hospital.

Decedent arrived at the hospital at 6:22 p.m. He was seen by intern John Knutson at 8:30. Knutson was the only intern on duty and there were no licensed physicians present. July 4 was Knutson's second day as an intern. Knutson examined decedent and ordered a blood test and throat culture. He then gave decedent a prescription for an antibiotic, erythromycin, and released him. Knutson did not use mirrors or a laryngoscope, even though these instruments were available to him. Use of such instruments would have allowed him to see beyond the soft palate to the epiglottis, tonsils, and trachea.

It was the policy of the hospital not to release emergency room patients until the on-call physician or the patient's local doctor had been contacted. Interns were to initiate a course of treatment only in emergencies, and they were not to prescribe drugs without consulting a licensed physician. Knutson attempted to contact the on-call physician for consultation in decedent's case, but was unable to do so for three and one-half to four hours. The hospital was responsible for assigning on-call physicians and assuring that they would be available when they were on call.

After Knutson released him, decedent returned to his motel. He took at least two of the antibiotic pills as directed by Knutson. When decedent's wife and children awoke the next morning, they found him dead. The autopsy indicated that death was caused by asphyxia resulting when his larnyx, tonsils, and epiglottis swelled, and the trachea was blocked.

. . . .

We conclude that the separate liability of Sioux Valley Hospital was not properly submitted to the jury.

. . . .

Under proper instructions, the jury could have found that Sioux Valley Hospital was negligent even if Knutson was not. Although it has been held that a hospital, even one operating an emergency room, has no duty to accept a patient for treatment, once it undertakes to render medical aid, the hospital is required to do so non-negligently. The duty arose in this case, since the hospital undertook, through its nurses and intern, to render treatment to decedent. Decedent had a right to expect that the treatment rendered by a hospital which maintains and staffs an emergency room would be commensurate with that available in the same or similar communities or in hospitals generally.

On this record, however, we find it unnecessary to evaluate the evidence in light of one of these standards, since the evidence of the hospital's breach of its own standards is sufficient to create a jury issue. The medical director of laboratories at the hospital, Dr. John Barlow, testified that the emergency room on-call doctor is to be available for consultation and that he is assigned that duty by the hospital. Dr. Richard Friess, director of the hospital's medical education, program, testified that interns could see the patients, but that the on-call physician, according to hospital policy, had to be contacted before treatment in all but serious emergencies. It is uncontroverted that the emergency room doctor was not available for consultation, and that Knutson rendered treatment without such consultation.

The failure to have an emergency room doctor available and failing to consult with him violated the hospital's own standard for treatment. This failure was attributable to the hospital in several ways independent of any negligence by Knutson. The jury could have believed, from the above evidence, that the hospital failed to properly assign an emergency room on-call physician, or that Knutson was not properly trained by the hospital to consult with a physician before releasing an emergency room patient. In addition, the actions of the on-call doctor in not being available for call to the emergency room are attributable to the hospital. In his capacity as on-call physician, he was acting on behalf of the hospital, and emergency patients could properly assume that the hospital would be responsible for the actions of its on-call physician.

Defendants insist that failure to have the on-call physician available was not the cause of decedent's death. Several expert defense witnesses so testified. There was, however, testimony from Dr. John Gregg that proper diagnostic procedures would have revealed the seriousness of decedent's condition. Dr. Gregg also testified that someone with decedent's symptoms should have been hospitalized, and that proper hospitalization would probably have saved decedent's life. The jury thus could have believed that an experienced physician would have taken the necessary steps to save decedent's life.

We must next consider whether the instructions as given were prejudicial to plaintiff. The verdict cannot be set aside if the instructions, considered as a whole, give a full and correct statement of the law applicable to the case. We conclude that instruction five, however, gave "undue emphasis to [a] phase of the case favorable to [one] side," and thus constituted reversible error. The instruction stated, without any limitation, that the jury could not find against the hospital if it found for Dr. Knutson. Although later instructions seem to refer to the hospital's separate liability, they do not eliminate the error of instruction five. This is particularly the case where the trial court refused to instruct the jury to consider the instructions as a whole. We therefore conclude that a new trial is required on the issue of the hospital's separate liability.

. . . .

Discussion Questions

1. Why has this court determined that the hospital could be separately liable for the death of the patient?

2. What is the effect of the hospital's rules and standards on its own liability?

3. Why do you suppose Dr. Knutson was found not liable?

4. How would you formulate a statement of the hospital's duty to patients such as Mr. Csoka?

Owens v. Nacogdoches County Hosp. Dist.
741 F. Supp. 1269 (E.D. Tex. 1990)

Justice, J.

On August 3, 1987, Rebecca Owens, a sixteen year old indigent resident of Nacogdoches County whose pregnancy was full term, began to experience labor pains. She went to the emergency room at Memorial Hospital in Nacogdoches at approximately 3:00 p.m. After initial processing, she was taken to the Labor and Delivery room, where she was examined by Dr. Bruce Thompson, who was under contract with Memorial Hospital to provide obstetric and gynecological care to indigent pregnant women. After approximately one-half hour, Dr. Thompson discharged Ms. Owens with instructions that she go to John Sealy Hospital in Galveston, Texas—a facility approximately two hundred miles and four hours driving time away—to deliver her baby. On the night of August 3, this court, upon the petition of Rebecca Owen's mother and next friend Betty Owens, issued a temporary restraining order enjoining Memorial Hospital from refusing to admit Rebecca Owens for the purpose of delivering her baby. On August 7, 1987, four days after the issuance of the temporary restraining order, Rebecca Owens was admitted to Memorial Hospital, where Dr. Bruce Thompson delivered her baby. Plaintiff has brought suit against the hospital and its board of directors in their official capacities, seeking damages, and declaratory and injunctive relief pursuant to 42 U.S.C. § 1395dd, the Emergency Medical Treatment and Active Labor Act, which forms part of the Consolidated Omnibus Budget Reconciliation Act of 1986 (COBRA).

It is clear beyond peradventure first, that no attempt was made by defendant hospital to comply with the transfer requirements of § 1395dd; second, that the sole reason for the instruction to Rebecca Owens to go to John Sealy Hospital was that she was without funds; third, that this action constituted "dumping," the very evil which § 1395dd was designed to prevent; fourth, that this incident was not an isolated one, but part of a pattern of dumpings of indigent patients that continued virtually until the time of trial in this civil action—a pattern caused by the unwillingness of defendant hospital to take the steps requisite for adequate performance of its statutory responsibilities for the care of indigent patients under both federal and state law; and finally, that what occurred to Rebecca Owens is capable of repetition, yet might evade review. Accordingly, judgment in this civil action will be entered for plaintiff, damages and attorney's fees in accordance with the stipulation of the parties will be awarded to her, and defendant hospital will be permanently enjoined from refusing her delivery in any future pregnancy in violation of 42 U.S.C. § 1395dd.

I. Background—42 U.S.C. § 1395dd

The Emergency Medical Treatment and Active Labor Act, sometimes referred to as the Anti-Dumping Act, was enacted by Congress as part of the Consolidated Omnibus Budget Reconciliation Act of 1986 (COBRA), and codified at 42 U.S.C. § 1395dd. The Act was a response to a national epidemic of "dumping," the practice by hospitals of refusing emergency care to indigent patients outright or of transferring such patients, without regard to the necessity for stabilizing their condition, to other—typically public—hospitals.

. . . .

To address these problems, 42 U.S.C. § 1395dd requires that any hospital with an emergency room must provide a medical screening examination to any patient who appears complaining of an emergency medical condition. It further provides that such patients cannot be transferred to another facility in an unstable condition, and requires that such a transfer be "appropriate." The guidelines for an appropriate transfer are that the physician certify in writing that the benefits of such transfer outweigh the risk, that the transferring hospital provide the medical treatment necessary to minimize the risk to the health of the patient (which includes, in the case of a woman in labor, the health of the child as well as the mother), that the transferring hospital send the relevant records in its possession with the patient, that the transferring hospital obtain the assurance of the receiving hospital that the receiving hospital has space and facilities for the patient and has accepted the transfer, and that the transfer "is effected through qualified personnel and transportation equipment, as required including the use of necessary and medically appropriate life support measures."

In order to make clear what the responsibilities of the physician and the transferring hospital are, the act includes definitional sections which establish what is meant by an "emergency medical condition" and "active labor." For the purpose of this civil action, the relevant section is 42 U.S.C. § 1395dd(e)(2), and particularly 42 U.S.C. § 1395dd(e)(2)(C):

(2)   The term "active labor" means labor at a time at which—

(A)   delivery is imminent,

(B)   there is inadequate time to effect safe transfer to another hospital prior to delivery, or

(C)   a transfer may pose a threat to the health or safety of the patient or the unborn child.

The definitional section of the act clearly establishes the basis for judging the acts of the physician and hospital. That is, the physician cannot, by a mere assertion that in his judgment neither an emergency medical situation nor active labor exists, evade or negate the plain intent of the statute. To hold otherwise would render the statutory scheme merely precatory, which, as the above citation of the history of the act makes clear, is not what Congress intended.

The act provides for a variety of sanctions to enforce its provisions, including termination or suspension of the defendant hospital's medicare [*sic*] provider agreement, civil monetary penalties, and the establishment of causes of action for both patients who are dumped and hospitals which receive dumped patients. . . .

. . . .

III. Transfer Requirements Under 42 U.S.C. § 1395dd

Defendants urge that Rebecca Owens was not "transferred" within the meaning of 42 U.S.C. § 1395dd. At first glance, this argument conflicts with the statutory language. The definitional section of the Anti-Dumping Act defines "transfer" as follows:

(5) The term "transfer" means the movement (including the discharge) of a patient outside a hospital's facilities at the direction of any person employed by (or affiliated or associated, directly or indirectly with) the hospital, but does not include such a movement of a patient who (A) has been declared dead, or (B) leaves the facility without the permission of any such person.

The contractual affiliation of Dr. Bruce Thompson and Memorial Hospital is uncontested. Dr. Thompson admits that he directed Rebecca Owens to go to Galveston, and the records so indicate. Rebecca Owens is not dead, and did not leave Memorial Hospital without permission on the night of August 3, 1987. That the order to go to Galveston constituted a transfer appears plain.

Defendants, however, appear to be of a different view. They contend that because Rebecca Owens was a M.I.H.I.A. [Maternal and Infant Health Improvement Act] patient, and because the University of Texas-Medical Branch at John Sealy Hospital in Galveston had, as Memorial Hospital did not, a contract to provide delivery services under M.I.H.I.A., Rebecca Owens was a patient of John Sealy Hospital; hence, they argue that the direction to go to John Sealy cannot be a transfer.

. . . .

Contrary to defendants' assertions, however, Rebecca Owens was not a patient of John Sealy Hospital on August 3, 1987. She had not presented herself for admission to John Sealy Hospital. She had come to Nacogdoches Memorial Hospital. She was obviously Memorial's patient, and defendants' artful quibbling on this point avails them nothing. The definition of "transfer" unquestionably encompasses the direction to proceed to Galveston.

. . . .

Given that the order to go to Galveston was a transfer order, it is apparent that it violated all the standards set down for a transfer in the act, as the narrative of events has already noted. Dr. Thompson was, by his own admission, aware of the procedural and substantive requirements for a transfer, though uncertain that those were legal requirements. He knew he was supposed to call the receiving hospital to get permission for the transfer. He knew he was supposed to make copies of the relevant records. He did, as a matter of routine, write a memorandum outlining the benefits versus the risks of a transfer. Yet he drafted no such transfer memorandum in the case of Rebecca Owens. Nor does the record reflect that he took any other action which was required by 42 U.S.C. § 1395dd.

As to the requirement of providing adequate transportation for the transfer, it is uncontroverted that no transport was provided. At best, the defendants rely on a document which asserts that according to Rebecca Owens, she had a car. Even were one willing to accept the assertions of this document, a 1976 Ford Pinto with no medical equipment, whose only other occupant besides the patient is her boyfriend, is not the equivalent of an ambulance for the purposes of the Anti-Dumping Act.

IV. Reasons for the Transfer

Defendants offer two arguments as reasons for the transfer of Rebecca Owens on August 3, 1987. First, they argue that Rebecca Owens announced that it was her intent to go to John Sealy Hospital when she came to Memorial. Second, they argue that it was preferable for Rebecca Owens, because she was a M.I.H.I.A. patient, to deliver at John Sealy Hospital since it is a Level-III hospital with a neonatal unit. Neither of these arguments is availing.

Rebecca Owens, in both her direct and her cross-examination, repeatedly and strenuously denied having told anyone at Memorial Hospital that she was on her way to Galveston. Nor, despite the assertions of defense counsel, is her testimony inconsistent with the previous deposition testimony. Moreover, her testimony is entirely consistent with her actions . . . .

. . . .

Given the relative credibility of the witnesses and the inferences that may be drawn from the behavior of Rebecca Owens on August 3, 1987, the court finds that as a matter of fact, Rebecca Owens expressed no intent to go to Galveston, Texas to deliver her child, but rather requested that she be delivered at Memorial Hospital.

Defendants' other principal argument is that the decision to send Rebecca Owens to Galveston was justified in light of the fact that the facilities of John Sealy Hospital, particularly the neonatal unit, were more appropriate for Rebecca Owen's delivery than those of Memorial Hospital. According to the testimony of Dr. Bruce Thompson, it was

for this reason that he felt the benefits of sending Rebecca Owens to Galveston outweighed the risks of sending her.

. . . .

In this case, the risks of the transportation were severe. According to the testimony of all the medical witnesses, including Dr. Thompson, there was a risk that, had the baby been born on the side of the road, both mother and child might have died. The transfer was wholly without supervision; so far as can be determined, nobody in the 1976 Pinto knew the faintest thing [about delivering babies]. Had the child been born in the car, and had the cord been wrapped around its neck on August 3, as it was on August 7, Christopher Dempsey might well have strangled at birth.

There is no reason to recite yet again the dangers which all the physicians agreed would have attended a birth somewhere on the two hundred miles of highway between Nacogdoches and Galveston. They are all a matter of record. Not even Dr. Thompson, when pressed, denies that they exist. It is found that, as a matter of fact, the transfer by private car of plaintiff Rebecca Owens from Nacogdoches to Galveston while she was undergoing labor pains on the night of August 3, 1987, did pose significant and wholly unnecessary risks to both Rebecca Owens and her unborn child.

Moreover, it is transparent that the sole reason for the illegal transfer was Rebecca Owens's indigency. Dr. Thompson repeatedly admitted that, had Rebecca Owens not been a M.I.H.I.A. patient, she would not have been sent to Galveston. . . .

. . . It is found, as a matter of fact, that the reason for the transfer was that Rebecca Owens was without funds. The flimsiness of the pretense that there was any reason other than her poverty to send the plaintiff to Galveston is apparent.

Further, since under substantive Texas personal injury law, which governs pursuant to 42 U.S.C. § 1395dd, proof of physical injury is not a prerequisite for recovery for negligent infliction of mental anguish, and since it has already been found that the decision to transfer her to Galveston caused Rebecca Owens severe mental anguish, it is found that the violation of the Anti-Dumping Act by Memorial Hospital through its agents Dr. Bruce Thompson caused Rebecca Owens personal injury within the meaning of the statute.

Pursuant to the joint stipulation of the parties regarding damages entered into on the morning trial commenced, the court assesses against Memorial Hospital the sum of $25,000.00 in damages and the sum of $25,000.00 in attorneys' fees.

V. Declaratory and Injunctive Relief

By its terms, the Anti-Dumping Act provides not only for damages for personal injury, but also for "such equitable relief as is appropriate." Accordingly, plaintiff Rebecca Owens has moved for injunctive relief as well as declaratory relief . . . .

Defendants demur, arguing that the relief sought is based upon speculation, and that there is no "real or immediate threat" of future injury by the defendants. The defendants argue that, since Rebecca Owens is not now pregnant, she has no standing to maintain her claims and there is no justiciable controversy in this regard.

Defendants' argument is unavailing. As plaintiff correctly points out, the appropriate standard here is whether the complained of acts are capable of repetition, yet may evade review. Given that the wrongs sought to be addressed by the Anti-Dumping Act are precisely not continuing but episodic, since that is the nature of emergency medical conditions and of childbirth, it simply does not make sense to assert that Rebecca Owens ceased to have standing for equitable relief when she gave birth. To so hold would render the inclusion of equitable relief in the statute mere surplusage. In any event, defendants are wrong as a matter of fact regarding the claim that plaintiff has not shown a real and immediate threat of future injury. Plaintiff's evidence demonstrates a long-standing pattern of patient dumping, caused by staffing policies that in the opinion of a series of medical experts would inevitably lead to standards of care at Memorial Hospital that patently did not meet state or federal statutory requirements. Bluntly stated, Memorial Hospital has callously and negligently allowed a situation to develop in which all emergency obstetric and gynecological services to indigent patients—an enormous and ever-increasing load—have been left to on-call private physicians like Dr. Thompson, and the dumping of pregnant women has been the inevitable result.

Plaintiff's counsel introduced testimony from Vera Brown, Lacreta Mergerson, Wanda Saxton, and Werdner Simmons which indicated a long-standing pattern of dumping from 1984 on; that testimony was essentially unrefuted by Memorial Hospital. The rebuttal testimony of Elaine Salisbury, who first became aware of this civil action during the course of its trial, indicated that this practice continued through 1989. There was no serious contest as to the credibility of these witnesses, and their statements are accepted as true. It is found, as a fact, that for at least five years, Memorial Hospital has flagrantly been engaged in patient dumping.

The evidence given by plaintiff's expert Dr. F. Barry Roberts, who practiced for nine and one-half years at Memorial Hospital, that Memorial has been continuously obstructionist whenever physicians attempted to bring the problem of indigent health care to the attention of the Board, is also found credible. The weight of the evidence—especially considering the fact that when this civil action came on for trial, a private practitioner was the only OB-GYN delivering poor babies at Memorial—convincingly establishes a disturbing pattern of negligent behavior on the part of the administrators of Memorial Hospital which has inevitably led to the pattern of patient dumping.

In the light of this pattern of either negligent or deliberate flouting by Memorial Hospital of its obligations under the Anti-Dumping Act, plaintiff Rebecca Owens has amply demonstrated that she has standing, and that there is a real threat of injury to her. The complained of acts are capable of repetition, and indeed have been repeated. Plaintiff is awarded permanent injunctive relief to prevent these egregious acts from evading review in the future.

VI. Conclusion

The purpose of the Anti-Dumping Act is to end the national scandal, as Senator Durenberger described it, of "rejecting indigent patients in life threatening situations for economic reasons alone[.]"

By terms of the Anti-Dumping Act, hospitals with emergency facilities cannot deny those facilities to the poor. They cannot shrug their shoulders and send children in rickety cars on four-hour drives, simply because they do not make the same money for treating such children as they do for paying customers. They may not wantonly turn their backs on the indigent.

Discussion Questions

1. The plaintiff was awarded $25,000 in damages and an additional $25,000 in attorney fees; what good will it do her also to have "permanent injunctive relief to prevent these egregious acts from evading review in the future"?

2. What actual damages did the plaintiff suffer to justify an award of $25,000?

3. The statute defines "emergency medical condition." By your interpretation, did Rebecca Owens meet the criteria of emergency medical condition to fall within the anti-dumping statute? Note: The full text of the statute is reproduced on pages 98–100.

Jones v. Wake County Hosp. Sys., Inc.
786 F. Supp. 538 (E.D. N.C. 1991)

Vastine Jones, Administratrix of the estate of Philip Jones, brings this action pursuant to the Federal Examination and Treatment for Emergency Medical Conditions and Women in Labor Act, part of the Consolidated Omnibus Budget Reconciliation Act, 42 U.S.C. § 1395dd . . . . Wake Medical Center, Gregory Solovieff, M.D. and Kevin Nolan, M.D. are named as defendants. As relief, she seeks compensatory damages, punitive damages, attorneys' fees, and injunctive relief. . . .

On or about September 6, 1988, at approximately 5:30 p.m., plaintiff's intestate, Philip Jones, was admitted to the emergency room of Wake Medical Center complaining of pain and weakness stemming from bodily burns received on September 4, 1988. He was examined by defendant Solovieff, an emergency room physician on duty that day. Jones' vital signs were checked, blood work was performed, and a dressing was applied. Defendant Solovieff, apparently concerned about the possibility of an infection, consulted defendant Nolan, another physician on duty in the emergency room. After consultation, they decided that further treatment was not necessary and discharged Jones at approximately 10:30 p.m. that same night. Within hours of his discharge, Jones began complaining of severe pain, paralysis, and a sense of disorientation. Plaintiff took Jones back to Wake Medical Center at approximately 5:30 p.m. on September 7, 1988. Shortly afterward, Jones suffered septic shock, respiratory arrest, and renal failure. He died at approximately 2:15 a.m. on September 8, 1988 from cardiac arrest. Plaintiff alleges that Jones was suffering from a potentially fatal systemic infection known as sepsis at the time of his visit to the emergency room on September 6 and that if defendants had exercised reasonable care and performed additional tests on Jones instead of discharging him, Jones' condition could have been diagnosed and treated.

Plaintiff filed her original complaint on September 5, 1990, which charged simply that the treatment of Jones violated COBRA. The original complaint did not include any allegations that plaintiff's treatment at the hospital was due to indigency, lack of medical insurance, or race.

However, on April 19, 1991, just as these motions became ripe for adjudication by this court, plaintiff was granted leave to file an amended complaint. Her amended complaint rehashed the allegations in her original complaint but included the additional allegations that Jones had received unfavorable treatment by the defendants because of his race and socioeconomic status.

By an order filed on May 28, 1991, this court denied defendant's motion to dismiss the original complaint as moot. Defendants then filed motions to dismiss the amended complaint on the same grounds as in their previous motions. Additionally, defendants motioned to strike those allegations in plaintiff's amended complaint pertaining to racism, arguing that plaintiff inserted these charges merely as a last minute attempt to survive the motion to dismiss.

COBRA was enacted by Congress primarily in response to concerns about the practice of "patient dumping", the refusal of a hospital emergency room to treat a person who does not have medical insurance. . . .

COBRA authorizes a private cause of action for any individual who suffers personal harm from the violation of the statute against the violating hospital. In addition, civil monetary penalties may be levied against the hospital and the responsible physicians.

. . . .

The few courts that have interpreted COBRA have split as to the scope of the act. The legislative history of the statute is predominated by concern over "patient dumping". This has led several courts to hold that COBRA applies only to instances where a plaintiff can show he was refused treatment due to indigency. However, the fact that the plain language of the statute does not limit COBRA to only situations where patients are denied treatment for economic reasons has led other courts to rule that no such showing is necessary. The Sixth Circuit has adopted a middle approach, holding . . . that for COBRA to apply, plaintiff must allege that the hospital failed to give him appropriate emergency treatment based on some impermissible motive such as indigency, dislike of the patient, or distaste for the patient's physical condition.

After careful consideration of the wisdom of these various approaches, the court concludes that COBRA does not apply strictly to acts of patient dumping by hospitals for economic reasons. The analyses engaged in by the Sixth Circuit and the District of Columbia Circuit are instructive. While the legislative history makes it abundantly clear that patient dumping was the primary evil Congress sought to curtail by its enactment of COBRA, it is no less true that the statute Congress wrote and enacted does not in any way restrict its application to such instances. Instead, COBRA plainly states that it applies to "any individual" who requests emergency room treatment. While defendants argue that this type of broad interpretation of COBRA would go beyond what Congress intended, the United States Supreme Court has stated that a "law need not be in every respect logically consistent with its aims to be constitutional. It is enough that there is an evil at hand for correction, and that it might be thought that the particular legislative measure was a rational way to correct it."

As a matter of statutory construction, federal courts are not free to rewrite statutes simply because Congress could have acted with greater clarity. Given the fact that Congressmen vote on the actual language of a bill, courts must be cautious in going beyond the plain words of the statute in an attempt to be true to the legislative intent. It is true that courts should not interpret laws in a way that would lead to unreasonable or absurd results. However, given Congress' stated concern over individuals being denied emergency treatment by hospitals, the broad interpretation given COBRA in *Cleland* and *Gatewood* cannot be labeled unreasonable or absurd. Had Congress desired to enact a more restrictive statute, presumably it would have done so. . . .

[The text of the antidumping statute is reproduced on pages 98–100. The court proceeds to analyze whether the plaintiff had stated a claim for relief under the statute.

First, the court considers the term "appropriate medical screening" in § 1395dd(a). In this case the hospital applied its customary screening procedures, but they turned out to result in an erroneous diagnosis. The court held that the term "is not designed to redress an incorrect diagnosis; instead it is merely an entitlement to receive the same treatment that is accorded to others similarly situated. Since plaintiff alleged that Mr. Jones was not given the same examination that would be given to other patients, she is entitled to present proof on whether the hospital did violate § 1935dd(a).

Second, because plaintiff did not allege that the defendants had determined that an "emergency medical condition" existed under § 1395dd(b), the allegation that they failed to stabilize his condition did not state a valid cause of action.

Third, the court holds that § 1395dd(d) does not provide for a private cause of action against individual physicians; therefore, the claims against the defendant physicians are dismissed.

Fourth, the court finds that § 1395dd(d)(2)(A)'s provision for injunctive relief covers the plaintiff's request for a permanent injunction. Thus Mrs. Jones is entitled to pre-sent evidence tending to show a pattern of deliberate violations of the act by the defendant hospital.

Fifth, the court upholds the constitutionality of the antidumping statute, holding that it is not unconstitutionally vague.

Finally, the court finds it premature to hold, as defendants requested, that punitive damages would be inappropriate. The matter was left for the trial court to decide.]

Discussion Questions

1. Based on *Owens* and *Jones*, do you believe the courts are appropriately applying the federal antidumping statute?

2. At the end of this excerpt, the court explains what it believes are some principles for judicial interpretation of congressional enactments. For example, it quotes with favor a Supreme Court opinion that stated, "a law need not be in every respect logically consistent with its aims to be constitutional." In addition, this court argues that its own "broad interpretation" of the antidumping law is reasonable because "[h]ad Congress desired to enact a more restrictive statute, presumably it would have done so." Are these reasonable interpretations or just another example of judge-made law?

Note

The full text of 42 U.S.C. § 1395dd is as follows:

§ 1395dd. Examination and treatment for emergency medical conditions and women in labor

(a) Medical screening requirement. In the case of a hospital that has a hospital emergency department, if any individual (whether or not eligible for benefits under this title [42 USCS §§ 1395 et seq.]) comes to the emergency department and a request is made on the individual's behalf for examination or treatment for a medical condition, the hospital must provide for an appropriate medical screening examination within the capability of the hospital's emergency department, including ancillary services routinely available to the emergency department, to determine whether or not an emergency medical condition (within the meaning of subsection (e)(1)) exists.

(b) Necessary stabilizing treatment for emergency medical conditions and labor. (1) In general. If any individual (whether or not eligible for benefits under this title [42 USCS §§ 1395 et seq.]) comes to a hospital and the hospital determines that the individual has an emergency medical condition, the hospital must provide either—

(A) within the staff and facilities available at the hospital, for such further medical examination and such treatment as may be required to stabilize the medical condition, or

(B) for transfer of the individual to another medical facility in accordance with subsection (c).

(2) Refusal to consent to treatment. A hospital is deemed to meet the requirement of paragraph (1)(A) with respect to an individual if the hospital offers the individual the further medical examination and treatment described in that paragraph and informs the individual (or a person acting on the individual's behalf) of the risks and benefits to the individual of such examination and treatment, but the individual (or a person acting on the individual's behalf) refuses to consent to the examination and treatment. The hospital shall take all reasonable steps to secure the individual's (or person's) written informed consent to refuse such examination and treatment.

(3) Refusal to consent to transfer. A hospital is deemed to meet the requirement of paragraph (1) with respect to an individual if the hospital offers to transfer the individual to another medical facility in accordance with subsection (c) and informs the individual (or a person acting on the individual's behalf) of the risks and benefits to the individual of such transfer, but the individual (or a person acting on the individual's behalf) refuses to consent to the transfer. The hospital shall take all reasonable steps to secure the individual's (or person's) written informed consent to refuse such transfer.

(c) Restricting transfers until individual stabilized. (1) Rule. If an individual at a hospital has an emergency medical condition which has not been stabilized (within the meaning of subsection (e)(3)(B)), the hospital may not transfer the individual unless—

(A)(i) the individual (or a legally responsible person acting on the individual's behalf) after being informed of the hospital's obligations under this section and of the risk of transfer, in writing requests transfer to another medical facility,

(ii) a physician (within the meaning of section 1861(r)(1) [42 USCS § 1395x(r)(1)]) has signed a certification that, based upon the information available at the time of transfer, the medical benefits reasonably expected from the provision of appropriate medical treatment at another medical facility outweigh the increased risks to the individual and, in the case of labor, to the unborn child from effecting the transfer, or

(iii) if a physician is not physically present in the emergency department at the time an individual is transferred, a qualified medical person (as defined by the Secretary in regulations) has signed a certification described in clause (ii) after a physician (as defined in section 1861(r)(1) [42 USCS § 1395x(r)(1)]), in consultation with the person, has made the determination described in such clause, and subsequently countersigns the certification; and

(B) the transfer is an appropriate transfer (within the meaning of paragraph (2)) to that facility.

A certification described in clause (ii) or (iii) of subparagraph (A) shall include a summary of the risks and benefits upon which the certification is based.

(2) Appropriate transfer. An appropriate transfer to a medical facility is a transfer—

(A) in which the transferring hospital provides the medical treatment within its capacity which minimizes the risks to the individual's health and, in the case of a woman in labor, the health of the unborn child;

(B) in which the receiving facility—

(i) has available space and qualified personnel for the treatment of the individual, and

(ii) has agreed to accept transfer of the individual and to provide appropriate medical treatment;

(C) in which the transferring hospital sends to the receiving facility with all medical records (or copies thereof), related to the emergency condition for which the individual has presented, available at the time of the transfer, including records related to the individual's emergency medical condition, observations of signs or symptoms, preliminary diagnosis, treatment provided, results of any tests and the informed written consent or certification (or copy thereof) provided under paragraph (1)(A), and the name and address of any on-call physician (described in subsection (d)(1)(C)) who has refused or failed to appear within a reasonable time to provide necessary stabilizing treatment;

(D) in which the transfer is effected through qualified personnel and transportation equipment, as required including the use of necessary and medically appropriate life support measures during the transfer; and

(E) which meets such other requirements as the Secretary may find necessary in the interest of the health and safety of individuals transferred.

(d) **Enforcement.** (1) Civil monetary penalties. (A) A participating hospital that negligently violates a requirement of this section is subject to a civil money penalty of not more than $50,000 (or not more than $25,000 in the case of a hospital with less than 100 beds) for each such violation. The provisions of section 1128A [42 USCS § 1320a-7a] (other than subsections (a) and (b)) shall apply to a civil money penalty under this subparagraph in the same manner as such provisions apply with respect to a penalty or proceeding under section 1128A(a) [42 USCS § 1320a-7a(a)].

(B) Subject to subparagraph (C), any physician who is responsible for the examination, treatment, or transfer of an individual in a participating hospital, including a physician on-call for the care of such an individual, and who negligently violates a requirement of this section, including a physician who—

(i) signs a certification under subsection (c)(1)(A) that the medical benefits reasonably to be expected from a transfer to another facility outweigh the risks associated with the transfer, if the physician knew or should have known that the benefits did not outweigh the risks, or

(ii) misrepresents an individual's condition or other information, including a hospital's obligations under this section,

is subject to a civil money penalty of not more than $50,000 for each such violation and, if the violation is gross and flagrant or is repeated, to exclusion from participation in this title and State health care programs. The provisions of section 1128A [42 USCS § 1320a-7a] (other than the first and second sentences of subsection (a) and subsection (b)) shall apply to a civil money penalty and exclusion under this subparagraph in the same manner as such provisions apply with respect to a penalty, exclusion, or proceeding under section 1128A(a) [42 USCS § 1320a-7a(a)].

(C) If, after an initial examination, a physician determines that the individual requires the services of a physician listed by the hospital on its list of on-call physicians (required to be maintained under section 1866(a)(1)(I) [42 USCS § 1395cc(a)(1)(I)]) and notifies the on-call physician and the on-call physician fails or refuses to appear within a reasonable period of time, and the physician orders the transfer of the individual because the physician determines that without the services of the on-call physician the benefits of transfer outweigh the risks of transfer, the physician authorizing the transfer shall not be subject to a penalty under subparagraph (B). However, the previous sentence shall not apply to the hospital or to the on-call physician who failed or refused to appear.

(2) Civil enforcement. (A) Personal harm. Any individual who suffers personal harm as a direct result of a participating hospital's violation of a requirement of this section may, in a civil action against the participating hospital, obtain those damages available for personal injury under the law of the State in which the hospital is located, and such equitable relief as is appropriate.

(B) Financial loss to other medical facility. Any medical facility that suffers a financial loss as a direct result of a participating hospital's violation of a requirement of this section may, in a civil action against the participating hospital, obtain those damages available for financial loss, under the law of the State in which the hospital is located, and such equitable relief as is appropriate.

(C) Limitations on actions. No action may be brought under this paragraph more than two years after the date of the violation with respect to which the action is brought.

(3) Consultation with peer review organizations. In considering allegations of violations of the requirements of this section in imposing sanctions under paragraph (1), the Secretary shall request the appropriate utilization and quality control peer review organization (with a contract under part B of title XI [42 USCS §§ 1320c et seq.]) to assess whether the individual involved had an emergency medical condition which had not been stabilized, and provide a report on its findings. Except in the case in which a delay would jeopardize the health or safety of individuals, the Secretary shall request such a review before effecting a sanction under paragraph (1) and shall provide a period of at least 60 days for such review.

(e) **Definitions.** In this section:

(1) The term "emergency medical condition" means—

(A) a medical condition manifesting itself by acute symptoms of sufficient severity (including severe pain) such that the absence of immediate medical attention could reasonably be expected to result in—

(i) placing the health of the individual (or, with respect to a pregnant woman, the health of the woman or her unborn child) in serious jeopardy,

(ii) serious impairment to bodily functions, or

(iii) serious dysfunction of any bodily organ or part; or

(B) with respect to a pregnant woman who is having contractions—

(i) that there is inadequate time to effect a safe transfer to another hospital before delivery, or

(ii) that transfer may pose a threat to the health or safety of the woman or the unborn child.

(2) The term "participating hospital" means hospital that has entered into a provider agreement under section 1866 [42 USCS § 1395cc].

(3)(A) The term "to stabilize" means, with respect to an emergency medical condition described in paragraph (1)(A), to provide such medical treatment of the condition as may be necessary to assure, within reasonable medical probability, that no material deterioration of the condition is likely to result from or occur during the transfer of the individual from a facility, or, with respect to an emergency medical condition described in paragraph (1)(B), to deliver (including the placenta).

(B) The term "stabilized" means, with respect to an emergency medical condition described in paragraph (1)(A), that no material deterioration of the condition is likely, within reasonable medical probability, to result from or occur during the transfer of the individual from a facility, or, with respect to an emergency medical condition described in paragraph (1)(B), that the woman has delivered (including the placenta).

(4) The term "transfer" means the movement (including the discharge) of an individual outside a hospital's facilities at the direction of any person employed by (or affiliated or associated, directly or indirectly, with) the hospital, but does not include such a movement of an individual who (A) has been declared dead, or (B) leaves the facility without the permission of any such person.

(5) [Redesignated]

(6) The term "hospital" includes a rural primary care hospital (as defined in section 1861(mm)(1) [42 USCS § 1395x (mm)(1)]).

(f) Preemption. The provisions of this section do not preempt any State or local law requirement, except to the extent that the requirement directly conflicts with a requirement of this section.

(g) Nondiscrimination. A participating hospital that has specialized capabilities or facilities (such as burn units, shock-trauma units, neonatal intensive care units, or (with respect to rural areas) regional referral centers as identified by the Secretary in regulation) shall not refuse to accept an appropriate transfer of an individual who requires such specialized capabilities or facilities if the hospital has the capacity to treat the individual.

(h) No delay in examination or treatment. A participating hospital may not delay provision of an appropriate medical screening examination required under subsection (a) or further medical examination and treatment required under subsection (b) in order to inquire about the individual's method of payment or insurance status.

(i) Whistleblower protections. A participating hospital may not penalize or take adverse action against a qualified medical person described in subsection (c)(1)(A)(iii) or a physician because the person or physician refuses to authorize the transfer of an individual with an emergency medical condition that has not been stabilized or against any hospital employee because the employee reports a violation of a requirement of this section.

10

Consent for Treatment and the Withholding of Consent

The United States is enthralled with the concept of individual rights: free speech; a fair trial; privacy; freedom of religion; free assembly; due process of law; cruel and unusual punishments; protection against unreasonable searches and seizures; the right to bear arms; pro-choice on abortion; pro-life of the unborn fetus; nondiscrimination on the basis of race, color, creed, national origin, gender, or sexual orientation; death with dignity—all these and many more public policy issues are commonly argued (especially in the political arena) with "rights" language: "I/we have a *right* to/not to _____."

Rights language has a strong popular appeal: it harkens back to the American Revolution, the glory days of history books when heroes like Washington, Jefferson, and Madison founded this country on the "self-evident" truths of "certain unalienable rights." And rights language has a practical advantage: convince someone that what you want is a *right*, and you have won the argument. This is because rights language is absolute; it is not concerned with such niceties as cost, practicality, the common good, or the reasonableness of others' viewpoints.

But therein lies the problem with rights language: precisely because it is absolute, it is harder to deal with; because it applies sledgehammer force to every concept, it can do violence to the more fragile issues.

The first amendment says "Congress shall make *no law* respecting an establishment of religion, or prohibiting the free exersise thereof; or abridging the freedom of speech; or of the press . . . " (italics added.) Some scholars, including the late, respected Supreme Court Justice Hugo Black, argue that "no law" means exactly that: *absolutely no law* of any kind limiting freedom of religion and freedom of expression in

this country. The Court has not taken this literal a reading of the amendment, but it is not hard to imagine the difficulty involved in deciding important, delicate issues in the face of the absolute language of the Constitution.

For example, given that "Congress shall make no law" on certain topics, could Congress pass any of these kinds of statutes:

- A law prohibiting a religious sect from practicing polygamy if it is a deeply held tenet of their beliefs?
- A law prohibiting Native Americans from using peyote in religious ceremonies?
- A law punishing newspaper reporters for disclosing classified information during war time?
- A law banning the burning of the U.S. flag as a form of political speech and protest?
- A law providing criminal or civil penalties for speech that incites a riot?
- A law allowing public officials to sue newspapers for libel because of critical editorials?
- A law prohibiting pornography?
- A law allowing civil penalties against one who falsely shouts "fire" in a crowded theater thereby causing injury?

The complexities of these issues are apparent on even the most superficial consideration. How difficult it is to address their delicate nuances in light of the apparently absolute standard of the first amendment!

Before proceeding, a brief pause to underscore the following point: the above is not intended as a criticism of the

First Amendment; it is merely meant to illustrate the difficulty of dealing with issues in terms of "rights language."

Having said that, we note that the subject of this chapter is strongly affected with rights language. As Southwick points out, with certain exceptions, "it is a fundamental principle that the consent of the patient, or of someone authorized to act for a legally incompetent patient, must be obtained before any medical or surgical treatment is undertaken . . . ." Justice Cardozo made the classic statement supporting this principle in 1914 in *Schloendorff v. Society of New York Hospital*, 211 N.Y. 125, 105 N.E. 92 (1914):

Every human being of adult years and sound mind has a right to determine what shall be done with his own body; and a surgeon who performs an operation without his patient's consent commits an assault for which he is liable in damages. This is true except in cases of emergency, where the patient is unconscious and where it is necessary to operate before consent can be obtained.

Even though this principle was asserted nearly eight decades ago, it was not until the late 1960s that decisions regarding the need to obtain the patient's informed consent began to receive intense judicial scrutiny. Interestingly, and perhaps not coincidentally, it was at this same time that the right of access to health care and other rights when receiving treatment also began receiving a high level of judicial and legislative attention.

Implicit in the right to consent to medical treatment is the right to refuse to consent. Thus, in the absence of extraordinary circumstances a competent person may refuse medical care even if the likely result of that refusal is the person's own death. (See, for example, *Shorter v. Drury*, excerpted in Chapter 3 of this book.) The right to refuse treatment is not absolute, as Southwick points out (see p. 377), but the exceptions are limited, and their application has been so narrowed by recent case law that they seldom apply. This right to refuse treatment, then, is the foundation for the so-called right to die, a concept interwoven with moral and religious beliefs, constitutional due process principles, and assertions of a right of privacy.

Although the legal maxim that one can refuse life-saving treatment is the natural extension of the law of battery, it has been extremely difficult for many health care providers (and others) to accept. The refusal of care seems contrary to one's natural instincts. It certainly runs counter to the basic purpose of the medical profession. In addition, a paternalistic attitude pervaded the physician community until recent years, and informed consent and the right to refuse to consent challenged the traditional notion, "doctor knows best."

The first case in this section contains classic and fundamental discussions of the issues surrounding consent and informed consent and has formed the basis for much of the related litigation of the past two decades. For these reasons, it is set forth at considerable length. The other selections address related issues, including the difficult medical-ethical issues

surrounding the right to refuse treatment, both by competent and incompetent individuals; the termination of life-sustaining treatment, and conflicting rights of the mother and her unborn child. In so doing we may shed some light on the professional, practical and emotional aspects of these difficult decisions.

Cobbs v. Grant
8 Cal. 3d 229, 502 P.2d 1, 104 Cal. Rptr. 505 (1972)

Mosk, J.

This medical malpractice case involves two issues: first, whether there was sufficient evidence of negligence in the performing of surgery to sustain a jury verdict for plaintiff; second, whether, under plaintiff's alternative theory, the instructions to the jury adequately set forth the nature of a medical doctor's duty to obtain the informed consent of a patient before undertaking treatment. We conclude there was insufficient evidence to support the jury's verdict under the theory that the defendant was negligent during the operation. Since there was a general verdict and we are unable to ascertain upon which of the two concepts the jury relied, we must reverse the judgment and remand for a new trial. To assist the trial court upon remand we analyze the doctor's duty to obtain the patient's informed consent and suggest principles for guidance in drafting new instructions on this question.

Plaintiff was admitted to the hospital in August 1964 for treatment of a duodenal ulcer. He was given a series of tests to ascertain the severity of his condition and, though administered medication to ease his discomfort, he continued to complain of lower abdominal pain and nausea. His family physician, Dr. Jerome Sands, concluding that surgery was indicated, discussed prospective surgery with plaintiff and advised him in general terms of the risks of undergoing a general anesthetic. Dr. Sands called in defendant, Dr. Dudley F. P. Grant, a surgeon, who after examining plaintiff, agreed with Dr. Sands that plaintiff had an intractable peptic duodenal ulcer and that surgery was indicated. Although Dr. Grant explained the nature of the operation to plaintiff, he did not discuss any of the inherent risks of the surgery.

A two-hour operation was performed the next day, in the course of which the presence of a small ulcer was confirmed. Following the surgery the ulcer disappeared. Plaintiff's recovery appeared to be uneventful, and he was permitted to go home eight days later. However, the day after he returned home, plaintiff began to experience intense pain in his abdomen. He immediately called Dr. Sands who advised him to return to the hospital. Two hours after his readmission plaintiff went into shock and emergency surgery was performed. It was discovered plaintiff was bleeding internally as a result of a severed artery at the hilum of his spleen. Because of the seriousness of the hemorrhaging and since the spleen of an adult may be removed without adverse effects, defendant decided to remove the spleen. Injuries to the spleen that compel a subsequent operation are a risk inherent in the type of surgery performed on plaintiff and occur in approximately 5 percent of such operations.

After removal of his spleen, plaintiff recuperated for two weeks in the hospital. A month after discharge he was readmitted because of sharp pains in his stomach. X-rays disclosed plaintiff was developing a gastric ulcer. The evolution of a new ulcer is another risk inherent in surgery performed to relieve a duodenal ulcer. Dr. Sands initially decided to attempt to treat this nascent gastric ulcer with antacids and a strict diet. However, some four months later plaintiff was again hospitalized when the gastric ulcer continued to deteriorate and he experienced severe pain. When plaintiff began to vomit blood the defendant and Dr. Sands concluded that a third operation was indicated: a gastrectomy with removal of 50 percent of plaintiff's stomach to reduce its acid-producing capacity. Some time after the surgery, plaintiff was discharged, but subsequently had to be hospitalized yet again when he began to bleed internally due to the premature absorption of a suture, another inherent risk of surgery. After plaintiff was hospitalized, the bleeding began to abate and a week later he was finally discharged.

Plaintiff brought this malpractice suit against his surgeon, Dr. Grant. The action was consolidated for trial with a similar action against the hospital. The jury returned a general verdict against the hospital in the amount of $45,000. This judgment has been satisfied. The jury also returned a general verdict against defendant Grant in the amount of $23,800. He appeals.

The jury could have found for plaintiff either by determining that defendant negligently performed the operation, or on the theory that defendant's failure to disclose the inherent risks of the initial surgery vitiated plaintiff's consent to operate. Defendant attacks both possible grounds of the verdict. He contends, first, [that] there was insufficient evidence to sustain a verdict of negligence, and, second, [that] the [trial] court committed prejudicial error in its instruction to the jury on the issue of informed consent.

I

[The appellate court agrees with the defendant's first argument (i.e., that the evidence did not justify a verdict of negligence). Because of the general verdict, the court could not determine on which basis the jury found for the plaintiff. Accordingly, the court reverses the judgment and orders a retrial.]

II

Since the question of informed consent is likely to arise on retrial, we address ourselves to that issue. In giving its instruction the trial court relied upon . . . a case in which it was held that if the defendant failed to make a sufficient disclosure of the risks inherent in the operation, he was guilty of a "technical battery." While a battery instruction may have been warranted under the facts alleged in [that case], in the case before us the instruction should have been framed in terms of negligence.

Where a doctor obtains consent of the patient to perform one type of treatment and subsequently performs a substantially different treatment for which consent was not obtained, there is a clear case of battery. . . .

However, when an undisclosed potential complication results, the occurrence of which was not an integral part of the treatment procedure but merely a known risk, the courts are divided on the issue of whether this should be deemed to be a battery or negligence. . . .

Dean Prosser surveyed the decisions in this area and concluded, "The earliest cases treated this as a matter of vitiating the consent, so that there was liability for battery. Beginning with a decision in Kansas in 1960 [*Natanson v. Kline*], it began to be recognized that this was really a matter of the standard of professional conduct * * * . [T]he prevailing view now is that the action * * * is in reality one for negligence in failing to conform to the proper standard * * * ."

Although this is a close question, either prong of which is supportable by authority, the trend appears to be towards categorizing failure to obtain informed consent as negligence. That this result now appears with growing frequency is of more than academic interest; it reflects an appreciation of the several significant consequences of favoring negligence over a battery theory. As will be discussed *infra*, most jurisdictions have permitted a doctor in an informed consent action to interpose a defense that the disclosure he omitted to make was not required within his medical community. However, expert opinion as to community standard is not required in a battery count, in which the patient must merely prove failure to give informed consent and a mere touching absent consent. Moreover a doctor could be held liable for punitive damages under a battery count, and if held liable for the intentional tort of battery he might not be covered by his malpractice insurance. Additionally, in some jurisdictions the patient has a longer statute of limitations if he sues in negligence.

We agree with the majority trend. The battery theory should be reserved for those circumstances when a doctor performs an operation to which the patient has not consented. When the patient gives permission to perform one type of treatment and the doctor performs another, the requisite element of deliberate intent to deviate from the consent given is present. However, when the patient consents to certain treatment and the doctor performs that treatment but an undisclosed inherent complication with a low probability occurs, no intentional deviation from the consent given appears; rather, the doctor in obtaining consent may have failed to meet his due care duty to disclose pertinent information. In that situation the action should be pleaded in negligence.

The facts of this case constitute a classic illustration of an action that sounds in negligence. Defendant performed the identical operation to which plaintiff had consented. The spleen injury, development of the gastric ulcer, gastrectomy and internal bleeding as a result of the premature absorption of a suture, were all links in a chain of low probability events inherent in the initial operation.

III

Since this is an appropriate case for the application of a negligence theory, it remains for us to determine [whether] the standard of care described in the jury instruction on this subject properly delineates defendant's duty to inform plaintiff of the inherent risks of the surgery. In pertinent part, the court gave the following instruction: "A physician's duty to disclose is not governed by the standard practice in the community; rather it is a duty imposed by law. A physician violates his duty to his patient and subjects himself to liability if he withholds any facts which are necessary to form the basis of an intelligent consent by the patient to the proposed treatment."

Defendant raises two objections to the foregoing instruction. First, he points out that the majority of the California cases have measured the duty to disclose not in terms of an absolute, but as a duty to reveal such information as would be disclosed by a doctor in good standing within the medical community. . . . One commentator has imperiously declared that "good medical practice is good law." Moreover, with one state and one federal exception every jurisdiction that has considered this question has adopted the community standard as the applicable test. Defendant's second contention is that this near unanimity reflects strong policy reasons for vesting in the medical community the unquestioned discretion to determine [whether] the withholding of information by a doctor from his patient is justified at the time the patient weighs the risks of the treatment against the risks of refusing treatment.

The thesis that medical doctors are invested with discretion to withhold information from their patients has been frequently ventilated in both legal and medical literature. . . . Despite what defendant characterizes as the prevailing rule, it has never been unequivocally adopted by an authoritative source. Therefore we probe anew into the rationale which purportedly justifies, in accordance with medical rather than legal standards, the withholding of information from a patient.

Preliminarily we employ several postulates. The first is that patients are generally persons unlearned in the medical sciences and therefore, except in rare cases, courts may safely assume the knowledge of patient and physician are not in parity. The second is that a person of adult years and in sound mind has the right, in the exercise of control over his own body, to determine whether or not to submit to lawful medical treatment. The third is that the patient's consent to treatment, to be effective, must be an informed consent. And the fourth is that the patient, being unlearned in medical sci-

ences, has an abject dependence upon and trust in his physician for the information upon which he relies during the decisional process, thus raising an obligation in the physician that transcends arms-length transactions.

From the foregoing axiomatic ingredients emerges a necessity, and a resultant requirement, for divulgence by the physician to his patient of all information relevant to a meaningful decisional process. In many instances, to the physician, whose training and experience enable a self-satisfying evaluation, the particular treatment which should be undertaken may seem evident, but it is the prerogative of the patient, not the physician, to determine for himself the direction in which he believes his interests lie. To enable the patient to chart his course knowledgeably, reasonable familiarity with the therapeutic alternatives and their hazards becomes essential.

Therefore, we hold, as an integral part of the physician's overall obligation to the patient there is a duty of reasonable disclosure of the available choices with respect to proposed therapy and of the dangers inherently and potentially involved in each.

A concomitant issue is the yardstick to be applied in determining reasonableness of disclosure. This defendant and the majority of courts have related the duty to the custom of physicians practicing in the community. The majority rule is needlessly overbroad. Even if there can be said to be a medical community standard as to the disclosure requirement for any prescribed treatment, it appears so nebulous that doctors become, in effect, vested with virtual absolute discretion. Unlimited discretion in the physician is irreconcilable with the basic right of the patient to make the ultimate informed decision regarding the course of treatment to which he knowledgeably consents to be subjected.

A medical doctor, being the expert, appreciates the risks inherent in the procedure he is prescribing, the risks of a decision not to undergo the treatment, and the probability of a successful outcome of the treatment. But once this information has been disclosed, that aspect of the doctor's expert function has been performed. The weighing of these risks against the individual subjective fears and hopes of the patient is not an expert skill. Such evaluation and decision is a nonmedical judgment reserved to the patient alone. A patient should be denied the opportunity to weigh the risks only where it is evident he cannot evaluate the data, as for example, where there is an emergency or the patient is a child or incompetent. For this reason, the law provides that in an emergency consent is implied, and if the patient is a minor or incompetent, the authority to consent is transferred to the patient's legal guardian or closest available relative. In all cases other than the foregoing, the decision whether or not to undertake treatment is vested in the party most directly affected: the patient.

The scope of the disclosure required of physicians defies simple definition. Some courts have spoken of "full disclosure" and others refer to "full and complete" disclosure, but such facile expressions obscure common practicalities. Two qualifications to a requirement of "full disclosure" need little explication. First, the patient's interest in information does not extend to a lengthy polysyllabic discourse on all possible complications. A mini-course in medical science is not required; the patient is concerned with the risk of death or bodily harm, and problems of recuperation. Second, there is no physician's duty to discuss the relatively minor risks inherent in common procedures, when it is common knowledge that such risks inherent in the procedure are of very low incidence. When there is a common procedure a doctor must, of course, make such inquiries as are required to determine if for the particular patient the treatment under consideration is contraindicated—for example, to determine if the patient has had adverse reactions to antibiotics; but no warning beyond such inquiries is required as to the remote possibility of death or serious bodily harm.

However, when there is a more complicated procedure, as the surgery in the case before us, the jury should be instructed that when a given procedure inherently involves a known risk of death or serious bodily harm, a medical doctor has a duty to disclose to his patient the potential of death or serious harm, and to explain in lay terms the complications that might possibly occur. Beyond the foregoing minimal disclosure, a doctor must also reveal to his patient such additional information as a skilled practitioner of good standing would provide under similar circumstances.

In sum, the patient's right of self-decision is the measure of the physician's duty to reveal. That right can be effectively exercised only if the patient possesses adequate information to enable an intelligent choice. The scope of the physician's communications to the patient, then, must be measured by the patient's need, and that need is whatever information is material to the decision. Thus the test for determining whether a potential peril must be divulged is its materiality to the patient's decision.

We point out, for guidance on retrial, an additional problem which suggests itself. There must be a causal relationship between the physician's failure to inform and the injury to the plaintiff. Such causal connection arises only if it is established that had revelation been made consent to treatment would not have been given. Here the record discloses no testimony that had plaintiff been informed of the risks of surgery he would not have consented to the operation.

The patient-plaintiff may testify on this subject but the issue extends beyond his credibility. Since at the time of trial the uncommunicated hazard has materialized, it would be surprising if the patient-plaintiff did not claim that had he been informed of the dangers he would have declined treatment. Subjectively he may believe so, with the 20/20 vision of hindsight, but we doubt that justice will be served by placing the physician in jeopardy of the patient's bitterness and disillusionment. Thus an objective test is preferable: i.e., what would a prudent person in the patient's position have decided if adequately informed of all significant perils.

. . . .

Whenever appropriate, the court should instruct the jury on the defenses available to a doctor who has failed to make the disclosure required by law. Thus, a medical doctor need not make disclosure of risks when the patient requests that he not be so informed. Such a disclosure need not be made if the procedure is simple and the danger remote and commonly appreciated to be remote. A disclosure need not be made beyond that required within the medical community when a doctor can prove . . . [that] he relied upon facts which would demonstrate to a reasonable man the disclosure would have so seriously upset the patient that the patient would not have been able to dispassionately weigh the risks of refusing to undergo the recommended treatment. Any defense, of course, must be consistent with what has been termed the "fiducial qualities" of the physician-patient relationship.

The judgment is reversed.

Discussion Questions

1. Sociologically speaking, what longstanding physician practice and attitude is being challenged here?

2. Does the manner in which the California Supreme Court imposes a new requirement on physicians remind you of any other case discussed in this book? What are the similarities and differences between the two cases?

3. What do you suppose were the reasons for the verdict against the hospital, and why did it not appeal that decision?

4. How effective do you suppose the principles of "informed consent" have been in enabling patients to make knowledgeable decisions?

5. How large would a risk of death or serious bodily harm have to be to influence a reasonable person's decision? One percent? Five? Ten? If you were a juror, how would you decide what is a material enough risk to require disclosure?

Comment

Courts have often held that it is not a hospital's duty to obtain informed consent. Hospitals are not licensed to practice medicine, and gaining informed consent requires delicate medical judgment, to paraphrase a Missouri court in *Roberson v. Menorah Medical Center*, 588 S.W.2d 134 (Mo. Ct. App. 1979). Even though the hospital may furnish the consent form, and even though as a practical matter it is nurses (hospital employees) who often secure the patient's signature, the hospital has no right to interfere in the physician-patient relationship. It is the physician's duty to inform the patient of risks and alternatives.

In *Roberson* the consent form (provided by the hospital) contained the following disclaimer:

The nature and purpose of the cited procedure, possible alternative methods of treatment, the risks involved, and the possibility of complications have been explained to me. I acknowledge that no Guarantee or assurance of the results that may be attained has been given by anyone.

Id. at 136–37. The form also contained language in which the signer agreed that he had read and understood the contents of the form. The *Roberson* court held that the hospital had no duty to inquire about the accuracy of these assertions in the form and no duty to check whether in fact the risks of and alternatives to the proposed treatment had in fact been explained.

Truman v. Thomas
27 Cal. 3d 285, 611 P.2d 902, 165 Cal. Rptr. 308 (1980)

Bird, C.J.

This court must decide whether a physician's failure to inform a patient of the material risks of not consenting to a recommended pap smear, so that the patient might make an informed choice, may have breached the physician's duty of due care to his patient, who died from cancer of the cervix.

I

Respondent, Dr. Claude R. Thomas, is a family physician engaged in a general medical practice. He was first contacted in April 1963 by appellants' mother, Rena Truman, in connection with her second pregnancy. He continued to act as the primary physician for Mrs. Truman and her two children until March 1969. During this six-year period, Mrs. Truman not only sought his medical advice, but often discussed personal matters with him.

In April 1969, Mrs. Truman consulted Dr. Casey, a urologist, about a urinary tract infection which had been treated previously by Dr. Thomas. While examining Mrs. Truman, Dr. Casey discovered that she was experiencing heavy vaginal discharges and that her cervix was extremely rough. Mrs. Truman was given a prescription for the infection and advised to see a gynecologist as soon as possible. When Mrs. Truman did not make an appointment with a gynecologist, Dr. Casey made an appointment for her with a Dr. Ritter.

In October 1969, Dr. Ritter discovered that Mrs. Truman's cervix had been largely replaced by a cancerous tumor. Too far advanced to be removed by surgery, the tumor was unsuccessfully treated by other methods. Mrs. Truman died in July 1970 at the age of 30.

Appellants are Rena Truman's two children. They brought this wrongful death action against Dr. Thomas for his failure to perform a pap smear test on their mother. At the trial, expert testimony was presented which indicated that if Mrs. Truman had undergone a pap smear at any time between 1964 and 1969, the cervical tumor probably would have been discovered in time to save her life. There was disputed expert testimony that the standard of medical practice required a physician to explain to women patients that it is important to have a pap smear each year to "pick up early lesions that are treatable rather than having to deal with [more developed] tumor[s] that very often aren't treatable * * * ."

Although Dr. Thomas saw Mrs. Truman frequently between 1964 and 1969, he never performed a pap smear test on her. Dr. Thomas testified that he did not "specifically" inform Mrs. Truman of the risk involved in any failure to undergo the pap smear test. Rather, "I said, 'You should have a pap smear.' We don't say by now it can be Stage Two [in the development of cervical cancer] or go through all of the different lectures about cancer. I think it is a widely known and generally accepted manner of treatment and I think the patient has a high degree of responsibility. We are not enforcers, we are advisors." However, Dr. Thomas' medical records contain no reference to any discussion or recommendation that Mrs. Truman undergo a pap smear test.

For the most part, Dr. Thomas was unable to describe specific conversations with Mrs. Truman. For example, he testified that during certain periods he "saw Rena very frequently, approximately once a week or so, and I am sure my opening remark was, 'Rena, you need a pap smear,' * * * I am sure we discussed it with her so often that she couldn't [have] fail[ed] to realize that we wanted her to have a complete examination, breast examination, ovaries and pap smear." Dr. Thomas also testified that on at least two occasions when he performed pelvic examinations of Mrs. Truman she refused him permission to perform the test, stating she could not afford the cost. Dr. Thomas offered to defer payment, but Mrs. Truman wanted to pay cash.

Appellants argue that the failure to give a pap smear test to Mrs. Truman proximately caused her death. Two instructions requested by appellants described alternative theories under which Dr. Thomas could be held liable for this failure. First, they asked that the jury be instructed that it "is the duty of a physician to disclose to his patient all relevant information to enable the patient to make an informed decision regarding the submission to or refusal to take a diagnostic test. [¶] Failure of the physician to disclose to his patient all relevant information including the risks to the patient if the test is refused renders the physician liable for any injury legally resulting from the patient's refusal to take the test if a reasonably prudent person in the patient's position would not have refused the test if she had been adequately informed of all the significant perils." Second, they requested that the jury be informed that "as a matter of law * * * a physician who fails to perform a Pap smear test on a female patient over the age of 23 and to whom the patient has entrusted her general physical care is liable for injury or death proximately caused by the failure to perform the test." Both instructions were refused.

The jury rendered a special verdict, finding Dr. Thomas free of any negligence that proximately caused Mrs. Truman's death. This appeal followed.

II

The central issue for this court is whether Dr. Thomas breached his duty of care to Mrs. Truman when he failed to inform her of the potentially fatal consequences of allowing cervical cancer to develop undetected by a pap smear.

In *Cobbs v. Grant*, this court considered the scope of a physician's duty to disclose medical information to his or her patients in discussing proposed medical procedures. Certain basic characteristics of the physician-patient relationship were identified. "The first is that patients are generally persons unlearned in the medical sciences and therefore, except in rare cases, courts may safely assume the knowledge of patient and physician are not in parity. The second is that a person of adult years and in sound mind has the right, in the exercise of control over his own body, to determine whether or not to submit to lawful medical treatment. The third is that the patient's consent to treatment, to be effective, must be an informed consent. And the fourth is that the patient, being unlearned in medical sciences, has an abject dependence upon and trust in his physician for the information upon which he relies during the decisional process, thus raising an obligation in the physician that transcends arms-length transactions."

In light of these factors, the court held that "as an integral part of the physician's overall obligation to the patient there is a duty of reasonable disclosure of the available choices with respect to proposed therapy and of the dangers inherently and potentially involved in each." The scope of a physician's duty to disclose is measured by the amount of knowledge a patient needs in order to make an informed choice. All information material to the patient's decision should be given.

Material information is that which the physician knows or should know would be regarded as significant by a reasonable person in the patient's position when deciding to accept or reject the recommended medical procedure. To be material, a fact must also be one which is not commonly appreciated. If the physician knows or should know of a patient's unique concerns or lack of familiarity with medical procedures, this may expand the scope of required disclosure.

Applying these principles, the court in *Cobbs* stated that a patient must be apprised not only of the "risks inherent in the procedure [prescribed, but also] the risks of a decision not to undergo the treatment, and the probability of a successful outcome of the treatment." This rule applies whether the procedure involves treatment or a diagnostic test. On the one hand, a physician recommending a risk-free procedure may safely forego discussion beyond that necessary to conform to competent medical practice and to obtain the patient's con-

sent. If a patient indicates that he or she is going to decline the risk-free test or treatment, then the doctor has the additional duty of advising of all material risks of which a reasonable person would want to be informed before deciding not to undergo the procedure. On the other hand, if the recommended test or treatment is itself risky, then the physician should always explain the potential consequences of declining to follow the recommended course of action.

Nevertheless, Dr. Thomas contends that *Cobbs* does not apply to him because the duty to disclose applies only where the patient consents to the recommended procedure. He argues that since a physician's advice may be presumed to be founded on an expert appraisal of the patient's medical needs, no reasonable patient would fail to undertake further inquiry before rejecting such advice. Therefore, patients who reject their physician's advice should shoulder the burden of inquiry as to the possible consequences of their decision.

This argument is inconsistent with *Cobbs*. The duty to disclose was imposed in *Cobbs* so that patients might meaningfully exercise their right to make decisions about their own bodies. The importance of this right should not be diminished by the manner in which it is exercised. Further, the need for disclosure is not lessened because patients reject a recommended procedure. Such a decision does not alter "what has been termed the 'fiducial qualities' of the physician-patient relationship," since patients who reject a procedure are as unskilled in the medical sciences as those who consent. To now hold that patients who reject their physician's advice have the burden of inquiring as to the potential consequences of their decisions would be to contradict *Cobbs*. It must be remembered that Dr. Thomas was not engaged in an arms-length transaction with Mrs. Truman. Clearly, under *Cobbs*, he was obligated to provide her with all the information material to her decision.

Dr. Thomas next contends that, as a matter of law, he had no duty to disclose to Mrs. Truman the risk of failing to undergo a pap smear test because "the danger [is] remote and commonly appreciated to be remote." The merit of this contention depends on whether a jury could reasonably find that knowledge of this risk was material to Mrs. Truman's decision.

The record indicates that the pap smear test is an accurate detector of cervical cancer. Although the probability that Mrs. Truman had cervical cancer was low, Dr. Thomas knew that the potential harm of failing to detect the disease at an early stage was death. This situation is not analogous to one which involves, for example, "relatively minor risks inherent in [such] common procedures" as the taking of blood samples. These risks are not central to the decision to administer or reject the procedure. In contrast, the risk which Mrs. Truman faced from cervical cancer was not only significant, it was the principal reason why Dr. Thomas recommended that she undergo a pap smear.

Little evidence was introduced on whether this risk was commonly known. Dr. Thomas testified that the risk would be known to a reasonable person. Whether such evidence is sufficient to establish that there was no general duty to disclose this risk to patients is a question of fact for the jury. Moreover, even assuming such disclosure was not generally required, the circumstances in this case may establish that Dr. Thomas did have a duty to inform Mrs. Truman of the risks she was running by not undergoing a pap smear.

Dr. Thomas testified he never specifically informed her of the purpose of a pap smear test. There was no evidence introduced that Mrs. Truman was aware of the serious danger entailed in not undergoing the test. However, there was testimony that Mrs. Truman said she would not undergo the test on certain occasions because of its cost or because "she just didn't feel like it." Under these circumstances, a jury could reasonably conclude that Dr. Thomas had a duty to inform Mrs. Truman of the danger of refusing the test because it was not reasonable for Dr. Thomas to assume that Mrs. Truman appreciated the potentially fatal consequences of her conduct. Accordingly, this court cannot decide as a matter of law that Dr. Thomas owed absolutely no duty to Mrs. Truman to make this important disclosure that affected her life.

The instruction proposed by appellants was a modification of [a standard instruction], which was adopted to describe a physician's duty of reasonable disclosure as established by this court in *Cobbs*. Appellants' instruction correctly indicated that a physician has a duty to disclose all material information to a patient. The instruction also stated that breach of this duty renders the physician liable for any "legally resulting [injury] * * * if a reasonably prudent person in the patient's position would not have refused the test if she had been adequately informed of all the significant perils."

The term "legally resulting" was defined for the jury . . . . The jury was instructed that a "proximate cause of an injury is a cause which, in natural and continuous sequence, produces the injury, and without which the injury would not have occurred." Obviously, this test could not be satisfied if the jury were to conclude that even given adequate disclosure Mrs. Truman would have refused to take the recommended test in time to save her life. Thus, the rejected instruction would have correctly indicated that satisfaction of the prudent person test for causation established in *Cobbs* was necessary but not sufficient for plaintiffs to recover. If the jury were to reasonably conclude that Mrs. Truman would have unreasonably refused a pap smear in the face of adequate disclosure, there could be no finding of proximate cause. Though awkwardly phrased, the rejected instruction accurately reflected the law and a theory of liability applicable to the facts of this case.

Refusal to give the requested instruction meant that the jury was unable to consider whether Dr. Thomas breached a duty by not disclosing the danger of failing to undergo a pap smear. Since this theory finds support in the record, it was error for the court to refuse to give the requested instruction. If the jury had been given this instruction and had found in favor

of the appellants, such a finding would have had support in the record before us. Reversal is therefore required. . . .

. . . .

The judgment is reversed.
TOBRINER, MOSK and NEWMAN, JJ., concur.
CLARK, Justice, dissenting.
I dissent.

The consent instruction demanded by plaintiffs will impose upon doctors the intolerable burden of having to explain diagnostic tests to healthy patients. To meet their new burden doctors will have to spend the greater part of their day not examining or treating patients, but explaining to them all information relevant to the purposes of diagnostic examinations and tests. Such burden is unreasonable, and the trial court properly refused the instruction. . . .

. . . .

A primary consideration in determining whether a new duty should be imposed upon a defendant is the "extent of the burden to the defendant and consequences to the community" in imposing the duty.

The burden of explaining the purposes of a pap smear and the potential risks in failing to submit to one may not appear to be great, but the newly imposed duty upon physicians created by today's majority opinion goes far beyond. The instruction requires disclosure of all "relevant information to enable the patient to make an informed decision regarding the submission to or refusal to take a diagnostic test." In short, it applies not only to pap smears, but to all diagnostic procedures allegedly designed to detect illness which could lead to death or serious complication if not timely treated.

Carried to its logical end, the majority decision requires physicians to explain to patients who have not had a recent general examination the intricacies of chest examinations, blood analyses, X-ray examinations, electrocardiograms, urine analyses and innumerable other procedures. In short, today's ruling mandates doctors to provide each such patient with a summary course covering most of his or her medical education. Most medical tests—like pap smears—are designed to detect illness which might prove fatal absent timely treatment. Explaining the purposes of each procedure to each such patient will obviously take hours if not days.

Few, if any, people in our society are unaware that a general examination is designed to discover serious illness for timely treatment. While a lengthy explanation may result in general examinations for some patients who would otherwise decline or defer them, the onerous duty placed upon doctors by today's decision will result in reduced care for others. Requiring physicians to spend a large portion of their time teaching medical science before practicing it will greatly increase the cost of medical diagnosis—a cost ultimately paid by an unwanting public. Persons desiring treatment for specific complaints will be deterred from seeking medical advice once they realize they will be charged not only for treatment but also for lengthy lectures on the merits of their examination.

The great educational program the majority embark upon, even if justifiable, is a question of public policy for the Legislature to determine: whether the cost warrants the burden, and whether the duty to educate rests with doctors, schools or health departments. Requiring individual doctors to enlighten the public may be found through legislative hearings to be inefficient, not reaching those who need it most—the ones hesitant to consult doctors.

When a patient chooses a physician, he or she obviously has confidence in the doctor and intends to accept proffered medical advice. When the doctor prescribes diagnostic tests, the patient is aware the tests are intended to discover illness. It is therefore reasonable to assume that a patient who refuses advice is aware of potential risk.

Moreover, the physician-patient relationship is based on trust, and forcing the doctor into a hard sell approach to his services can only jeopardize that relationship.

The new duty to explain, imposed by the majority as a matter of law, creates an undue burden on both the doctor and society and should be rejected. Strict tort liability does not extend to professional services. The ordinary duty in medical practice cases calls for determining the community standard of care, the appropriate duty in the instant case. Doctors—or at least the Legislature—rather than judges are in the best position to balance the professional relationship between doctors and patients, to determine how far a doctor should go in selling his services without alienating the patient from all medical care, and to promote the highest level of diagnostic care for the community. In the instant case, evidence as to community medical standard was appropriately received, the case was tried on this basis, and we should not reverse the judgment.

. . . .

Discussion Questions

1. If you were a physician in this situation, how would you decide what information is material to your patient's decision?

2. Given Dr. Thomas' long-standing relationship with Mrs. Truman, including the fact that she "often discussed [nonmedical] personal matters with him," was it reasonable for Dr. Thomas not to explain the risks of refusal with her? Why or why not?

3. In Part II of the opinion, the court provides its formulation of the central issue. Do you agree with that statement of the issue in this case?

4. Based on the result of this appeal, has Dr. Thomas breached his duty of care to Mrs. Truman?

Gray v. Director of the Dep't. of Mental Health, Retardation and Hosps.
697 F. Supp. 580 (D. R.I. 1988)

Boyle, C.J.

The Plaintiff Glenn Gray seeks a declaratory judgment authorizing him to direct the removal of a feeding tube and further life support administered to his wife Marcia Gray, who is presently a patient at Rhode Island Medical Center [RIMC], General Hospital. The effect of removal of the feeding tube or closing off of the feeding tube would be to bring about the death of Marcia Gray.

[The 49-year-old patient was in a persistent vegetative state due to an intracranial hemorrhage suffered on January 4, 1986. She had been at RIMC since June of that year.]

The court appointed Guardian *Ad Litem* described her condition as follows:

Marcia Gray has been diagnosed as being in "persistent vegetative state" (PVS). PVS is a type of comatose state in which the cerebral functioning has ceased but in which the brain stem functioning is fully or partially intact. The brain stem controls primitive reflexes, including heart activity, breathing, the sleep/wake cycle, reflexive activity in upper and lower extremities, some swallowing motions and eye movements. Marcia shows signs of each of these activities. The cerebrum, on the other hand, controls sensation and voluntary and conscious activities. Marcia's cerebrum has been damaged severely, and as a result she displays no voluntary or conscious movements, nor does she display any awareness or sensation. This combination of reflexive activity in the absence of sensation or conscious activity is characteristic of PVS. PVS is generally a permanent condition.

At the present time Marcia is fed a liquid formula every four hours which passes through the G-tube and water is provided by the tube in-between feedings. In spite of her "comfort only status" as a patient she is in need of constant attention.

On May 20, 1987, the family, including her husband, her two children, her mother and her sister-in-law requested that her attending physician order that feeding be stopped and that Marcia Gray be permitted to die. The family's request was denied by the hospital. The neurosurgeon who performed the craniotomy and the consulting physician hired by the family agree that there is no "reasonable likelihood of returning to a conscious state" and that there is "no chance" of Maria Gray's recovery. In addition, Mrs. Gray's treating physician since 1986 at the General Hospital states that her chances of recovery to conscious state are "close to zero." Her neurosurgeon expressed the opinion that Marcia Gray's brain stem functions are primarily intact, although not entirely, but she exhibits no conscious, cognitive, sentient responses which would indicate functioning cerebral hemisphere activity. He suggests that her response to noxious stimuli was of questionable significance given the primitive nature of the startle reflex. He does not believe that she will experience hunger, thirst or pain should the feeding be stopped. He states that because her conscious faculties have ceased to function, she would not experience, in his opinion, that sensory recognition. The consulting physician engaged by Mrs. Gray's family also believes strongly that there is no sensation and hence no pain, thirst, or hunger recognition.

The Guardian *Ad Litem* has reported to the Court that the hospital as an institution is opposed to denying Mrs. Gray nutrition and hydration because it is tantamount to euthanasia, inconsistent with the physician's role as safekeeper of his or her patient's well being, the fear that the hospital has of civil or criminal responsibility and the reputation which the hospital has [as] an institution for long-term care and the treatment of chronic care patients. Those professional health care personnel who administer to Mrs. Gray's needs presently are unanimous in their adamant opposition to the proposal to remove nutrition and hydration.

Mrs. Gray's family, including her husband, her two children, her mother and her sister-in-law are convinced that it would be her desire not to be sustained with artificial measures if her life were otherwise hopeless. The Guardian *Ad Litem* reports conversations between Mr. and Mrs. Gray concerning the plight of Karen Ann Quinlan. Mr. Gray states that on one occasion Mrs. Gray required that he promise not to keep her alive by artificial means should she ever be in a circumstance similar to Karen Ann Quinlan. The same sentiments were also expressed to him on other occasions by his wife. Her sister-in-law, who was at the time Director of Social Services of a hospice in Chapel Hill, North Carolina, states that Mrs. Gray discussed the plight of Karen Ann Quinlan and was critical of the fact that she was fed artificially and said that she would not want a respirator or a feeding tube if she were in the same circumstances.

. . . .

Although it has been customary to cast actions such as this in the light of raising the issue of a right to die[,] this shorthand expression does not in any sense communicate effectively the nature of this controversy. Essentially this controversy concerns the question of whether or not the State can insist that a person in a vegetative state incapable of intelligent sensation, whose condition is irreversible, may be required to submit to medical care under circumstances in which the patient prefers not to do so. In this light the issues presented do not essentially involve death but essentially relate to life and its circumstances. Due to advances in medical care, it is possible in some circumstances to sustain the body's biological functions for extended periods of time while the patient has no sense of pain or pleasure, fear or joy, love or hate, understanding or appreciation, taste or touch or smell or any other aspect of life's experience, with no realistic possibility of sentient life.

Given the tragic circumstances of Mrs. Gray's condition, the question is who has the right to determine her course of care. She is unable to make a decision. Her family clearly wishes that she should not be further sustained by the provision of nourishment and hydration. The State has its right and, indeed, it may well be said, its duty to continue to provide nourishment and hydration. The issue is how and under what circumstances should either point of view prevail. How is Marcia Gray to be protected?

I

The first question to be resolved is whether Marcia Gray has a federal constitutional right to refuse life-sustaining medical treatment. Put another way, the question is whether the right of privacy, from either the Fourteenth Amendment's due process clause or other constitutional guarantees' penumbras, is broad enough to include a person's right to refuse medical treatment which will result in death.

. . . .

. . . [A]lthough the Supreme Court has never directly addressed the issue of a person's federal constitutional right to refuse life-sustaining medical treatment, the Court's decisions have repeatedly affirmed the principle of individual self-determination. A person has the right, subject to important state interest, to control fundamental medical decisions that affect his or her own body. This right, whether described as the principle of personal autonomy, the right of self-determination, or the right of privacy, is properly grounded in the liberties protected by the Fourteenth Amendment's due process clause. This right is also grounded in the notion of an individual's dignity and interest in bodily integrity.

The right to control fundamental medical decisions is similar in nature to the abortion decision, the contraceptive decision, and the surgical decision. These decisions are extremely personal and the consequences of such decisions may literally be life or death. Decisions concerning medical treatment, therefore, bear little connection to the claimed constitutional right to engage in consensual homosexual acts rejected in *Bowers*. Instead, the right to control fundamental medical decisions is an aspect of the right of self-determination and personal autonomy that is "deeply rooted in this Nation's history and tradition."

Indeed, the right to control medical decisions affecting one's body can hardly be questioned. "The root premise is the concept, fundamental in American jurisprudence, that '[e]very human being of adult years and sound mind has a right to determine what shall be done with his own body * * * .' " In a recent case involving an individual compelled to take antipsychotic drugs, the Fourth Circuit Court of Appeals reiterated this principle:

The right to be free of unwanted physical invasions has been recognized as an integral part of the individual's constitutional freedoms, whether termed a liberty interest protected by the Due Process Clause, or an aspect of the right to privacy contained in the notions of personal freedom which underwrote the Bill of Rights. The right to refuse medical treatment has been specifically recognized as a subject of constitutional protections.

The right to control fundamental medical decisions, which includes the right to refuse treatment, reaches its extreme when the decision results in the individual's death. Nevertheless, a person "has a paramount right to control the disposition to be made of his or her body, absent a compelling countervailing governmental interest," even if the decision results in that person's death. In [a 1985 case from the District of Columbia], the [court] ordered, in accordance with the patient's wishes, the removal of her life-support system, although such an action would likely result in her immediate death. Marcia Gray's right to privacy encompasses the same right to refuse life-sustaining medical treatment.

II

The next issue is whether nutrition and hydration supplied through a gastrostomy tube are a form of medical treatment that Marcia Gray may properly refuse. Courts addressing this issue have concluded that analytically no difference exists between artificial feeding and other life support measures. Although an emotional symbolism attaches itself to artificial feeding, there is no legal difference between a mechanical device that allows a person to breathe artificially and a mechanical device that artificially allows a person nourishment. If a person has the right to decline life on a respirator, then a person has the equal right to decline a gastrostomy tube. Accordingly, Marcia Gray's right to refuse medical treatment includes the right to have the G-tube removed.

III

Although Marcia Gray is now rendered incompetent, she still retains her right to decide whether the G-tube remains implanted or is removed. The right to refuse medical treatment " 'must extend to the case of an incompetent, as well as a competent, patient because the value of human dignity extends to both.' " [Quoting *Brophy*, a leading case from Massachusetts.] " 'Any other view would permit obliteration of an incompetent's panoply of rights merely because the patient could no longer sense the violation of those rights.' " [Quoting a New Jersey decision, *In re Conroy*.] Indeed, the United States Supreme Court has recognized that the "law must often adjust the manner in which it affords rights to those whose status renders them unable to exercise choice freely," noting that "those who are irreversibly ill with loss of brain function * * * retain 'rights,' to be sure, but often such rights are only meaningful as they are exercised by agents acting with the best interests of their principals in mind."

. . . .

It is unnecessary to determine in this action how the decision should be made. All are in agreement, including the

Court, her husband and her court-appointed guardian, her family, and the Guardian *Ad Litem* appointed by this Court. The evidence clearly supports a finding that Marcia Gray, if competent, would exercise her right to refuse the life-sustaining medical treatment.

The court-appointed Guardian *Ad Litem* concluded that Marcia Gray, if competent, would support her guardian's and family's decision to cease the artificial feeding. First, Marcia Gray's conversations concerning the termination of life-sustaining treatment, especially that with her sister-in-law, clearly indicate Marcia Gray's intent. Second, the depth, quality, and reasoning of the family's prediction of Marcia Gray's intent is impressive. The family speaks with one voice and no apparent conflict of interest exists. The Guardian *Ad Litem*, summing up his discussion of the substituted judgment approach, stated:

[u]nder this approach, it is rather clear that the substituted judgment decision would be to withhold treatment. Not only is the family unanimous in this prediction, but their reasons are enlightening. They describe Marcia as a very private and dignified woman, and as one who loved life dearly. They feel strongly that she would not want merely to exist as she does now, with frequent handling and manipulation, with no control over her most personal and private functions, with no hope of ever enjoying, appreciating or even experiencing life. They also feel that her commitment to her family would lead her to want to spare the family the great pain which it is enduring during this attenuated dying process.

A decision such as this is not to be made lightly. Yet Marcia Gray's conversations with her husband and sister-in-law and the Guardian *Ad Litem*'s thorough and careful consideration of Marcia Gray's wishes emphasize that Marcia Gray, were she competent, would decline life-sustaining apparatus.

IV

Although Marcia Gray has a constitutional right to refuse life-sustaining medical treatment, no right is absolute. Accordingly, Marcia Gray's right must be balanced against competing governmental interests that include: the preservation of life, the prevention of suicide, the protection of innocent third parties, and the integrity of medical ethics. Upon examination, Marcia Gray's interest in self-determination outweighs all governmental interests.

The preservation of life is, of course, the greatest governmental interest. But, governmental interests, like constitutional rights, are not always overriding.

The duty of the State to preserve life must encompass a recognition of an individual's right to avoid circumstances in which the individual himself would feel that efforts to sustain life demean or degrade his humanity. It is antithetical to our scheme of ordered liberty and to our respect for the autonomy of the individual for the State to make decisions regarding the individual's quality of life. It is for the patient to decide such issues. Our role is limited to ensuring that a refusal of treatment does not violate legal norms. [Quoting the *Brophy* decision again.]

The stated role is not a matter of crossing t's and dotting i's. A serious inquiry is demanded. A judicial determination concerning life is imminently more significant [than] a determination of dollar damages. These "legal norms" are standards of the highest order. The facts in Marcia Gray's case support the finding that she would consider that efforts now to sustain her life demean her humanity.

Amici argues that in balancing the individual's and the state's interests, courts have distinguished between ordinary and extraordinary medical treatment. While this is a factor to be considered, recent decisions have criticized the distinction as one without meaning. Although the maintenance of the G-tube may not be extraordinary or invasive, the initial insertion of the G-tube certainly was. Moreover, the *Brophy* court reasoned that maintaining a person by artificial feeding "over an extended period is not only intrusive but extraordinary." . . .

However the maintenance of the G-tube is characterized, its continued use, against Marcia Gray's wishes, robs her of the right to determine her course of care. A state's interest in the preservation of life is highest when the state seeks to protect an individual who may potentially be the subject of abuse because he or she cannot protect his or her own interests. That clearly is not the situation here; rather, a number of persons are attempting to ensure that Marcia Gray's wishes are respected. In this situation, therefore, Marcia Gray's right to self-determination must prevail over the state's interest in preserving life for all.

The other state interests that are implicated also do not override Marcia Gray's rights. The state interest in preventing suicide is not an issue as there is an obvious distinction between deliberately ending a life by artificial means and allowing nature to take its course.

. . . .

The state's interest in protection of innocent third parties also does not overcome Marcia Gray's right to self-determination. As the *Tune* court noted, "[c]onsideration of the rights of innocent third parties is generally limited to situations in which the interests of the patient's dependents may be adversely affected." The rights of Marcia Gray's family will not be adversely affected by allowing her to exercise her right to refuse medical treatment, as they have sought and endorsed that right.

Finally, consideration of the integrity of medical ethics does not present a compelling justification to refuse Marcia Gray's wishes. Indeed, medical ethics incorporates the principle that the patient, not the health care provider, determines what the course of care should be. . . .

Marcia Gray's right to refuse medical treatment therefore overrides any countervailing state interests.

V

The final issue to be resolved is whether the Rhode Island Medical Center should be required to carry out Marcia Gray's wishes or whether the Medical Center and its personnel may refuse to participate in such a procedure.

First, in the context of individual rights, the Constitution rarely commands an affirmative obligation on the government's part; instead, individual rights are stated in the negative, instructing the government on what it cannot do. For example, a State may not under the Fourteenth Amendment deny life or liberty. Thus, the right of procreational autonomy is grounded in the right to make the childbearing decision without governmental interference. Similarly, the right of personal autonomy is the right to make medical decisions affecting oneself free from unwarranted governmental intrusion. In both situations, however, the government is under no constitutional obligation to provide resources to enable an individual to take full advantage of his or her rights.

As mentioned earlier, Rhode Island legislation guarantees a patient the right to refuse medical care. Rhode Island case law also expressly recognizes a patient's right to refuse treatment. Implicit in this right is that the patient should not be penalized for exercising his or her judgment. " 'A decision to forego life-sustaining treatment is not a ground to withdraw all care—nor should care givers treat it in this way * * * .' " Patients who have decided to forego life-sustaining treatment may still opt for "supportive care—pain control, skin care, and personal hygiene."

The defendants argue that the principle underlying [the Rhode Island statute], which states that a person associated with a health care facility may refuse on moral or religious grounds to participate in an abortion or sterilization procedure, should apply in this situation. The statute is clearly limited to procedures involving abortion and sterilization. It does not apply to the circumstances of [these] actions.

Marcia Gray and her family had no reason to believe that they were giving up her right to determine her course of care by entering the Rhode Island Medical Center. The Rhode Island Medical Center apparently did not articulate or notify the Grays of its policy of refusing to participate in a patient's decision to terminate a G-tube's use until after Glenn Gray, on behalf of Marcia, had made such a request. Under these facts, Marcia Gray and her family "were entitled to rely on the * * * [hospital's] willingness to defer to their choice among courses of medical treatment."

Recognition of Marcia Gray's right to terminate nutrition and hydration obviously places a great burden on health care professionals who rank giving food and water to the sick as one of their highest duties. It is fortunate that they are so concerned. Yet, even though Marcia Gray has decided to forego the use of the G-tube, she still needs medical attention. As unsettling as it must be to them, health care professionals must acknowledge Marcia Gray's right of self-determination. Accordingly, if Marcia Gray cannot be promptly transferred to a health care facility that will respect her wishes, the Rhode Island Medical Center must accede to her requests.

ORDERED, that judgment will be granted for the Plaintiff, as prayed.

Discussion Questions

1. How would you articulate what the precise issue was in this case? Do you agree with the way the court has decided that issue? Do you agree with the ultimate result, allowing Mrs. Gray to die by withholding artificially supplied nutrition and hydration?

2. Note the quotation from Justice Cardozo, quoted with favor by this court on page 110. Do you feel it should apply to decisions of artificial nutrition and hydration, which, after all, were unanticipated in 1914 when Cardozo wrote the *Schloendorff* decision?

3. Do you understand the distinction between *ordinary* and *extraordinary* treatments? Do you agree that it is a "distinction . . . without meaning," as the court states?

4. Who should make termination-of-treatment decisions for an infant, for an adult who has not expressed any opinion on the matter, or for an adult who has never been competent? What standards should be used for making such decisions? How can society protect such a person against decisions made for motives other than the patient's best interests?

5. Do the health care providers have rights in these matters too? If so, how can those rights be protected? Has this court adequately protected those rights?

Cruzan v. Director, Mo. Dep't. of Health
497 U.S. 261 (1990)

Rehnquist, C.J.

Petitioner Nancy Beth Cruzan was rendered incompetent as a result of severe injuries sustained during an automobile accident. Co-petitioners Lester and Joyce Cruzan, Nancy's parents and co-guardians, sought a court order directing the withdrawal of their daughter's artificial feeding and hydration equipment after it became apparent that she had virtually no chance of recovering her cognitive faculties. The Supreme Court of Missouri held that because there was no clear and convincing evidence of Nancy's desire to have life-sustaining treatment withdrawn under such circumstances, her parents lacked authority to effectuate such a request. We granted certiorari, and now affirm.

On the night of January 11, 1983, Nancy Cruzan lost control of her car as she traveled down Elm Road in Jasper County, Missouri. The vehicle overturned, and Cruzan was discovered lying face down in a ditch without detectable respiratory or cardiac function. Paramedics were able to restore her breathing and heartbeat at the accident site, and she was transported to a hospital in an unconscious state. An attending neurosurgeon diagnosed her as having sustained probable cerebral contusions compounded by significant anoxia (lack of oxygen). The Missouri trial court in this case found that permanent brain damage generally results after 6 minutes in an anoxic state; it was estimated that Cruzan was deprived of oxygen from 12 to 14 minutes. She remained in a coma for approximately three weeks and then progressed to an unconscious state in which she was able to orally ingest some nutrition. In order to ease feeding and further the recovery, surgeons implanted a gastrostomy feeding and hydration tube in Cruzan with the consent of her then husband. Subsequent rehabilitative efforts proved unavailing. She now lies in a Missouri state hospital in what is commonly referred to as a persistent vegetative state: generally, a condition in which a person exhibits motor reflexes but evinces no indications of significant cognitive function. The State of Missouri is bearing the cost of her care.

After it had become apparent that Nancy Cruzan had virtually no chance of regaining her mental faculties her parents asked hospital employees to terminate the artificial nutrition and hydration procedures. All agree that such a removal would cause her death. The employees refused to honor the request without court approval. The parents then sought and received authorization from the state trial court for termination. The court found that a person in Nancy's condition had a fundamental right under the State and Federal Constitutions to refuse or direct the withdrawal of "death prolonging procedures." The court also found that Nancy's "expressed thoughts at age twenty-five in somewhat serious conversation with a housemate friend that if sick or injured she would not wish to continue her life unless she could live at least halfway normally suggests that given her present condition she would not wish to continue on with her nutrition and hydration."

The Supreme Court of Missouri reversed by a divided vote. The court recognized a right to refuse treatment embodied in the common-law doctrine of informed consent, but expressed skepticism about the application of that doctrine in the circumstances of this case. The court also declined to read a broad right of privacy into the State Constitution which would "support the right of a person to refuse medical treatment in every circumstance," and expressed doubt as to whether such a right existed under the United States Constitution. It then decided that the Missouri Living Will statute embodied a state policy strongly favoring the preservation of life. The court found that Cruzan's statements to her roommate regarding her desire to live or die under certain conditions were "unreliable for the purpose of determining her intent," "and thus insufficient to support the co-guardians['] claim to exercise substituted judgment on Nancy's behalf." It rejected the argument that Cruzan's parents were entitled to order the termination of her medical treatment, concluding that "no person can assume that choice for an incompetent in the absence of the formalities required under Missouri's Living Will statutes or the clear and convincing, inherently reliable evidence absent here." The court also expressed its view that "[b]road policy questions bearing on life and death are more properly addressed by representative assemblies" than judicial bodies.

We granted certiorari to consider the question of whether Cruzan has a right under the United States Constitution which would require the hospital to withdraw life-sustaining treatment from her under these circumstances.

At common law, even the touching of one person by another without consent and without legal justification was a battery. Before the turn of the century, this Court observed that "[n]o right is held more sacred, or is more carefully guarded, by the common law, than the right of every individual to the possession and control of his own person, free from all restraint or interference of others, unless by clear and unquestionable authority of law." This notion of bodily integrity has been embodied in the requirement that informed consent is generally required for medical treatment.

The logical corollary of the doctrine of informed consent is that the patient generally possesses the right not to consent, that is, to refuse treatment. Until about 15 years ago and the seminal decision in *In re Quinlan*, the number of right-to-refuse-treatment decisions were relatively few. Most of the earlier cases involved patients who refused medical treatment forbidden by their religious beliefs, thus implicating First Amendment rights as well as common-law rights of self-determination. More recently, however, with the advance of medical technology capable of sustaining life well past the point where natural forces would have brought certain death in earlier times, cases involving the right to refuse life-sustaining treatment have burgeoned.

In the *Quinlan* case, young Karen Quinlan suffered severe brain damage as the result of anoxia, and entered a persistent vegetative state. Karen's father sought judicial approval to disconnect his daughter's respirator. The New Jersey Supreme Court granted the relief, holding that Karen had a right of privacy grounded in the Federal Constitution to terminate treatment. Recognizing that this right was not absolute, however, the court balanced it against asserted state interests. Noting that the State's interest "weakens and the individual's right to privacy grows as the degree of bodily invasion increases and the prognosis dims," the court concluded that the state interests had to give way in that case. The court also concluded that the "only practical way" to prevent the loss of Karen's privacy right due to her incompetence was to allow her guardian and family to decide "whether she would exercise it in these circumstances."

After *Quinlan*, however, most courts have based a right to refuse treatment either solely on the common-law right to informed consent or on both the common-law right and a constitutional privacy right. [Here the court undertakes an extensive review of prior cases in this area.]

As these cases demonstrate, the common-law doctrine of informed consent is viewed as generally encompassing the right of a competent individual to refuse medical treatment. Beyond that, these decisions demonstrate both similarity and diversity in their approach to decision of what all agree is a perplexing question with unusually strong moral and ethical overtones. State courts have available to them for decision a number of sources—state constitutions, statutes, and common law—which are not available to us. In this Court, the question is simply and starkly whether the United States Constitution prohibits Missouri from choosing the rule of decision which it did. This is the first case in which we have been squarely presented with the issue of whether the United States Constitution grants what is in common parlance referred to as a "right to die." We follow the judicious counsel of our decision in *Twin City Bank v. Nebeker* (1897), where we said that in deciding "a question of such magnitude and importance * * * it is the [better] part of wisdom not to attempt, by any general statement, to cover every possible phase of the subject."

The Fourteenth Amendment provides that no State shall "deprive any person of life, liberty, or property, without due process of law." The principle that a competent person has a constitutionally protected liberty interest in refusing unwanted medical treatment may be inferred from our prior decisions. In *Jacobson v. Massachusetts* (1905), for instance, the Court balanced an individual's liberty interest in declining an unwanted smallpox vaccine against the State's interest in preventing disease. Decisions prior to the incorporation of the Fourth Amendment into the Fourteenth Amendment analyzed searches and seizures involving the body under the Due Process Clause and were thought to implicate substantial liberty interests.

Just this Term, in the course of holding that a State's procedures for administering antipsychotic medication to prisoners were sufficient to satisfy due process concerns, we recognized that prisoners possess "a significant liberty interest in avoiding the unwanted administration of antipsychotic drugs under the Due Process Clause of the Fourteenth Amendment." Still other cases support the recognition of a general liberty interest in refusing medical treatment.

But determining that a person has a "liberty interest" under the Due Process Clause does not end the inquiry; "whether respondent's constitutional rights have been violated must be determined by balancing his liberty interests against the relevant state interests."

Petitioners insist that under the general holdings of our cases, the forced administration of life-sustaining medical treatment, and even of artificially delivered food and water essential to life, would implicate a competent person's liberty interest. Although we think the logic of the cases discussed above would embrace such a liberty interest, the dramatic consequences involved in refusal of such treatment would inform the inquiry as to whether the deprivation of that interest is constitutionally permissible. But for purposes of this case, we assume that the United States Constitution would grant a competent person a constitutionally protected right to refuse lifesaving hydration and nutrition.

Petitioners go on to assert that an incompetent person should possess the same right in this respect as is possessed by a competent person. . . .

The difficulty with petitioners' claim is that in a sense it begs the question: an incompetent person is not able to make an informed and voluntary choice to exercise a hypothetical right to refuse treatment or any other right. Such a "right" must be exercised for her, if at all, by some sort of surrogate. Here, Missouri has in effect recognized that under certain circumstances a surrogate may act for the patient in electing to have hydration and nutrition withdrawn in such a way as to cause death, but it has established a procedural safeguard to assure that the action of the surrogate conforms as best it may to the wishes expressed by the patient while competent. Missouri requires that evidence of the incompetent's wishes as to the withdrawal of treatment be proved by clear and convincing evidence. The question, then, is whether the United States Constitution forbids the establishment of this procedural requirement by the State. We hold that it does not.

Whether or not Missouri's clear and convincing evidence requirement comports with the United States Constitution depends in part on what interests the State may properly seek to protect in this situation. Missouri relies on its interest in the protection and preservation of human life, and there can be no gainsaying this interest. As a general matter, the States—indeed, all civilized nations—demonstrate their commitment to life by treating homicide as serious crime. Moreover, the majority of States in this country have laws imposing criminal penalties on one who assists another to commit suicide. We do not think a State is required to remain neutral in the face of an informed and voluntary decision by a physically-able adult to starve to death.

But in the context presented here, a State has more particular interests at stake. The choice between life and death is a deeply personal decision of obvious and overwhelming finality. We believe Missouri may legitimately seek to safeguard the personal element of this choice through the imposition of heightened evidentiary requirements. It cannot be disputed that the Due Process Clause protects an interest in life as well as an interest in refusing life-sustaining medical treatment. Not all incompetent patients will have loved ones available to serve as surrogate decisionmakers. And even where family members are present, "[t]here will, of course, be some unfortunate situations in which family members will not act to protect a patient." A State is entitled to guard against potential abuses in such situations. Similarly, a State is entitled to consider that a judicial proceeding to make a determination regarding an incompetent's wishes may very well not be an adversarial one, with the added guarantee of accurate factfinding that the adversary process brings with it. Finally, we think a State may properly decline to make judgments about the "quality" of life that a particular individual may enjoy, and simply assert an unqualified interest in the preservation of human life to be weighed against the constitutionally protected interests of the individual.

In our view, Missouri has permissibly sought to advance these interests through the adoption of a "clear and convincing" standard of proof to govern such proceedings. . . .

We think it self-evident that the interests at stake in the instant proceedings are more substantial, both on an individual and societal level, than those involved in a run-of-the-mine civil dispute. But not only does the standard of proof reflect the importance of a particular adjudication, it also serves as "a societal judgment about how the risk of error should be distributed between the litigants." The more stringent the burden of proof a party must bear, the more that party bears the risk of an erroneous decision. We believe that Missouri may permissibly place an increased risk of an erroneous decision on those seeking to terminate an incompetent individual's life-sustaining treatment. An erroneous decision not to terminate results in a maintenance of the status quo; the possibility of subsequent developments such as advancements in medical science, the discovery of new evidence regarding the patient's intent, changes in the law, or simply the unexpected death of the patient despite the administration of life-sustaining treatment, at least create the potential that a wrong decision will eventually be corrected or its impact mitigated. An erroneous decision to withdraw life-sustaining treatment, however, is not susceptible of correction.

In sum, we conclude that a State may apply a clear and convincing evidence standard in proceedings where a guardian seeks to discontinue nutrition and hydration of a person diagnosed to be in a persistent vegetative state. We note that many courts which have adopted some sort of substituted judgment procedure in situations like this, whether they limit consideration of evidence to the prior expressed wishes of the incompetent individual, or whether they allow more general proof of what the individual's decision would have been, require a clear and convincing standard of proof for such evidence.

The Supreme Court of Missouri held that in this case the testimony adduced at trial did not amount to clear and convincing proof of the patient's desire to have hydration and nutrition withdrawn. In so doing, it reversed a decision of the Missouri trial court which had found that the evidence "suggest[ed]" Nancy Cruzan would not have desired to continue such measures, but which had not adopted the standard of "clear and convincing evidence" enunciated by the Supreme Court. The testimony adduced at trial consisted primarily of Nancy Cruzan's statements made to a housemate about a year before her accident that she would not want to live should she face life as a "vegetable," and other observations to the same effect. The observations did not deal in terms with withdrawal of medical treatment or of hydration and nutrition. We cannot say that the Supreme Court of Missouri committed constitutional error in reaching the conclusion that it did. . . .

. . . .

The judgment of the Supreme Court of Missouri is *Affirmed.*

[The concurring opinion of Justice O'Connor is omitted.]
JUSTICE SCALIA, concurring.

The various opinions in this case portray quite clearly the difficult, indeed agonizing, questions that are presented by the constantly increasing power of science to keep the human body alive for longer than any reasonable person would want to inhabit it. The States have begun to grapple with these problems through legislation. I am concerned, from the tenor of today's opinions, that we are poised to confuse that enterprise as successfully as we have confused the enterprise of legislating concerning abortion—requiring it to be conducted against a background of federal constitutional imperatives that are unknown because they are being newly crafted from Term to Term. That would be a great misfortune.

While I agree with the Court's analysis today, and therefore join in its opinion, I would have preferred that we announce, clearly and promptly, that the federal courts have no business in this field; that American law has always accorded the State the power to prevent, by force if necessary, suicide—including suicide by refusing to take appropriate measures necessary to preserve one's life; that the point at which life becomes "worthless," and the point at which the means necessary to preserve it become "extraordinary" or "inappropriate," are neither set forth in the Constitution nor known to the nine Justices of this Court any better than they are known to nine people picked at random from the Kansas City telephone directory; and hence, that even when it is demonstrated by clear and convincing evidence that a patient no longer wishes certain measures to be taken to preserve her life, it is up to the citizens of Missouri to decide, through their elected representatives, whether that wish will be honored. It is quite impossible (because the Constitution says nothing about the matter) that those citizens will decide upon a line less lawful than the one we would choose; and it is unlikely (because we know no more about "life-and-death" than they do) that they will decide upon a line less reasonable. . . .

Justice BRENNAN, with whom Justice MARSHALL and Justice BLACKMUN join, dissenting.

"Medical technology has effectively created a twilight zone of suspended animation where death commences while life, in some form, continues. Some patients, however, want no part of a life sustained only by medical technology. Instead, they prefer a plan of medical treatment that allows nature to take its course and permits them to die with dignity."

Nancy Cruzan has dwelt in that twilight zone for six years. She is oblivious to her surroundings and will remain so. Her body twitches only reflexively, without consciousness. The areas of her brain that once thought, felt, and experienced sensations have degenerated badly and are continuing to do so. The cavities remaining are filling with cerebrospinal fluid. The " 'cerebral cortical atrophy is irreversible, permanent, progressive and ongoing.' " "Nancy will never interact meaningfully with her environment again. She will remain in a persistent vegetative state until her death." Because she cannot swallow, her nutrition and hydration are delivered through a tube surgically implanted in her stomach.

A grown woman at the time of the accident, Nancy had previously expressed her wish to forgo continuing medical care under circumstances such as these. Her family and her friends are convinced that this is what she would want. A guardian ad litem appointed by the trial court is also convinced that this is what Nancy would want. Yet the Missouri Supreme Court, alone among state courts deciding such a question, has determined that an irreversibly vegetative patient will remain a passive prisoner of medical technology—for Nancy, perhaps for the next 30 years.

Today the Court, while tentatively accepting that there is some degree of constitutionally protected liberty interest in avoiding unwanted medical treatment, including life-sustaining medical treatment such as artificial nutrition and hydration, affirms the decision of the Missouri Supreme Court. The majority opinion, as I read it, would affirm that decision on the ground that a State may require "clear and convincing" evidence of Nancy Cruzan's prior decision to forgo life-sustaining treatment under circumstances such as hers in order to ensure that her actual wishes are honored. Because I believe that Nancy Cruzan has a fundamental right to be free of unwanted artificial nutrition and hydration, which right is not outweighed by any interests of the State, and because I find that the improperly biased procedural obstacles imposed by the Missouri Supreme Court impermissibly burden that right, I respectfully dissent. Nancy Cruzan is entitled to choose to die with dignity. . . .

JUSTICE STEVENS, dissenting.

Our Constitution is born of the proposition that all legitimate governments must secure the equal right of every person to "Life, Liberty, and the pursuit of Happiness." In the ordinary case we quite naturally assume that these three ends are compatible, mutually enhancing, and perhaps even coincident.

The Court would make an exception here. It permits the State's abstract, undifferentiated interest in the preservation of life to overwhelm the best interests of Nancy Beth Cruzan, interests which would, according to an undisputed finding, be served by allowing her guardians to exercise her constitutional right to discontinue medical treatment. Ironically, the Court reaches this conclusion despite endorsing three significant propositions which should save it from any such dilemma. First, a competent individual's decision to refuse life-sustaining medical procedures is an aspect of liberty protected by the Due Process Clause of the Fourteenth Amendment. Second, upon a proper evidentiary showing, a qualified guardian may make that decision on behalf of an incompetent ward. Third, in answering the important question presented by this tragic case, it is wise "not to attempt by any general statement, to cover every possible phase of the subject." Together, these considerations suggest that Nancy Cruzan's liberty to be free from medical treatment must be understood in light of the facts and circumstances particular to her.

I would so hold: in my view, the Constitution requires the State to care for Nancy Cruzan's life in a way that gives appropriate respect to her own best interests.

. . . .

Discussion Questions

1. *Cruzan* created a furor when decided by the Missouri Supreme Court. The Missouri court's opinion is replete with citations to 54 other right-to-die cases that—as the court admitted—uniformly allow nutrition and hydration to be withdrawn under these circumstances. Nevertheless, the Missouri decision came out against ending the treatment. How much do you believe a court should defer to overwhelming authority from other states?

2. Based on the U.S. Supreme Court's decision in *Cruzan*, what do you believe it would say about a less stringent burden of proof (i.e., "preponderance of evidence") that another state might adopt? Would the Court approve a state ruling that a surrogate (e.g., a spouse or family member) could make the life-or-death decision without *any* evidence of the patient's wishes?

3. The Missouri court put considerable emphasis on whether the continuation of the artificial nutrition and hydration was burdensome to Nancy (holding that it was not). Is this a valid consideration? Are there others? What should the ethical standard be for making judgments about the termination of treatment?

4. The majority of the Missouri court made a point of deferring to the legislature for making the public policy decisions required in this area, yet one of the dissenters considered this an abdication of judicial responsibility. Which of these positions is more persuasive to you?

5. Suppose the Cruzan family had foreseen the agony they would have to go through and had refused to consent to the initial surgery that implanted the gastrostomy tube. Could the state have required the surgery to be performed? Do you think it matters (medically, ethically, or legally) whether the refusal relates to starting a treatment or discontinuing a treatment already begun?

Comment

Following the U.S. Supreme Court's decision, the *Cruzan* case returned to the trial court in Missouri. After hearing additional testimony, the court judge ruled that the evidence was clear and convincing, and he again ruled that Nancy Cruzan's artificially supplied nutrition and hydration could be withdrawn. The state attorney general declined to appeal, the treatment was terminated, and Nancy Cruzan died in a matter of days.

In re A.C.
533 A.2d 611 (D.C. 1987)

Nebeker, J.

This appeal presented an emergency request for a stay of a Superior Court order permitting a Caesarean section on a terminally ill woman who was *in extremis*. This opinion is written after the fact; its purpose is to assist others and to test this court's decision with analysis of precedent—some of which was not considered at the time of decision. Counsel are commended for their assistance to the courts—trial and appellate. Condolences are extended to those who lost the mother and child.

History tells us that innumerable health care emergency issues used to be decided within the family and medical circle. In the past few decades, for reasons similar to many of those prompting expanded recourse to the courts generally, health care providers have sought equitable or declaratory action approving or directing active or passive treatment of ill or injured patients. These patients—sometimes with family or friends in attendance—are often *in extremis*; some are not conscious or are otherwise unable to express present desire; some are minors or, as here, in fetal state.

Complex issues—legal, moral and religious—are presented, and courts, though they must under present circumstances, are often hard pressed to arrive at a right answer. The courts do, however, make the final mortal decision. That is, in itself, probably the best that can be said of the process. It would be far better if, by legislation, these bio-ethical decisions could be made by duly constituted and informed ethical groups within the health care system, and if desired, appellate review as provided in other administrative proceedings. In this way, the need to attempt to inform judges of, to them, complex medical facts on very short notice could be eliminated.

On June 16, 1987, George Washington University and George Washington University Hospital (the hospital) sought a declaratory order from the Superior Court "as to what it should do in terms of the fetus, whether to intervene [by Caesarean section] and save its life." The trial court, after a hearing at the hospital, determined that the hospital should proceed with the operation, and an appeal was taken and a stay sought. Later that day, after a telephone conference call hearing, this court issued an order denying the motion for stay. That order effectively ended the appeal; the operation was performed, and the child and mother died soon thereafter.

I.

A.C. was diagnosed with leukemia when she was thirteen years old. As part of her treatment, she underwent a number of major surgical procedures, therapy, and chemotherapy. When she was twenty-seven years old, after her cancer had been in remission for three years, A.C. married. At the time she became pregnant, she had not undergone chemotherapy for more than a year. In her fifteenth week of pregnancy, she was referred to the hospital's high-risk pregnancy clinic.

When A.C. was approximately twenty-five weeks pregnant, she went to her regularly scheduled prenatal visit complaining of shortness of breath and some pain in her back. Her physicians subsequently discovered that she had a tumor mass in her lung which was most likely a metastatic oxygenic carcinoma. She was admitted to the hospital on June 11 and her prognosis was terminal.

On June 15, during A.C.'s twenty-sixth week of pregnancy, A.C., her physicians, her mother, and her husband discussed the possibility of providing A.C. with radiation therapy or chemotherapy to relieve her pain and to continue her pregnancy. Her physicians believed that her unborn child's chances of viability would be greatly increased if it were delivered when it had reached twenty-eight weeks gestational age. By June 16, the date on which the hospital sought the declaratory order in the Superior Court, A.C. had been heavily sedated so that she could continue to breathe. Her condition was declining, and the attending medical staff concluded that passive treatment was appropriate because the mother would not survive and the child's chances of survival were grim. The hospital administration then decided to test this decision in the Superior Court.

The trial court appointed counsel for A.C. and the fetus, respectively. The District of Columbia was permitted to intervene for the fetus as *parens patriae*. A hearing was held at the hospital and was transcribed.

There was some dispute about whether A.C. would have chosen to have a Caesarean section on June 16. Before she was sedated, A.C. indicated that she would choose to relinquish her life so that the fetus could survive should such a choice present itself at the fetus' gestational age of twenty-eight weeks. Her physicians never discussed with her what her choice would be if such a choice had to be made before the fetus reached the twenty-eight-week point. The fetus was suffering oxygen starvation and resultant rapid heart rate. There was at that point less than 20 percent chance that it would be afflicted with cerebral palsy, neurological defects, deafness and blindness. There was not a clear medical consensus on the course of A.C.'s treatment. Those physicians who objected to the proposed surgery did so because A.C. refused her consent to the procedure, not because the surgery was medically objectionable. One physician testified that he believed that A.C. would not have wanted to deliver a baby that might have to undergo the pain of having handicaps that are associated with premature delivery. Another physician believed that A.C. would not have refused permission for the Caesarean section to be performed. During the course of her pregnancy, however, A.C. was aware that a number of medications she was taking might harm the fetus. Nevertheless, she expressed a desire to her physicians to be kept as comfortable as possible throughout her pregnancy and to maintain the quality of her life.

The trial court determined that the fetus was viable and that the District of Columbia had an interest in protecting the potential life of the fetus. Relying on an earlier Superior Court decision, the court decided that the Caesarean section should be performed.

Shortly after the trial judge made his decision, A.C. was informed of it. She stated, during a period of lucidity, that she would agree to the surgery although she might not survive it. When another physician went to A.C. to verify her decision, she apparently changed her mind, mouthing the words, "I don't want it done." There was no explanation for either decision.

After our Clerk was advised of the desire to appeal, a telephonic hearing was had before a hastily assembled division of the court. The trial judge's findings were read to us, and we heard from counsel and an attending physician. The latter answered questions respecting the relative chances of survival of both A.C. and the fetus with and without the surgery. He also informed us of the rapid decline of A.C. and the need to proceed promptly with the surgery, if it was decided to do so. There was no time to have the transcript read or to do effective research. The atypical nature of the appellate hearing included our hearing directly from one of the physicians.

The court based its decision to deny a stay on the medical judgment that A.C would not survive for a significant time after the surgery and that the fetus had a better, though slim, chance if taken before A.C.'s imminent death. If A.C. died before delivery, the fetus would die as well. Though A.C. might have lived twenty-four to forty-eight hours, the surgery might have hastened her death. The ordinary question of likelihood of ultimate success on the merits was deemed subsumed in the immediate necessity to balance the delicate interests of fetus survival with the other's condition and options on her behalf.

In retrospect, we must acknowledge that any attempt to use rules on stay procedures places appellate form over substance. No appeal in this case could mature. We decided the entire matter when we denied the stay.

II.

We could begin our analysis of the law, which some may reasonably hold to be self-justifying, by testing ordinary rules for a stay against these facts. And we well know that we may have shortened A.C.'s life span by a few hours. We do not think we should opine whether the decision would have or should have been different if her quality of life during that period had been better than it was.

In recent years, a number of commentators have written on the propriety of court-ordered Caesarean sections. These articles and notes demonstrate the difficult task a court faces when presented with a woman whose significant interest in her bodily integrity must be balanced against the state's interest in potential human life. It is, of course, always preferable to avoid a court order at odds with the medical judgment of the doctor who will carry it out.

This is a case of first impression for this court. In fact, only one other appellate court in the nation has reported that it squarely addressed the issue of whether and when a court should order or permit that a Caesarean section be performed on a woman. *Jefferson* is of limited help for our purposes. Here, the mother was not near term for delivery; in *Jefferson*, the mother was at term. Furthermore, the performance of a Caesarean section would not clearly prevent the death of the mother or the child in this case; in *Jefferson*, both the mother and child would almost certainly have survived the performance of a Caesarean section.

It is appropriate here to state that this case is not about abortion. The Supreme Court has made clear that state legislation may not altogether prohibit a woman from making the decision to terminate her pregnancy. However, when a fetus becomes viable, that is, when the fetus is "potentially able to live outside the mother's womb albeit with artificial aid," the state had a compelling interest in protecting the "potentiality of human life," as well as the life and health of the mother. Thus, as a matter of law, the right of a woman to an abortion is different and distinct from her obligations to the fetus once she has decided not to timely terminate her pregnancy. With a viable fetus, a balancing of interests must replace the single interest of the mother, and as in this case, time can be a critical factor.

We next view this case within the context of its closest legal analogues: the right of an adult to refuse medical treatment and the right of a parent to refuse medical treatment on behalf of offspring.

A number of courts have explicitly or implicitly recognized the right of individuals to bodily integrity. The right to bodily integrity exists within the penumbral right to privacy guaranteed by the Ninth and Fourteenth Amendments to the United States Constitution.

The fundamental right to bodily integrity encompasses an adult's right to refuse medical treatment, even if the refusal will result in death. . . . The right of an adult to refuse medical treatment is not absolute, however. The state has four countervailing interests in sustaining a person's life: preserving life, preventing suicide, maintaining the integrity of the medical profession, and protecting innocent third parties. The state's interest in preventing suicide is not relevant here, nor is safeguarding the integrity of the medical profession.

The state's interest in preserving life usually will not override an adult's right to refuse medical treatment. In most cases where a court orders an adult to receive medical treatment against his consent, it will be to protect innocent third parties who would be harmed by the adult's decision.

The conclusion we draw from these cases is that in most circumstances, an adult's right to bodily integrity precludes the state from intervening in the adult's decision to refuse medical treatment. The state's interest in the preservation of life, the prevention of suicide, and the integrity of the medical profession, while significant, usually will not overcome the individual's right to bodily integrity.

The state's interest in protecting innocent third parties from an adult's decision to refuse medical treatment, however, may override the interest in bodily integrity. In *Prince v. Massachusetts* (1944), the Supreme Court stated:

Parents may be free to become martyrs themselves. But it does not follow that they are free, in identical circumstances, to make martyrs of their children before they have reached the age of full and legal discretion when they can make that choice for themselves.

Courts have used this reasoning to hold that parents may not withhold life-saving treatment from their children because of the parents' religious beliefs. . . . The state may intervene even when a parent's refusal of medical treatment for his or her child does not place the child in danger of imminent death. . . .

Some jurisdictions have held that the doctrine is equally applicable to unborn children. . . .

There is a significant difference, however, between a court authorizing medical treatment for a child already born and a child who is yet unborn, although the state has compelling interests in protecting the life and health of both children and viable unborn children. Where birth has occurred, the medical treatment does not infringe on the mother's right to bodily integrity. With an unborn child, the state's interest in preserving the health of the child may run squarely against the mother's interest in her bodily integrity.

It can be argued that the state may not infringe upon the mother's right to bodily integrity to protect the life or health of her unborn child unless to do so will not significantly affect the health of the mother and unless the child has a significant chance of being alive. Performing Caesarean sections will, in most instances, have an effect on the condition of the mother. That effect may be temporary in otherwise normal patients. The surgery presents a number of common complications, including infection, hemorrhage, gastric aspiration of the stomach contents, and postoperative embolism. It also produces considerable discomfort. In some cases, the surgery will result in the mother's death.

Even though we recognize these considerations, we think they should not have been dispositive here. The Caesarean section would not significantly affect A.C.'s condition because she had, at best, two days left of sedated life; the complications arising from the surgery would not significantly alter that prognosis. The child, on the other hand, had a chance of surviving delivery, despite the possibility that it would be born handicapped. Accordingly, we concluded that the trial judge did not err in subordinating A.C.'s right against bodily intrusion to the interests of the unborn child and the state, and hence we denied the motion for stay.

In conclusion, we observe that the judicial process in this case did not require a physician or the hospital as a separate entity to perform a procedure against an expressed medical judgment. The hospital had sought a declaratory order whether to intervene with surgery given the mother's last-minute objection, an objection for which there may have been one or more reasons. There were physicians willing to operate and staff able to care for the fetus as needed. With the competing legal interests of the mother (some of which would survive her), and those of the fetus or child, it is understandable why the hospital sought before-the-fact judicial pronouncement of its duties. The balancing of the many factors presented ought, however, to be left to a sort of quasi-official body where the judiciary plays an appropriate and limited reviewing role, rather than the primary adjudicator in a highly charged and short time frame.

Finally, we wish to express our appreciation to counsel and the trial judge for a difficult task well done despite the pressures created by time and tragic circumstances.

Discussion Questions

1. Why is the patient identified only as A.C.?

2. The court states, "It would be far better [than litigating the issues] if, by legislation, these bio-ethical decisions could be made by duly constituted and informed ethical groups within the health care system . . . ." Do you agree? How would such groups be chosen? By whom? Using what standards? And on what basis would they make their decisions? And why would their decisions be any more likely to be "correct" than those of the courts?

3. The facts of the case are somewhat uncertain, especially regarding A.C.'s intent. How significant is this for the court?

4. How important should it be that the fetus might be born with handicaps?

5. How would you frame the issue in this case? How well has the court dealt with that issue?

6. Do you agree that, "as a matter of law, the right of a woman to an abortion is different and distinct from her obligations to the fetus once she has decided not to timely terminate her pregnancy"? Is it legally consistent and logical to say that a woman cannot be forced to bear a child when she wants to have an abortion but can be forced to do so when someone wants her to submit to a Caesarean section? Why or why not?

11

Family Planning

Courts of law today are asked to decide many of society's most perplexing problems. The judicial system of this country is daily asked to apply Solomonic wisdom to virtually intractable social, moral, ethical, and economic controversies, all of which are masked in the guise of legal principles. Although the system seems often imperfectly constructed to do so, it must make a decision in every justiciable case.

Much of the litigation involving these kinds of issues has arisen along with increases in scientific and medical technology. For example, as doctors develop advanced reproductive techniques such as *in vitro* fertilization, questions will inevitably continue to surface regarding parental and custodial rights. For lack of any traditional or alternative forums for such disputes, the questions often find their way into a courtroom. Similarly, as societal attitudes and mores change, the courts will likely be asked to determine the boundaries of the sort contemplated by the *Baby M* case. Finally, as medical technology expands, particularly in the area of neonatal care and treatment, courts have been asked to reevaluate past decisions in light of changing conditions. The extent to which such decisions can or should be modified remains a continual source of judicial inquiry, particularly in the area of abortion.

As long as society wants, needs, or is required to have such family planning matters resolved and as long as reasonable alternative forums are not developed, these issues will continue to be heard in our country's courtrooms. This state of affairs is likely to persist well into the future.

As to the nation's health care providers, judicial decisions in this area will influence both the nature and the extent of the services they are able and willing to provide. With hospital policies being the subject of frequent litigation in one aspect or another, health care leaders will need to be cognizant of potential legal liability.

The liability of health care institutions, generally, will be further explored in Chapter 13. In the meantime, the difficulty courts have with these kinds of issues is seen in this chapter titled "Family Planning." The student will readily appreciate that the cases present not so much an appreciation of legal points but the tensions between profound human emotions. The following cases, perhaps more so than others in this book, should be understood for their underlying real-life stories as much as for their precedent value.

Buck v. Bell
274 U.S. 200 (1927)

Holmes, J.

This is a writ of error to review a judgment of the Supreme Court of Appeals of the State of Virginia, affirming a judgment of the Circuit Court of Amherst County, by which the defendant in error, the superintendent of the State Colony for Epileptics and Feeble Minded, was ordered to perform the operation of salpingectomy upon Carrie Buck, the plaintiff in error, for the purpose of making her sterile. The case comes here upon the contention that the statute authorizing the judgment is void under the Fourteenth Amendment as denying to the plaintiff in error due process of law and the equal protection of the laws.

Carrie Buck is a feeble minded white woman who was committed to the State Colony above mentioned in due form. She is the daughter of a feeble minded mother in the same institution, and the mother of an illegitimate feeble minded child. She was eighteen years old at the time of the trial of her case in the Circuit Court, in the latter part of 1924. An Act of

Virginia, approved March 20, 1924, recites that the health of the patient and the welfare of society may be promoted in certain cases by the sterilization of mental defectives, under careful safeguard, &c.; that the sterilization may be effected in males by vasectomy and in females by salpingectomy, without serious pain or substantial danger to life; that the Commonwealth is supporting in various institutions many defective persons who if now discharged would become a menace but if incapable of procreating might be discharged with safety and become self-supporting with benefit to themselves and to society; and that experience has shown that heredity plays an important part in the transmission of insanity, imbecility, &c. The statute then enacts that whenever the superintendent of certain institutions including the above named State Colony shall be of opinion that it is for the best interests of the patients and of society that an inmate under his care should be sexually sterilized, he may have the operation performed upon any patient afflicted with hereditary forms of insanity, imbecility, &c., on complying with the very careful provisions by which the act protects the patients from possible abuse.

The superintendent first presents a petition to the special board of directors of his hospital or colony, stating the facts and the grounds for his opinion, verified by affidavit. Notice of the petition and of the time and place of the hearing in the institution is to be served upon the inmate, and also upon his guardian, and if there is no guardian the superintendent is to apply to the Circuit Court of the County to appoint one. If the inmate is a minor notice also is to be given to his parents if any with a copy of the petition. The board is to see to it that the inmate may attend the hearings if desired by him or his guardian. The evidence is all to be reduced to writing, and after the board has made its order for or against the operation, the superintendent, or the inmate, or his guardian, may appeal to the Circuit Court of the County. The Circuit Court may consider the record of the board and the evidence before it and such other admissible evidence as may be offered, and may affirm, revise, or reverse the order of the board and enter such order as it deems just. Finally any party may apply to the Supreme Court of Appeals, which, if it grants the appeal, is to hear the case upon the record of the trial in the Circuit Court and may enter such order as it thinks the Circuit Court should have entered. There can be no doubt that so far as procedure is concerned the rights of the patient are most carefully considered, and as every step in this case was taken in scrupulous compliance with the statute and after months of observation, there is no doubt that in that respect the plaintiff in error has had due process of law.

The attack is not upon the procedure but upon the substantive law. It seems to be contended that in no circumstances could such an order be justified. It certainly is contended that the order cannot be justified upon the existing grounds. The judgment finds the facts that have been recited and that Carrie Buck "is the probable potential parent of so-

cially inadequate offspring, likewise afflicted, that she may be sexually sterilized without detriment to her general health and that her welfare and that of society will be promoted by her sterilization," and thereupon makes the order. In view of the general declarations of the legislature and the specific findings of the Court, obviously we cannot say as matter of law that the grounds do not exist, and if they exist they justify the result. We have seen more than once that the public welfare may call upon the best citizens for their lives. It would be strange if it could not call upon those who already sap the strength of the State for these lesser sacrifices, often not felt to be such by those concerned, in order to prevent our being swamped with incompetence. It is better for all the world, if instead of waiting to execute degenerate offspring for crime, or to let them starve for their imbecility, society can prevent those who are manifestly unfit from continuing their kind. The principle that sustains compulsory vaccination is broad enough to cover cutting the Fallopian tubes. Three generations of imbeciles are enough.

But, it is said, however it might be if this reasoning were applied generally, it fails when it is confined to the small number who are in the institutions named and is not applied to the multitudes outside. It is the usual last resort of constitutional arguments to point out shortcomings of this sort. But the answer is that the law does all that is needed when it does all that it can, indicates a policy, applies it to all within the lines, and seeks to bring within the lines all similarly situated so far and so fast as its means allow. Of course so far as the operations enable those who otherwise must be kept confined to be returned to the world, and thus open the asylum to others, the equality aimed at will be more nearly reached.

Judgment affirmed.

Skinner v. Oklahoma ex rel. Attorney Gen.
316 U.S. 535 (1942)

Douglas, J.

This case touches a sensitive and important area of human rights. Oklahoma deprives certain individuals of a right which is basic to the perpetuation of a race—the right to have offspring. Oklahoma has decreed the enforcement of its law against petitioner, overruling his claim that it violated the Fourteenth Amendment. Because that decision raised grave and substantial constitutional questions, we granted the petition for certiorari.

The statute involved is Oklahoma's Habitual Criminal Sterilization Act. That Act defines an "habitual criminal" as a person who, having been convicted two or more times for crimes "amounting to felonies involving moral turpitude," either in an Oklahoma court or in a court of any other State, is thereafter convicted of such a felony in Oklahoma and is sentenced to a term of imprisonment in an Oklahoma penal institution. Machinery is provided for the institution by the Attorney General of a proceeding against such a person in the Oklahoma courts for a judgment that such person shall be rendered sexually sterile. Notice, an opportunity to be heard, and the right to a jury trial are provided. The issues triable in such a proceeding are narrow and confined. If the court or jury finds that the defendant is an "habitual criminal" and that he "may be rendered sexually sterile without detriment to his or her general health," then the court "shall render judgment to the effect that said defendant be rendered sexually sterile" by the operation of vasectomy in case of a male, and of salpingectomy in case of a female. Only one other provision of the Act is material here, and that is [a section] which provides that "offenses arising out of the violation of the prohibitory laws, revenue acts, embezzlement, or political offenses, shall not come or be considered within the terms of this Act."

Petitioner was convicted in 1926 of the crime of stealing chickens, and was sentenced to the Oklahoma State Reformatory. In 1929 he was convicted of the crime of robbery with firearms, and was sentenced to the reformatory. In 1934 he was convicted again of robbery with firearms, and was sentenced to the penitentiary. He was confined there in 1935 when the Act was passed. In 1936 the Attorney General instituted proceedings against him. Petitioner in his answer challenged the Act as unconstitutional by reason of the Fourteenth Amendment. A jury trial was had. The court instructed the jury that the crimes of which petitioner had been convicted were felonies involving moral turpitude, and that the only question for the jury was whether the operation of vasectomy could be performed on petitioner without detriment to his general health. The jury found that it could be. A judgment directing that the operation of vasectomy be performed on petitioner was affirmed by the Supreme Court of Oklahoma by a five to four decision.

Several objections to the constitutionality of the Act have been pressed upon us. It is urged that the Act cannot be sustained as an exercise of the police power, in view of the state of scientific authorities respecting inheritability of criminal traits. It is argued that due process is lacking because, under this Act, unlike the Act upheld in *Buck v. Bell*, the defendant is given no opportunity to be heard on the issue as to whether he is the probable potential parent of socially undesirable offspring. . . . It is also suggested that the Act is penal in character and that the sterilization provided for is cruel and unusual punishment and violative of the Fourteenth Amendment. . . . We pass those points without intimating an opinion on them, for there is a feature of the Act which clearly condemns it. That is, its failure to meet the requirements of the equal protection clause of the Fourteenth Amendment.

We do not stop to point out all of the inequalities in this Act. A few examples will suffice. In Oklahoma, grand larceny is a felony. Larceny is grand larceny when the property taken exceeds $20 in value. Embezzlement is punishable "in the manner prescribed for feloniously stealing property of the value of that embezzled." Hence, he who embezzles property worth more than $20 is guilty of a felony. A clerk who appropriates over $20 from his employer's till and a stranger who steals the same amount are thus both guilty of felonies. If the latter repeats his act and is convicted three times, he may be sterilized. But the clerk is not subject to the pains and penalties of the Act no matter how large his embezzlements nor how frequent his convictions. A person who enters a chicken coop and steals chickens commits a felony and he may be sterilized if he is thrice convicted. If, however, he is a bailee of the property and fraudulently appropriates it, he is an embezzler. Hence, no matter how habitual his proclivities for embezzlement are and no matter how often his conviction, he may not be sterilized. Thus, the nature of the two crimes is intrinsically the same and they are punishable in the same manner. Furthermore, the line between them follows close distinctions—distinctions comparable to those highly technical ones which shaped the common law as to "trespass" or "taking." There may be larceny by fraud rather than embezzlement even where the owner of the personal property delivers it to the defendant, if the latter has at that time "a fraudulent intention to make use of the possession as a means of converting such property to his own use, and does so convert it." If the fraudulent intent occurs later and the defendant converts the property, he is guilty of embezzlement. Whether a particular act is larceny by fraud or embezzlement thus turns not on the intrinsic quality of the act but on when the felonious intent arose—a question for the jury under appropriate instructions.

It was stated in *Buck v. Bell* that the claim that state legislation violates the equal protection clause of the Fourteenth Amendment is "the usual last resort of constitutional arguments." Under our constitutional system the States in determining the reach and scope of particular legislation need not provide "abstract symmetry." They may mark and set apart the classes and types of problems according to the needs and as dictated or suggested by experience. It was in that connection that Mr. Justice Holmes . . . stated [in another case], "We must remember that the machinery of government would not work if it were not allowed a little play in its joints." . . .

But the instant legislation runs afoul of the equal protection clause, though we give Oklahoma that large deference which the rule of the foregoing cases requires. We are dealing here with legislation which involves one of the basic civil rights of man. Marriage and procreation are fundamental to the very existence and survival of the race. The power to sterilize, if exercised, may have subtle, far-reaching and devastating effects. In evil or reckless hands it can cause races or types which are inimical to the dominant group to wither and disappear. There is no redemption for the individual whom the law touches. Any experiment which the State conducts is to his irreparable injury. He is forever deprived of a basic liberty. We mention these matters not to reexamine the scope of the police power of the States. We advert to them merely in emphasis of our view that strict scrutiny of the classification which a State makes in a sterilization law is essential, lest unwittingly, or otherwise, invidious discriminations are made against groups or types of individuals in violation of the constitutional guaranty of just and equal laws. The guaranty of "equal protection of the laws is a pledge of the protection of equal laws." When the law lays an unequal hand on those who have committed intrinsically the same quality of offense and sterilizes one and not the other, it has made as invidious a discrimination as if it had selected a particular race or nationality for oppressive treatment. Sterilization of those who have thrice committed grand larceny, with immunity for those who are embezzlers, is a clear, pointed, unmistakable discrimination. Oklahoma makes no attempt to say that he who commits larceny by trespass or trick or fraud has biologically inheritable traits which he who commits embezzlement lacks. Oklahoma's line between larceny by fraud and embezzlement is determined, as we have noted, "with reference to the time when the fraudulent intent to convert the property to the taker's own use" arises. We have not the slightest basis for inferring that that line has any significance in eugenics, nor that the inheritability of criminal traits follows the neat legal distinctions which the law has marked between those two offenses. In terms of fines and imprisonment, the crimes of larceny and embezzlement rate the same under the Oklahoma code. Only when it comes to sterilization are the pains and penalties of the law different. The equal protection clause would indeed be a formula of empty words if such conspicuously artificial lines could be drawn. In *Buck v. Bell*, the Virginia statute was upheld though it applied only to feeble-minded persons in institutions of the State. But it was pointed out that "so far as the operations enable those who otherwise must be kept confined to be returned to the world, and thus open the asylum to others, the equality aimed at will be more nearly reached." Here there is no such saving feature. Embezzlers are forever free. Those who steal or take in other ways are not. If such a classification were permitted, the technical common law concept of a "trespass" based on distinctions which are "very largely dependent upon history for explanation" could readily become a rule of human genetics.

It is true that the Act has a broad severability clause. But we will not endeavor to determine whether its application would solve the equal protection difficulty. The Supreme Court of Oklahoma sustained the Act without reference to the severability clause. We have therefore a situation where the Act as construed and applied to petitioner is allowed to perpetuate the discrimination which we have found to be fatal. Whether the severability clause would be so applied as to remove this particular constitutional objection is a question which may be more appropriately left for adjudication by the Oklahoma court. That is reemphasized here by our uncertainty as to what excision, if any, would be made as a matter of Oklahoma law. It is by no means clear whether, if an exci-

sion were made, this particular constitutional difficulty might be solved by enlarging on the one hand or contracting on the other the class of criminals who might be sterilized.

Reversed.

Discussion Questions

1. Contrast the Holmes decision in *Buck v. Bell* with that of Douglas in *Skinner*. Is there a presumption that both health and criminal proclivity are inherited?

2. Are you persuaded by Justice Douglas's attempts to distinguish *Buck* from *Skinner*?

3. In the 1930's, Hereditary Health Courts were established in Nazi Germany to enforce sterilization laws on individuals suspected of heriditary diseases and other defects. *See generally* Litton, *The Nazi Doctors: Medical Killing and the Psychology of Genocide* 22–44 (1986). Should forced sterilization ever be allowed? If so, under what circumstances?

Griswold v. Connecticut
381 U.S. 479 (1965)

Douglas, J.

Appellant Griswold is Executive Director of the Planned Parenthood League of Connecticut. Appellant Buxton is a licensed physician and a professor at the Yale Medical School who served as Medical Director for the League at its Center in New Haven—a center open and operating from November 1 to November 10, 1961, when appellants were arrested.

They gave information, instruction, and medical advice to married persons as to the means of preventing conception. They examined the wife and prescribed the best contraceptive device or material for her use. Fees were usually charged, although some couples were serviced free.

The statutes whose constitutionality is involved in this appeal are §§ 53-32 and 54-196 of the General Statutes of Connecticut. The former provides:

"Any person who uses any drug, medicinal article or instrument for the purpose of preventing conception shall be fined not less than fifty dollars or imprisoned not less than sixty days nor more than one year or be both fined and imprisoned."

Section 54-196 provides:

"Any person who assists, abets, counsels, causes, hires or commands another to commit any offense may be prosecuted and punished as if he were the principal offender."

The appellants were found guilty as accessories and fined $100 each, against the claim that the accessory statute as so applied violated the Fourteenth Amendment. The Appellate Division of the Circuit Court affirmed. The Supreme Court of Errors affirmed that judgment. . . .

. . . .

Coming to the merits, we are met with a wide range of questions that implicate the Due Process Clause of the Fourteenth Amendment. . . . We do not sit as a super-legislature to determine the wisdom, need, and propriety of laws that touch economic problems, business affairs, or social conditions. This law, however, operates directly on an intimate relation of husband and wife and their physician's role in one aspect of that relation.

The association of people is not mentioned in the Constitution nor in the Bill of Rights. The right to educate a child in a school of the parents' choice—whether public or private or parochial—is also not mentioned. Nor is the right to study any particular subject or any foreign language. Yet the First Amendment has been construed to include certain of those rights.

By *Pierce v. Society of Sisters*, the right to educate one's children as one chooses is made applicable to the States by the force of the First and Fourteenth Amendments. By *Meyer v. Nebraska*, the same dignity is given the right to study the German language in a private school. In other words, the State may not, consistently with the spirit of the First Amendment, contract the spectrum of available knowledge. The right of freedom of speech and press includes not only the right to utter or to print, but the right to distribute, the right to receive, the right to read and freedom of inquiry, freedom of thought, and freedom to teach—indeed the freedom of the entire university community. Without those peripheral rights the specific rights would be less secure. And so we reaffirm the principle of the *Pierce* and the *Meyer* cases.

In *NAACP v. Alabama*, we protected the "freedom to associate and privacy in one's associations," noting that freedom of association was a peripheral First Amendment right. Disclosure of membership lists of a constitutionally valid association, we held, was invalid "as entailing the likelihood of a substantial restraint upon the exercise by petitioner's members of their right to freedom of association." In other words, the First Amendment has a penumbra where privacy is protected from governmental intrusion. In like context, we have protected forms of "association" that are not political in the customary sense but pertain to the social, legal, and economic benefit of the members. In *Schware v. Board of Bar Examiners*, we held it not permissible to bar a lawyer from practice, because he had once been a member of the Communist Party. The man's "association with that Party" was not shown to be "anything more than a political faith in a political party" and was not action of a kind proving bad moral character.

Those cases involved more than the "right of assembly"—a right that extends to all irrespective of their race or ideology. The right of "association," like the right of belief, is more than the right to attend a meeting; it includes the right to express one's attitudes or philosophies by membership in a group or by affiliation with it or by other lawful means. Association in that context is a form of expression of opinion; and while it is not expressly included in the First Amendment its existence is necessary in making the express guarantees fully meaningful.

The foregoing cases suggest that specific guarantees in the Bill of Rights have penumbras, formed by emanations from those guarantees that help give them life and substance. Various guarantees create zones of privacy. The right of association contained in the penumbra of the First Amendment is one, as we have seen. The Third Amendment in its prohibition against the quartering of soldiers "in any house" in time of peace without the consent of the owner is another facet of that privacy. The Fourth Amendment explicitly affirms the "right of the people to be secure in their persons, houses, papers, and effects, against unreasonable searches and seizures." The Fifth Amendment in its Self-Incrimination Clause enables the citizen to create a zone of privacy which government may not force him to surrender to his detriment. The Ninth Amendment provides: "The enumeration in the Constitution, of certain rights, shall not be construed to deny or disparage others retained by the people."

The Fourth and Fifth Amendments were described in *Boyd v. United States*, as protection against all governmental invasions "of the sanctity of a man's home and the privacies of life." We recently referred in *Mapp v. Ohio*, to the Fourth Amendment as creating a "right to privacy, no less important than any other right carefully and particularly reserved to the people."

We have had many controversies over these penumbral rights of "privacy and repose." These cases bear witness that the right of privacy which presses for recognition here is a legitimate one.

The present case, then, concerns a relationship lying within the zone of privacy created by several fundamental constitutional guarantees. And it concerns a law which, in forbidding the use of contraceptives rather than regulating their manufacture or sale, seeks to achieve its goals by means having a maximum destructive impact upon that relationship. Such a law cannot stand in light of the familiar principle, so often applied by this Court, that a "governmental purpose to control or prevent activities constitutionally subject to state regulation may not be achieved by means which sweep unnecessarily broadly and thereby invade the area of protected freedoms." Would we allow the police to search the sacred precincts of marital bedrooms for telltale signs of the use of contraceptives? The very idea is repulsive to the notions of privacy surrounding the marriage relationship.

We deal with a right of privacy older than the Bill of Rights—older than our political parties, older than our school system. Marriage is a coming together for better or for worse, hopefully enduring, and intimate to the degree of being sacred. It is an association that promotes a way of life, not causes; a harmony in living, not political faiths; a bilateral loyalty, not commercial or social projects. Yet it is an association for as noble a purpose as any involved in our prior decisions.

Reversed.

. . . .

MR. JUSTICE BLACK, with whom MR. JUSTICE STEWART joins, dissenting.

I agree with my Brother STEWART'S dissenting opinion. And like him I do not to any extent whatever base my view that this Connecticut law is constitutional on a belief that the law is wise or that its policy is a good one. In order that there may be no room at all to doubt why I vote as I do, I feel constrained to add that the law is every bit as offensive to me as it is to my Brethren of the majority and my Brothers HARLAN, WHITE and GOLDBERG who, reciting reasons why it is offensive to them, hold it unconstitutional. There is no single one of the graphic and eloquent strictures and criticisms fired at the policy of this Connecticut law either by the Court's opinion or by those of my concurring Brethren to which I cannot subscribe—except their conclusion that the evil qualities they see in the law make it unconstitutional.

Had the doctor defendant here, or even the nondoctor defendant, been convicted for doing nothing more than expressing opinions to persons coming to the clinic that certain contraceptive devices, medicines or practices would do them good and would be desirable, or for telling people how devices could be used, I can think of no reasons at this time why their expressions of views would not be protected by the First and Fourteenth Amendments, which guarantee freedom of speech. But speech is one thing; conduct and physical activities are quite another. The two defendants here were active participants in an organization which gave physical examinations to women, advised them what kind of contraceptive devices or medicines would most likely be satisfactory for them, and then supplied the devices themselves, all for a graduated scale of fees, based on the family income. Thus these defendants admittedly engaged with others in a planned course of conduct to help people violate the Connecticut law. Merely because some speech was used in carrying on that conduct—just as in ordinary life some speech accompanies most kinds of conduct—we are not in my view justified in holding that the First Amendment forbids the State to punish their conduct. Strongly as I desire to protect all First Amendment freedoms, I am unable to stretch the Amendment so as to afford protection to the conduct of these defendants in violating the Connecticut law. What would be the constitutional fate of the law if hereafter applied to punish nothing but speech is, as I have said, quite another matter.

The Court talks about a constitutional "right of privacy" as though there is some constitutional provision or provisions forbidding any law ever to be passed which might abridge the "privacy" of individuals. But there is not. There are, of course, guarantees in certain specific constitutional provisions which are designed in part to protect privacy at certain times and places with respect to certain activities. Such, for example, is the Fourth Amendment's guarantee against "unreasonable searches and seizures." But I think it belittles that Amendment to talk about it as though it protects nothing but "privacy." To treat it that way is to give it a niggardly interpretation, not the kind of liberal reading I think any Bill of Rights provision should be given. The average man would very likely not have his feelings soothed any more by having his property seized openly than by having it seized privately and by stealth. He simply wants his property left alone. And a person can be just as much, if not more, irritated, annoyed and injured by an unceremonious public arrest by a policeman as he is by a seizure in the privacy of his office or home.

One of the most effective ways of diluting or expanding a constitutionally guaranteed right is to substitute for the crucial word or words of a constitutional guarantee another word or words, more or less flexible and more or less restricted in meaning. This fact is well illustrated by the use of the term "right of privacy" as a comprehensive substitute for the Fourth Amendment's guarantee against "unreasonable searches and seizures." "Privacy" is a broad, abstract and ambiguous concept which can easily be shrunken in meaning but which can also, on the other hand, easily be interpreted as a constitutional ban against many things other than searches and seizures. I have expressed the view many times that First Amendment freedoms, for example, have suffered from a failure of the courts to stick to the simple language of the First Amendment in construing it, instead of invoking multitudes of words substituted for those the Framers used. For these reasons I get nowhere in this case by talk about a constitutional "right of privacy" as an emanation from one or more constitutional provisions. I like my privacy as well as the next one, but I am nevertheless compelled to admit that government has a right to invade it unless prohibited by some specific constitutional provision. For these reasons I cannot agree with the Court's judgment and the reasons it gives for holding this Connecticut law unconstitutional.

MR. JUSTICE STEWART, whom MR. JUSTICE BLACK joins, dissenting.

Since 1879 Connecticut has had on its books a law which forbids the use of contraceptives by anyone. I think this is an uncommonly silly law. As a practical matter, the law is obviously unenforceable, except in the oblique context of the present case. As a philosophical matter, I believe the use of contraceptives in the relationship of marriage should be left to personal and private choice, based upon each individual's moral, ethical, and religious beliefs. As a matter of social policy, I think professional counsel about methods of birth control should be available to all, so that each individual's choice can be meaningfully made. But we are not asked in this case to say whether we think this law is unwise, or even asinine. We are asked to hold that it violates the United States Constitution. And that I cannot do.

In the course of its opinion the Court refers to no less than six Amendments to the Constitution: the First, the Third, the Fourth, the Fifth, the Ninth, and the Fourteenth. But the Court does not say which of these Amendments, if any, it thinks is infringed by this Connecticut law.

We are told that the Due Process Clause of the Fourteenth Amendment is not, as such, the "guide" in this case. With that much I agree. There is no claim that this law, duly enacted by the Connecticut Legislature, is unconstitutionally vague. There is no claim that the appellants were denied any of the elements of procedural due process at their trial, so as to make their convictions constitutionally invalid. And, as the Court says, the day has long passed since the Due Process Clause was regarded as a proper instrument for determining "the wisdom, need, and propriety" of state laws. My Brothers HARLAN and WHITE to the contrary, "we have returned to the original constitutional proposition that courts do not substitute their social and economic beliefs for the judgment of legislative bodies, who are elected to pass laws."

As to the First, Third, Fourth, and Fifth Amendments, I can find nothing in any of them to invalidate this Connecticut law, even assuming that all those Amendments are fully applicable against the States.[1] It has not even been argued that this is a law "respecting an establishment of religion, or prohibiting the free exercise thereof." And surely, unless the solemn process of constitutional adjudication is to descend to the level of a play on words, there is not involved here any abridgment of "the freedom of speech, or of the press; or the right of the people peaceably to assemble, and to petition the Government for a redress of grievances." No soldier has been quartered in any house. There has been no search, and no seizure. Nobody has been compelled to be a witness against himself.

The Court also quotes the Ninth Amendment, and my Brother GOLDBERG's concurring opinion relies heavily upon it. But to say that the Ninth Amendment has anything to do with this case is to turn somersaults with history. The Ninth Amendment, like its companion the Tenth, which this Court held "states but a truism that all is retained which has not been surrendered," was framed by James Madison and adopted by the States simply to make clear that the adoption of the Bill of Rights did not alter the plan that the Federal Government was to be a government of express and limited powers, and that all rights and powers not delegated to it were retained by the people and the individual States. Until today no member of this Court has ever suggested that the Ninth Amendment meant anything else, and the idea that a federal court could ever use the Ninth Amendment to annul a law passed by the elected representatives of the people of the State of Connecticut would have caused James Madison no little wonder.

What provision of the Constitution, then, does make this state law invalid? The Court says it is the right of privacy "created by several fundamental constitutional guarantees." With all deference, I can find no such general right of privacy in the Bill of Rights, in any other part of the Constitution, or in any case ever before decided by this Court. At the oral argument in this case we were told that the Connecticut law does not "conform to current community standards." But it is not the function of this Court to decide cases on the basis of community standards. We are here to decide cases "agreeably to the Constitution and laws of the United States." It is the essence of judicial duty to subordinate our own personal views, our own ideas of what legislation is wise and what is not. If, as I should surely hope, the law before us does not reflect the standards of the people of Connecticut, the people of Connecticut can freely exercise their true Ninth and Tenth Amendment rights to persuade their elected representatives to repeal it. That is the constitutional way to take this law off the books.

Discussion Questions

1. This case presents an interesting contrast in judicial philosophies and temperaments, especially given that the Court was generally much more liberal and activist at the time than it has been in recent years. With which viewpoint—that of the majority opinion or the dissents—do you agree? Why?

2. What do you know of the judicial philosophies of Justices Douglas, Black, and Stewart? Which do you find most persuasive?

3. Is the result in this case an example of judge-made law and a failure to adhere to the original intent of the Framers? Or is it an example of the law's adaptability to unforeseen and unforeseeable circumstances within the general framework of the constitution?

4. How, do you suppose, the justices here would have decided a case involving the recent "gag rule" on abortion counseling in programs receiving federal financial assistance?

Planned Parenthood of S.E. Pa. v. Casey
112 S. Ct. 2791 (1992)

JUSTICE O'CONNOR, JUSTICE KENNEDY, and JUSTICE SOUTER announced the judgment of the Court and delivered the opinion of the Court with respect to Parts I, II, III, V-A, V-C, and VI, an opinion with respect to Part V-E, in

---

1. The Amendments in question were, as everyone knows, originally adopted as limitations upon the power of the newly created Federal Government, not as limitations upon the powers of the individual States. But the Court has held that many of the provisions of the first eight amendments are fully embraced by the Fourteenth Amendment as limitations upon state action, and some members of the Court have held the view that the adoption of the Fourteenth Amendment made every provision of the first eight amendments fully applicable against the States.

which JUSTICE STEVENS joins, and an opinion with respect to Parts IV, V-B, and V-D.

I

Liberty finds no refuge in a jurisprudence of doubt. Yet 19 years after our holding that the Constitution protects a woman's right to terminate her pregnancy in its early stages, *Roe v. Wade* (1973), that definition of liberty is still questioned. Joining the respondents as amicus curiae, the United States, as it has done in five other cases in the last decade, again asks us to overrule *Roe*.

At issue in these cases are five provisions of the Pennsylvania Abortion Control Act of 1982 as amended in 1988 and 1989. . . . The Act requires that a woman seeking an abortion give her informed consent prior to the abortion procedure, and specifies that she be provided with certain information at least 24 hours before the abortion is performed. For a minor to obtain an abortion, the Act requires the informed consent of one of her parents, but provides for a judicial bypass option if the minor does not wish to or cannot obtain a parent's consent. Another provision of the Act requires that, unless certain exceptions apply, a married woman seeking an abortion must sign a statement indicating that she has notified her husband of her intended abortion. The Act exempts compliance with these three requirements in the event of a "medical emergency," which is defined in . . . the Act. In addition to the above provisions regulating the performance of abortions, the Act imposes certain reporting requirements on facilities that provide abortion services.

. . . .

. . . [W]e find it imperative to review once more the principles that define the rights of the woman and the legitimate authority of the State respecting the termination of pregnancies by abortion procedures.

After considering the fundamental constitutional questions resolved by *Roe*, principles of institutional integrity, and the rule of stare decisis, we are led to conclude this: the essential holding of *Roe v. Wade* should be retained and once again reaffirmed.

It must be stated at the outset and with clarity that *Roe*'s essential holding, the holding we reaffirm, has three parts. First is a recognition of the right of the woman to choose to have an abortion before viability and to obtain it without undue interference from the State. Before viability, the State's interests are not strong enough to support a prohibition of abortion or the imposition of a substantial obstacle to the woman's effective right to elect the procedure. Second is a confirmation of the State's power to restrict abortions after fetal viability, if the law contains exceptions for pregnancies which endanger a woman's life or health. And third is the principle that the State has legitimate interests from the outset of the pregnancy in protecting the health of the woman and the life of the fetus that may become a child. These principles do not contradict one another; and we adhere to each.

II

Constitutional protection of the woman's decision to terminate her pregnancy derives from the Due Process Clause of the Fourteenth Amendment. It declares that no State shall "deprive any person of life, liberty, or property, without due process of law." The controlling word in the case before us is "liberty." Although a literal reading of the Clause might suggest that it governs only the procedures by which a State may deprive persons of liberty, for at least 105 years . . . the Clause has been understood to contain a substantive component as well, one "barring certain government actions regardless of the fairness of the procedures used to implement them." As Justice Brandeis (joined by Justice Holmes) observed, "despite arguments to the contrary which had seemed to me persuasive, it is settled that the due process clause of the Fourteenth Amendment applies to matters of substantive law as well as to matters of procedure. Thus all fundamental rights comprised within the term liberty are protected by the Federal Constitution from invasion by the States."

The most familiar of the substantive liberties protected by the Fourteenth Amendment are those recognized by the Bill of Rights. We have held that the Due Process Clause of the Fourteenth Amendment incorporates most of the Bill of Rights against the States. It is tempting, as a means of curbing the discretion of federal judges, to suppose that liberty encompasses no more than those rights already guaranteed to the individual against federal interference by the express provisions of the first eight amendments to the Constitution. But of course this Court has never accepted that view.

It is also tempting, for the same reason, to suppose that the Due Process Clause protects only those practices, defined at the most specific level, that were protected against government interference by other rules of law when the Fourteenth Amendment was ratified. But such a view would be inconsistent with our law. It is a promise of the Constitution that there is a realm of personal liberty which the government may not enter. We have vindicated this principle before. Marriage is mentioned nowhere in the Bill of Rights and interracial marriage was illegal in most States in the 19th century, but the Court was no doubt correct in finding it to be an aspect of liberty protected against state interference by the substantive component of the Due Process Clause . . . .

. . . .

In *Griswold* [*v. Connecticut*, a 1977 case], we held that the Constitution does not permit a State to forbid a married couple to use contraceptives. That same freedom was later guaranteed, under the Equal Protection Clause, for unmarried couples. Constitutional protection was extended to the sale and distribution of contraceptives in [a later case]. It is settled now, as it was when the Court heard arguments in *Roe v. Wade*, that the Constitution places limits on a State's right to interfere with a person's most basic decisions about family and parenthood[.]

The inescapable fact is that adjudication of substantive due process claims may call upon the Court in interpreting the Constitution to exercise that same capacity which by tradition courts always have exercised: reasoned judgment. Its boundaries are not susceptible of expression as a simple rule. That does not mean we are free to invalidate state policy choices with which we disagree; yet neither does it permit us to shrink from the duties of our office. As Justice Harlan observed:

> Due process has not been reduced to any formula; its content cannot be determined by reference to any code. The best that can be said is that through the course of this Court's decisions it has represented the balance which our Nation, built upon postulates of respect for the liberty of the individual, has struck between that liberty and the demands of organized society. If the supplying of content to this Constitutional concept has of necessity been a rational process, it certainly has not been one where judges have felt free to roam where unguided speculation might take them. The balance of which I speak is the balance struck by this country, having regard to what history teaches are the traditions from which it developed as well as the traditions from which it broke. That tradition is a living thing. A decision of this Court which radically departs from it could not long survive, while a decision which builds on what has survived is likely to be sound. No formula could serve as a substitute, in this area, for judgment and restraint.

Men and women of good conscience can disagree, and we suppose some always shall disagree, about the profound moral and spiritual implications of terminating a pregnancy, even in its earliest stage. Some of us as individuals find abortion offensive to our most basic principles of morality, but that cannot control our decision. Our obligation is to define the liberty of all, not to mandate our own moral code. The underlying constitutional issue is whether the State can resolve these philosophic questions in such a definitive way that a woman lacks all choice in the matter, except perhaps in those rare circumstances in which the pregnancy is itself a danger to her own life or health, or is the result of rape or incest.

. . . .

It was this dimension of personal liberty that *Roe* sought to protect, and its holding invoked the reasoning and the tradition of the precedents we have discussed, granting protection to substantive liberties of the person. *Roe* was, of course, an extension of those cases and, as the decision itself indicated, the separate States could act in some degree to further their own legitimate interests in protecting pre-natal life. The extent to which the legislatures of the States might act to outweigh the interests of the woman in choosing to terminate her pregnancy was a subject of debate both in *Roe* itself and in decisions following it.

While we appreciate the weight of the arguments made on behalf of the State in the case before us, arguments which in their ultimate formulation conclude that *Roe* should be overruled, the reservations any of us may have in reaffirming the central holding of *Roe* are outweighed by the explication

of individual liberty we have given combined with the force of stare decisis. We turn now to that doctrine.

III

A

The obligation to follow precedent begins with necessity, and a contrary necessity marks its outer limit. With Cardozo, we recognize that no judicial system could do society's work if it eyed each issue afresh in every case that raised it. Indeed, the very concept of the rule of law underlying our own Constitution requires such continuity over time that a respect for precedent is, by definition, indispensable. At the other extreme, a different necessity would make itself felt if a prior judicial ruling should come to be seen so clearly as error that its enforcement was for that very reason doomed.

Even when the decision to overrule a prior case is not, as in the rare, latter instance, virtually foreordained, it is common wisdom that the rule of stare decisis is not an "inexorable command," and certainly it is not such in every constitutional case. Rather, when this Court reexamines a prior holding, its judgment is customarily informed by a series of prudential and pragmatic considerations designed to test the consistency of overruling a prior decision with the ideal of the rule of law, and to gauge the respective costs of reaffirming and overruling a prior case.

So in this case we may inquire whether *Roe*'s central rule has been found unworkable; whether the rule's limitation on state power could be removed without serious inequity to those who have relied upon it or significant damage to the stability of the society governed by the rule in question; whether the law's growth in the intervening years has left *Roe*'s central rule a doctrinal anachronism discounted by society; and whether *Roe*'s premises of fact have so far changed in the ensuing two decades as to render its central holding somehow irrelevant or unjustifiable in dealing with the issue it addressed. [The opinion proceeds to discuss each of these questions and to answer each in the negative.]

. . . .

The sum of the precedential inquiry to this point shows *Roe*'s underpinnings unweakened in any way affecting its central holding. While it has engendered disapproval, it has not been unworkable. An entire generation has come of age free to assume *Roe*'s concept of liberty in defining the capacity of women to act in society, and to make reproductive decisions; no erosion of principle going to liberty or personal autonomy has left *Roe*'s central holding a doctrinal remnant; *Roe* portends no developments at odds with other precedent for the analysis of personal liberty; and no changes of fact have rendered viability more or less appropriate as the point at which the balance of interests tips. Within the bounds of normal stare decisis analysis, then, and subject to the considerations on which it customarily turns, the stronger argument is for affirming *Roe*'s central holding, with whatever degree of personal reluctance any of us may have, not for overruling it.

B

In a less significant case, *stare decisis* analysis could, and would, stop at the point we have reached. But the sustained and widespread debate *Roe* has provoked calls for some comparison between that case and others of comparable dimension that have responded to national controversies and taken on the impress of the controversies addressed. Only two such decisional lines from the past century present themselves for examination, and in each instance the result reached by the Court accorded with the principles we apply today.

[The court here discusses two examples of Supreme Court decisions overruled in subsequent cases. One was the early-twentieth-century line of cases striking down health and welfare regulations (such as minimum wage and child labor laws) in favor of laissez-faire economics. These cases were overturned in a 1937 decision, *West Coast Hotel Co. v. Parrish*; by this time the Great Depression had taught us that an unregulated economy could not be assumed to provide satisfactory levels of human welfare for the working class. The second example involved the "separate but equal" rule of racial segregation established by *Plessy v. Ferguson* in 1896. That case was the law of the land for more than half a century until it was overruled by the 1954 holding in *Brown v. Board of Education* that "separate but equal" is inherently unequal and hence unconstitutional.]

West Coast Hotel and *Brown* each rested on facts, or an understanding of facts, changed from those which furnished the claimed justifications for the earlier constitutional resolutions. Each case was comprehensible as the Court's response to facts that the country could understand, or had come to understand already, but which the Court of an earlier day, as its own declarations disclosed, had not been able to perceive. As the decisions were thus comprehensible they were also defensible, not merely as the victories of one doctrinal school over another by dint of numbers (victories though they were), but as applications of constitutional principle to facts as they had not been seen by the Court before. In constitutional adjudication as elsewhere in life, changed circumstances may impose new obligations, and the thoughtful part of the Nation could accept each decision to overrule a prior case as a response to the Court's constitutional duty.

Because the case before us presents no such occasion it could be seen as no such response. Because neither the factual underpinnings of *Roe*'s central holding nor our understanding of it has changed (and because no other indication of weakened precedent has been shown) the Court could not pretend to be reexamining the prior law with any justification beyond a present doctrinal disposition to come out differently from the Court of 1973. To overrule prior law for no other reason than that would run counter to the view repeated

in our cases, that a decision to overrule should rest on some special reason over and above the belief that a prior case was wrongly decided.

[Here the Court embarks on a lengthy description of "why overruling *Roe*'s central holding would not only reach an unjustifiable result under principles of *stare decisis* but would seriously weaken the Court's capacity to exercise the judicial power and to function as the Supreme Court of a Nation dedicated to the rule of law." This description is set forth in Chapter 1 of this book at pages 5–6 and need not be duplicated here.]

IV

From what we have said so far it follows that it is a constitutional liberty of the woman to have some freedom to terminate her pregnancy. We conclude that the basic decision in *Roe* was based on a constitutional analysis which we cannot now repudiate. The woman's liberty is not so unlimited, however, that from the outset the State cannot show its concern for the life of the unborn, and at a later point in fetal development the State's interest in life has sufficient force so that the right of the woman to terminate the pregnancy can be restricted.

That brings us, of course, to the point where much criticism has been directed at *Roe*, a criticism that always inheres when the Court draws a specific rule from what in the Constitution is but a general standard. We conclude, however, that the urgent claims of the woman to retain the ultimate control over her destiny and her body, claims implicit in the meaning of liberty, require us to perform that function. Liberty must not be extinguished for want of a line that is clear. And it falls to us to give some real substance to the woman's liberty to determine whether to carry her pregnancy to full term.

We conclude the line should be drawn at viability, so that before that time the woman has a right to choose to terminate her pregnancy. We adhere to this principle for two reasons. First, as we have said, is the doctrine of stare decisis. Any judicial act of line-drawing may seem somewhat arbitrary, but *Roe* was a reasoned statement, elaborated with great care. We have twice reaffirmed it in the face of great opposition. . . . [T]he central premise of those cases represents an unbroken commitment by this Court to the essential holding of *Roe*. It is that premise which we reaffirm today.

The second reason is that the concept of viability, as we noted in *Roe*, is the time at which there is a realistic possibility of maintaining and nourishing a life outside the womb, so that the independent existence of the second life can in reason and all fairness be the object of state protection that now overrides the rights of the woman. Consistent with other constitutional norms, legislatures may draw lines which appear arbitrary without the necessity of offering a justification. But courts may not. We must justify the lines we draw. And there is no line other than viability which is more workable. To be sure, as we have said, there may be some medical developments that affect the precise point of viability, but this is an imprecision within tolerable limits given that the medical community and all those who must apply its discoveries will continue to explore the matter. The viability line also has, as a practical matter, an element of fairness. In some broad sense it might be said that a woman who fails to act before viability has consented to the State's intervention on behalf of the developing child.

The woman's right to terminate her pregnancy before viability is the most central principle of *Roe v. Wade*. It is a rule of law and a component of liberty we cannot renounce.

On the other side of the equation is the interest of the State in the protection of potential life. The *Roe* Court recognized the State's "important and legitimate interest in protecting the potentiality of human life." The weight to be given this state interest, not the strength of the woman's interest, was the difficult question faced in *Roe*. We do not need to say whether each of us, had we been Members of the Court when the valuation of the State interest came before it as an original matter, would have concluded, as the *Roe* Court did, that its weight is insufficient to justify a ban on abortions prior to viability even when it is subject to certain exceptions. The matter is not before us in the first instance, and coming as it does after nearly 20 years of litigation in *Roe*'s wake we are satisfied that the immediate question is not the soundness of *Roe*'s resolution of the issue, but the precedential force that must be accorded to its holding. And we have concluded that the essential holding of *Roe* should be reaffirmed.

Yet it must be remembered that *Roe v. Wade* speaks with clarity in establishing not only the woman's liberty but also the State's "important and legitimate interest in potential life." That portion of the decision in *Roe* has been given too little acknowledgement and implementation by the Court in its subsequent cases. Those cases decided that any regulation touching upon the abortion decision must survive strict scrutiny, to be sustained only if drawn in narrow terms to further a compelling state interest. Not all of the cases decided under that formulation can be reconciled with the holding in *Roe* itself that the State has legitimate interests in the health of the woman and in protecting the potential life within her. In resolving this tension, we choose to rely upon *Roe*, as against the later cases.

Roe established a trimester framework to govern abortion regulations. Under this elaborate but rigid construct, almost no regulation at all is permitted during the first trimester of pregnancy; regulations designed to protect the woman's health, but not to further the State's interest in potential life, are permitted during the second trimester; and during the third trimester, when the fetus is viable, prohibitions are permitted provided the life or health of the mother is not at stake. Most of our cases since *Roe* have involved the application of rules derived from the trimester framework.

The trimester framework no doubt was erected to ensure that the woman's right to choose not become so subordinate to the State's interest in promoting fetal life that her choice exists in theory but not in fact. We do not agree, however, that the trimester approach is necessary to accomplish this objective. A framework of this rigidity was unnecessary and in its later interpretation sometimes contradicted the State's permissible exercise of its powers.

Though the woman has a right to choose to terminate or continue her pregnancy before viability, it does not at all follow that the State is prohibited from taking steps to ensure that this choice is thoughtful and informed. Even in the earliest stages of pregnancy, the State may enact rules and regulations designed to encourage her to know that there are philosophic and social arguments of great weight that can be brought to bear in favor of continuing the pregnancy to full term and that there are procedures and institutions to allow adoption of unwanted children as well as a certain degree of state assistance if the mother chooses to raise the child herself. " 'The Constitution does not forbid a State or city, pursuant to democratic processes, from expressing a preference for normal childbirth.' " It follows that States are free to enact laws to provide a reasonable framework for a woman to make a decision that has such profound and lasting meaning. This, too, we find consistent with *Roe*'s central premises, and indeed the inevitable consequence of our holding that the State has an interest in protecting the life of the unborn.

We reject the trimester framework, which we do not consider to be part of the essential holding of *Roe*. Measures aimed at ensuring that a woman's choice contemplates the consequences for the fetus do not necessarily interfere with the right recognized in *Roe*, although those measures have been found to be inconsistent with the rigid trimester framework announced in that case. A logical reading of the central holding in *Roe* itself, and a necessary reconciliation of the liberty of the woman and the interest of the State in promoting prenatal life, require, in our view, that we abandon the trimester framework as a rigid prohibition on all previability regulation aimed at the protection of fetal life. The trimester framework suffers from these basic flaws: in its formulation it misconceives the nature of the pregnant woman's interest; and in practice it undervalues the State's interest in potential life, as recognized in *Roe*.

As our jurisprudence relating to all liberties save perhaps abortion has recognized, not every law which makes a right more difficult to exercise is, ipso facto, an infringement of that right. An example clarifies the point. We have held that not every ballot access limitation amounts to an infringement of the right to vote.

The abortion right is similar. Numerous forms of state regulation might have the incidental effect of increasing the cost or decreasing the availability of medical care, whether for abortion or any other medical procedure. The fact that a law which serves a valid purpose, one not designed to strike at the right itself, has the incidental effect of making it more difficult or more expensive to procure an abortion cannot be enough to invalidate it. Only where state regulation imposes an undue burden on a woman's ability to make this decision does the power of the State reach into the heart of the liberty protected by the Due Process Clause.

. . . .

The very notion that the State has a substantial interest in potential life leads to the conclusion that not all regulations must be deemed unwarranted. Not all burdens on the right to decide whether to terminate a pregnancy will be undue. In our view, the undue burden standard is the appropriate means of reconciling the State's interest with the woman's constitutionally protected liberty.

The concept of an undue burden has been utilized by the Court as well as individual members of the Court, including two of us, in ways that could be considered inconsistent. Because we set forth a standard of general application to which we intend to adhere, it is important to clarify what is meant by an undue burden.

A finding of an undue burden is a shorthand for the conclusion that a state regulation has the purpose or effect of placing a substantial obstacle in the path of a woman seeking an abortion of a nonviable fetus. A statute with this purpose is invalid because the means chosen by the State to further the interest in potential life must be calculated to inform the woman's free choice, not hinder it. And a statute which, while furthering the interest in potential life or some other valid state interest, has the effect of placing a substantial obstacle in the path of a woman's choice cannot be considered a permissible means of serving its legitimate ends. To the extent that the opinions of the Court or of individual Justices use the undue burden standard in a manner that is inconsistent with this analysis, we set out what in our view should be the controlling standard. In our considered judgment, an undue burden is an unconstitutional burden. Understood another way, we answer the question, left open in previous opinions discussing the undue burden formulation, whether a law designed to further the State's interest in fetal life which imposes an undue burden on the woman's decision before fetal viability could be constitutional. The answer is no.

Some guiding principles should emerge. What is at stake is the woman's right to make the ultimate decision, not a right to be insulated from all others in doing so. Regulations which do no more than create a structural mechanism by which the State, or the parent or guardian of a minor, may express profound respect for the life of the unborn are permitted, if they are not a substantial obstacle to the woman's exercise of the right to choose. Unless it has that effect on her right of choice, a state measure designed to persuade her to choose childbirth over abortion will be upheld if reasonably related to that goal. Regulations designed to foster the health of a woman seeking an abortion are valid if they do not constitute an undue burden.

Even when jurists reason from shared premises, some disagreement is inevitable. That is to be expected in the application of any legal standard which must accommodate life's complexity. We do not expect it to be otherwise with respect to the undue burden standard. We give this summary:

(a) To protect the central right recognized by *Roe v. Wade* while at the same time accommodating the State's profound interest in potential life, we will employ the undue burden analysis as explained in this opinion. An undue burden exists, and therefore a provision of law is invalid, if its purpose or effect is to place a substantial obstacle in the path of a woman seeking an abortion before the fetus attains viability.

(b) We reject the rigid trimester framework of *Roe v. Wade*. To promote the State's profound interest in potential life, throughout pregnancy the State may take measures to ensure that the woman's choice is informed, and measures designed to advance this interest will not be invalidated as long as their purpose is to persuade the woman to choose childbirth over abortion. These measures must not be an undue burden on the right.

(c) As with any medical procedure, the State may enact regulations to further the health or safety of a woman seeking an abortion. Unnecessary health regulations that have the purpose or effect of presenting a substantial obstacle to a woman seeking an abortion impose an undue burden on the right.

(d) Our adoption of the undue burden analysis does not disturb the central holding of *Roe v. Wade*, and we reaffirm that holding. Regardless of whether exceptions are made for particular circumstances, a State may not prohibit any woman from making the ultimate decision to terminate her pregnancy before viability.

(e) We also reaffirm *Roe*'s holding that "subsequent to viability, the State in promoting its interest in the potentiality of human life may, if it chooses, regulate, and even proscribe, abortion except where it is necessary, in appropriate medical judgment, for the preservation of the life or health of the mother."

These principles control our assessment of the Pennsylvania statute, and we now turn to the issue of the validity of its challenged provisions.

V

The Court of Appeals applied what it believed to be the undue burden standard and upheld each of the provisions except for the husband notification requirement. We agree generally with this conclusion, but refine the undue burden analysis in accordance with the principles articulated above. We now consider the separate statutory sections at issue.

[The Court proceeds to evaluate specific provisions of the Pennsylvania statute in question. It decides (1) the "medical emergency" exception in the statute is not too narrowly defined, (2) the requirement of informed consent (done 24 hours in advance and containing certain specifics) is not an undue burden, (3) the requirement that a married woman's husband be notified in advance is an undue burden and hence invalid, and (4) the requirement of parental or judicial consent for unemancipated minors is not unduly burdensome and therefore is valid.]

VI

Our Constitution is a covenant running from the first generation of Americans to us and then to future generations. It is a coherent succession. Each generation must learn anew that the Constitution's written terms embody ideas and aspirations that must survive more ages than one. We accept our responsibility not to retreat from interpreting the full meaning of the covenant in light of all of our precedents. We invoke it once again to define the freedom guaranteed by the Constitution's own promise, the promise of liberty.

* * *

The judgment in No. 91-902 is affirmed. The judgment in No. 91-744 is affirmed in part and reversed in part, and the case is remanded for proceedings consistent with this opinion, including consideration of the question of severability.

It is so ordered.

Discussion Question

1. The divisiveness of the abortion issue has obviously divided even the U.S. Supreme Court. Are you persuaded by the logic of the decision? What do you think will come of the controversy in the coming years?

Note

Because of the length of the *Planned Parenthood* decision, it is not possible to present summaries of each of the concurring and dissenting opinions. The student must understand, however, the complexity of the case and the votes of the justices.

As noted in the excerpt given, the judgment of the Court was announced in an opinion authored primarily by Justices O'Connor, Kennedy, and Souter. Justices Blackmun and Stevens joined in portions of that opinion, thus providing the five votes necessary for the particular actions ultimately taken ("affirmed," "affirmed in part," "reversed in part," etc.). It is important to understand, however, that Blackmun and Stevens joined Chief Justice Rehnquist and Justices White, Scalia, and Thomas in dissenting to at least a part of the lead opinion. Furthermore, the latter four members of the Court would have reexamined *Roe*'s principle that abortion is a fundamental right, disagreed with the "undue burden" standard, concluded that the choice of an abortion is not a constitutional right at all, and urged that the Pennsylvania statute be upheld in its entirety.

It can be seen, therefore, that even though a majority of the Court voted for a particular action on each of the two cases decided here, there is no clear majority opinion of the Court.

Harbeson v. Parke-Davis, Inc.
98 Wash. 2d 460, 656 P.2d 483 (1983)

Pearson, J.

This case requires us to decide whether to recognize two new causes of action: "wrongful birth" and "wrongful life." We hold that, subject to the limitations set forth in this opinion, such actions may be brought in this state.

[The facts of the case involved the prescription of Dilantin, an anticonvulsive drug, to control the epilepsy of Mrs. Jean Harbeson, a military dependent. Military physicians at Madigan Army Medical Center in Washington prescribed the drug. Despite the Harbesons' inquiries about the risks of taking Dilantin during pregnancy, none of the physicians conducted literature searches or consulted other sources regarding the correlation between Dilantin and birth defects. Based on the doctors' assurances, Mrs. Harbeson continued to take the drug during two pregnancies and each time gave birth to daughters who suffer birth defects that include growth deficiencies, mild to moderate retardation, and other physical and developmental defects. The evidence shows that had they been informed of the risks, the Harbesons would not have had these children.

The plaintiffs brought an action against the United States for medical malpractice and failure to inform of the material risks of treatment. The U.S. District Court found that the actions of the Army physicians were negligent and the proximate cause of the birth defects. It then certified to the Washington Supreme Court the legal questions of whether Mr. and Mrs. Harbeson can maintain a "wrongful birth" action and whether the children can maintain a "wrongful life" claim.]

WRONGFUL BIRTH

The epithet wrongful birth has been used to describe several fundamentally different types of action. Many of the actions once entitled wrongful birth are now referred to as wrongful conception and wrongful pregnancy actions. A recent definition of a wrongful birth action is an action brought by parents against

a physician [who] failed to inform [them] of the increased possibility that the mother would give birth to a child suffering from birth defects * * * [thereby precluding] an informed decision about whether to have the child.

. . . .

[Recent cases from other jurisdictions] recognize the right of parents to prevent the conception or birth of children suffering defects. They recognize that physicians owe a duty to parents to preserve that right. Physicians may breach this duty either by failure to impart material information or by negligent performance of a procedure to prevent the birth of a defective child. The parents' right to prevent a defective child and the correlative duty flowing from that right is the heart of the wrongful birth action.

For the purposes of the analysis which follows, therefore, wrongful birth will refer to an action based on an alleged breach of the duty of a health care provider to impart information or perform medical procedures with due care, where the breach is a proximate cause of the birth of a defective child. We do not in this opinion address issues which may arise where the birth of a healthy child is allegedly caused by a breach of duty owed to the parents. Such actions are referred to as wrongful conception or wrongful pregnancy, rather than wrongful birth. Other jurisdictions have consistently treated such actions as different from, although related to, wrongful birth. We do likewise.

Having defined the scope of our inquiry, we now consider whether the wrongful birth action should be allowed in this state. We conclude that the action conforms comfortably to the structure of tort principles and that recognition of wrongful birth claims is a logical and necessary development. Accordingly, we hold that wrongful birth claims will be recognized in Washington.

. . . .

First, we measure the proposed wrongful birth action against the traditional concepts of duty, breach, injury, and proximate cause. The critical concept is duty. The core of our decision is whether we should impose upon health care providers a duty correlative to parents' right to prevent the birth of defective children.

Until recently, medical science was unable to provide parents with the means of predicting the birth of a defective child. Now, however, the ability to predict the occurrence and recurrence of defects has improved significantly. . . .

We believe we must recognize the benefits of these medical developments and therefore we hold that parents have a right to prevent the birth of a defective child and health care providers a duty correlative to that right. This duty requires health care providers to impart to their patients material information as to the likelihood of future children's [sic] being born defective, to enable the potential parents to decide whether to avoid the conception or birth of such children. If medical procedures are undertaken to avoid the conception or birth of defective children, the duty also requires that these procedures be performed with due care. This duty includes, therefore, the requirement that a health care provider who undertakes to perform an abortion use reasonable care in doing so. The duty does not, however, affect in any way the right of a physician to refuse on moral or religious grounds to perform an abortion. Recognition of the duty will "promote societal interests in genetic counseling and prenatal testing, deter medical malpractice, and at least partially redress a clear and undeniable wrong."

. . . .

Having recognized that a duty exists, we have taken the major step toward recognizing the wrongful birth action. The second element of the traditional tort analysis is more straightforward. Breach will be measured by failure to conform to the appropriate standard of skill, care, or learning.

More problematical is the question of whether the birth of a defective child represents an injury to the parents. The only case to touch on this question in this state did not resolve it. However, it is an inevitable consequence of recognizing the parents' right to avoid the birth of a defective child that we recognize that the birth of such a child is an actionable injury. The real question as to injury, therefore, is not the existence of the injury, but the extent of that injury. In other words, having recognized that the birth of the child represents an injury, how do we measure damages? [The court notes that other jurisdictions have taken widely divergent approaches but answers this question by referring to a Washington statute that allows parents to recover damages for other forms of injuries to a child. These damages include compensation "not only for pecuniary loss but also for emotional injury."] Accordingly, we hold that recovery may include the medical, hospital, and medication expenses attributable to the child's birth and to its defective condition, and in addition damages for the parents' emotional injury caused by the birth of the defective child. In considering damages for emotional injury, the jury should be entitled to consider the countervailing emotional benefits attributable to the birth of the child.

. . . .

We now turn to answer the first issue certified to us by the District Court. Our analysis leads us to conclude that plaintiffs . . . may maintain a cause of action for the wrongful births of Elizabeth and Christine. . . .

The final element which must be proved is that the negligence of the physicians was a proximate cause of this injury. The District Court concluded that Dilantin was the proximate cause of the birth defects suffered by the children . . . and that an adequate literature search would have revealed the risks associated with Dilantin . . . . The court made a finding of fact that had the Harbesons been informed of those risks they would not have had any other children. These conclusions and findings establish that the breach of duty was a cause in fact of the birth of Elizabeth and Christine, and therefore a proximate cause of the injury.

The parents may therefore recover damages for the wrongful births of Elizabeth and Christine. . . .

WRONGFUL LIFE

In a wrongful life claim,

[t]he child does not allege that the physician's negligence caused the child's deformity. Rather, the claim is that the physician's neg-

ligence—his failure to adequately inform the parents of the risk—has caused the *birth* of the deformed child. The child argues that *but for* the inadequate advice, it would not have been born to experience the pain and suffering attributable to the deformity.

To this definition we would add that the physician's negligence need not be limited to failure to adequately inform the parents of the risk. It may also include negligent performance of a procedure intended to prevent the birth of a defective child: sterilization or abortion.

Wrongful life is the child's equivalent of the parents' wrongful birth action. However, whereas wrongful birth actions have apparently been accepted by all jurisdictions to have considered the issue, wrongful life actions have been received with little favor. . . .

Two other jurisdictions have come closer to embracing the cause of action. In Pennsylvania, a trial court decision that the action was not legally cognizable was affirmed only as a result of the even division of the Supreme Court. The Supreme Court of California rejected the claim of a child for general damages, but allowed the recovery of extraordinary medical expenses occasioned by the child's defect. The court [in *Turpin v. Sortini*] acknowledges that "it would be illogical and anomalous to permit only parents, and not the child, to recover for the cost of the child's own medical care." We agree. The child's need for medical care and other special costs attributable to his defect will not miraculously disappear when the child attains his majority. In many cases, the burden of those expenses will fall on the child's parents or the state. Rather than allowing this to occur by refusing to recognize the cause of action, we prefer to place the burden of those costs on the party whose negligence was in fact a proximate cause of the child's continuing need for such special medical care and training.

We hold, accordingly, that a child may maintain an action for wrongful life in order to recover the extraordinary expenses to be incurred during the child's lifetime, as a result of the child's congenital defect. Of course, the costs of such care for the child's minority may be recovered only once. If the parents recover such costs for the child's minority in a wrongful birth action, the child will be limited to the costs to be incurred during his majority.

The analysis whereby we arrived at our holding is similar to that which we used in considering the parents' wrongful birth action. It is convenient therefore to consider wrongful life according to the four traditional tort concepts of duty, breach, injury, and proximate cause.

We begin with duty. The first potential difficulty with the element of a wrongful life action is that in every case the alleged negligent act will occur before the birth of the child, and in many cases (including the one before us) before the child is conceived. Prenatal injuries to a fetus have been recognized as actionable in this state for 20 years. We have not previously considered whether a duty could exist prior to conception. Other courts have recognized such a preconception duty. We now hold that a duty may extend to persons not yet conceived at the time of a negligent act or omission. Such a duty is limited, like any other duty, by the element of foreseeability. A provider of health care, or anyone else, will be liable only to those persons foreseeably endangered by his conduct. In most wrongful life cases it should not be difficult to establish foreseeability. In the case before us, for example, the parents informed the defendant physicians of their intention to have further children. Such future children were therefore foreseeably endangered by defendants' failure to take reasonable steps to determine the danger of prescribing Dilantin for their mother.

One reason for the reluctance of other jurisdictions to recognize a duty to the child appears to be the attitude that to do so would represent a disavowal of the sanctity of a less-than-perfect human life. This reasoning was rejected in *Turpin v. Sortini*:

[I]t is hard to see how an award of damages to a severely handicapped or suffering child would "disavow" the value of life or in any way suggest that the child is not entitled to the full measure of legal and nonlegal rights and privileges accorded to all members of society.

We agree.

Furthermore, the policies which persuaded us (along with several other jurisdictions) to recognize parents' claims of wrongful birth apply equally to recognition of claims of wrongful life. Imposition of a corresponding duty to the child will similarly foster the societal objectives of genetic counseling and prenatal testing, and will discourage malpractice. . . .

. . . .

This duty will be breached by failure to observe the appropriate standard of care.

The most controversial element of the analysis in other jurisdictions has been injury and the extent of damages. The New Jersey Supreme Court gave two reasons for rejecting a child's wrongful life claim in [its leading case]. First, the quantum of damages in such an action would be impossible to compute because the trier of fact would be required to "measure the difference in value between life in an impaired condition and the 'utter void of nonexistence.'" Second, to recognize life itself as an actionable injury would be inimical to deeply held beliefs that life is more precious than nonlife.

We agree with the New Jersey court that measuring the value of an impaired life as compared to nonexistence is a task that is beyond mortals, whether judges or jurors. However, we do not agree that the impossibility of valuing life and nonexistence precludes the action altogether. General damages are certainly beyond computation. They are therefore incapable of satisfying the requirement of Washington law that damages be established with "reasonable certainty." But one of the consequences of the birth of the child who claims wrongful life is the incurring of extraordinary expenses for medical care and special training. These expenses are calculable. . . .

The second objection advanced by the New Jersey court . . . we have already discussed. Suffice it to say here that we do not agree that requiring a negligent party to provide the costs of health care of a congenitally deformed child does not appear to us to be a disavowal of the sanctity of human life.

The final element which requires consideration is proximate cause.

The causation issue in a wrongful life claim is whether "[b]ut for the physician's negligence, the parents would have avoided conception, or aborted the pregnancy, and the child would not have existed." . . . It is clear in the case before us that, were it not for the negligence of the physicians, the minor plaintiffs would not have been born, and would consequently not have suffered [their disabilities]. . . . There appears to be no reason a finder of fact could not find that the physicians' negligence was a proximate cause of the plaintiffs' injuries.

For these reasons, we hold that a claim for wrongful life may be maintained in this state. . . .

Discussion Questions

1. Give some serious thought to the analysis and logic of this decision. Does anything about it bother you?

2. The U.S. Supreme Court in *Roe v. Wade* in effect held that a fetus (at least a nonviable fetus) is not a "person" within the meaning of the U.S. Constitution. How can a duty be said to exist in favor of a nonperson? How does one discharge such a duty?

3. Suppose the doctors in this case had warned the parents and they persisted with the pregnancy. Could the child then sue the parents for the alleged "wrongful life"?

4. Once the child is born, there is an ongoing injury that the court says is compensible. Do the plaintiffs have a duty to mitigate the damages being suffered?

5. The procedural aspects of this case are interesting. Why is the Supreme Court of Washington deciding issues in a case being tried in a U.S. district court?

6. The individual doctors involved in this case were not defendants. Why not?

7. At two points in the opinion, the court refers to societal objectives regarding genetic counseling and prenatal testing. What evidence is there about these objectives? Does society generally agree with them? Do you agree with the court that the decision will foster legitimate social ends, however described?

In re Baby M
109 N.J. 396, 537 A.2d 1227 (1988)

Wilentz, C.J.

In this matter the Court is asked to determine the validity of a contract that purports to provide a new way of bringing children into a family. For a fee of $10,000, a woman agrees to be artificially inseminated with the semen of another woman's husband; she is to conceive a child, carry it to term, and after its birth surrender it to the natural father and his wife. The intent of the contract is that the child's natural mother will thereafter be forever separated from her child. The wife is to adopt the child, and she and the natural father are to be regarded as its parents for all purposes. The contract providing for this is called a "surrogacy contract," the natural mother inappropriately called the "surrogate mother."

We invalidate the surrogacy contract because it conflicts with the law and public policy of this State. While we recognize the depth of the yearning of infertile couples to have their own children, we find the payment of money to a "surrogate" mother illegal, perhaps criminal, and potentially degrading to women. Although in this case we grant custody to the natural father, the evidence having clearly proved such custody to be in the best interests of the infant, we void both the termination of the surrogate mother's parental rights and the adoption of the child by the wife/stepparent. We thus restore the "surrogate" as the mother of the child. We remand the issue of the natural mother's visitation rights to the trial court, since that issue was not reached below and the record before us is not sufficient to permit us to decide it de novo.

We find no offense to our present laws where a woman voluntarily and without payment agrees to act as a "surrogate" mother, provided that she is not subject to a binding agreement to surrender her child. Moreover, our holding today does not preclude the Legislature from altering the current statutory scheme, within constitutional limits, so as to permit surrogacy contracts. Under current law, however, the surrogacy agreement before us is illegal and invalid.

I.
FACTS

In February 1985, William Stern and Mary Beth Whitehead entered into a surrogacy contract. It recited that Stern's wife, Elizabeth, was infertile, that they wanted a child, and that Mrs. Whitehead was willing to provide that child as the mother with Mr. Stern as the father. The contract provided that through artificial insemination using Mr. Stern's sperm, Mrs. Whitehead would become pregnant, carry the child to term, bear it, deliver it to the Sterns, and thereafter do whatever was necessary to terminate her maternal rights so that Mrs. Stern could thereafter adopt the child. . . .

[The court here restates the facts of the case in exhaustive detail, including the lower court's decision that the surrogacy contract is valid and that the eventual placement of the child must look to the best interest of the child.]

II.
INVALIDITY AND UNENFORCEABILITY OF SURROGACY CONTRACT

We have concluded that this surrogacy contract is invalid. Our conclusion has two bases: direct conflict with existing statutes and conflict with the public policies of this State, as expressed in its statutory and decisional law.

. . . .

A. Conflict with Statutory Provisions

The surrogacy contract conflicts with: (1) laws prohibiting the use of money in connection with adoptions; (2) laws requiring proof of parental unfitness or abandonment before termination of parental rights is ordered or an adoption is granted; and (3) laws that make surrender of custody and consent to adoption revocable in private placement adoptions.

[The court next provides a lengthy review of applicable New Jersey Statutes. In so doing, it comments that "considerable care was taken in this case to structure the surrogacy arrangement so as not to violate [the] prohibition" against "paying or accepting money in connection with any placement of a child for adoption." The court concludes, however, by saying, "Nevertheless, it seems clear that the money was paid and accepted in connection with an adoption."]

B. Public Policy Considerations

The surrogacy contract's invalidity, resulting from its direct conflict with the above statutory provisions, is further underlined when its goals and means are measured against New Jersey's public policy. The contract's basic premise, that the natural parents can decide in advance of birth which one is to have custody of the child, bears no relationship to the settled law that the child's best interests shall determine custody. . . .

Worst of all, however, is the contract's total disregard of the best interests of the child. There is not the slightest suggestion that any inquiry will be made at any time to determine the fitness of the Sterns as custodial parents, of Mrs. Stern as an adoptive parent, their superiority to Mrs. Whitehead, or the effect on the child of not living with her natural mother.

This is the sale of a child, or, at the very least, the sale of a mother's right to her child, the only mitigating factor being that one of the purchasers is the father. Almost every evil that prompted the prohibition on the payment of money in connection with adoptions exists here.

. . . .

The long-term effects of surrogacy contracts are not known, but feared—the impact on the child who learns her life was bought, that she is the offspring of someone who gave birth to her only to obtain money; the impact on the natural mother as the full weight of her isolation is felt along with the full reality of the sale of her body and her child; the impact on the natural father and adoptive mother once they realize the consequences of their conduct. Literature in related areas suggests these are substantial considerations, although, given the newness of surrogacy, there is little information. . . .

The surrogacy contract is based on principles that are directly contrary to the objectives of our laws. It guarantees the separation of a child from its mother; it looks to adoption regardless of suitability; it totally ignores the child; it takes the child from the mother regardless of her wishes and her maternal fitness; and it does all of this, it accomplishes all of its goals, through the use of money.

Beyond that is the potential degradation of some women that may result from this arrangement. In many cases, of course, surrogacy may bring satisfaction, not only to the infertile couple, but to the surrogate mother herself. The fact, however, that many women may not perceive surrogacy negatively but rather see it as an opportunity does not diminish its potential for devastation to other women.

In sum, the harmful consequences of this surrogacy arrangement appear to us all too palpable. In New Jersey the surrogate mother's agreement to sell her child is void. Its irrevocability infects the entire contract, as does the money that purports to buy it.

. . . .

IV.
CONSTITUTIONAL ISSUES

Both parties argue that the Constitutions—state and federal—mandate approval of their basic claims. The source of their constitutional arguments is essentially the same: the right of privacy, the right to procreate, the right to the companionship of one's child, those rights flowing either directly from the fourteenth amendment or by its incorporation of the Bill of Rights, or from the ninth amendment, or through the penumbra surrounding all of the Bill of Rights. They are the rights of personal intimacy, of marriage, of sex, of family, of procreation. Whatever their source, it is clear that they are fundamental rights protected by both the federal and state Constitutions. . . . The right asserted by the Sterns is the right of procreation; that asserted by Mary Beth Whitehead is the right to the companionship of her child. We find that the right of procreation does not extend as far as claimed by the Sterns. As for the right asserted by Mrs. Whitehead, since we uphold it on other grounds (i.e., we have restored her as mother and recognized her right, limited by the child's best interests, to her companionship), we need not decide that constitutional issue, and for reasons set forth below, we should not.

The right to procreate, as protected by the Constitution, has been ruled on directly only once by the United States Supreme Court. . . . The right to procreate very simply is the right to have natural children, whether through sexual intercourse or artificial insemination. It is no more than that. Mr. Stern has not been deprived of that right. Through artificial insemination of Mrs. Whitehead, Baby M is his child. The custody, care, companionship, and nurturing that follow birth are not parts of the right to procreation; they are rights that may also be constitutionally protected, but that involve many considerations other than the right of procreation. To assert that Mr. Stern's right of procreation gives him the right to the custody of Baby M would be to assert that Mrs. Whitehead's right of procreation does not give her the right to the custody of Baby M; it would be to assert that the constitutional right of procreation includes within it a constitutionally protected contractual right to destroy someone else's right of procreation.

We conclude that the right of procreation is best understood and protected if confined to its essentials, and that when dealing with rights concerning the resulting child, different interests come into play. There is nothing in our culture or society that even begins to suggest a fundamental right on the part of the father to the custody of the child as part of his right to procreate when opposed by the claim of the mother to the same child. We therefore disagree with the trial court: there is no constitutional basis whatsoever requiring that Mr. Stern's claim to the custody of Baby M be sustained. Our conclusion may thus be understood as illustrating that a person's rights of privacy and self-determination are qualified by the effect on innocent third persons of the exercise of those rights.

. . . .

Mrs. Whitehead, on the other hand, asserts a claim that falls within the scope of a recognized fundamental interest protected by the Constitution. As a mother, she claims the right to the companionship of her child. This is a fundamental interest, constitutionally protected. Furthermore, it was taken away from her by the action of the court below. Whether that action under these circumstances would constitute a constitutional deprivation, however, we need not and do not decide. By virtue of our decision Mrs. Whitehead's constitutional complaint—that her parental rights have been unconstitutionally terminated—is moot. We have decided that both the statutes and public policy of this state require that that termination be voided and that her parental rights be restored. It therefore becomes unnecessary to decide whether that same result would be required by virtue of the federal or state Constitutions. . . .

V.
CUSTODY

Having decided that the surrogacy contract is illegal and unenforceable, we now must decide the custody question without regard to the provisions of the surrogacy contract that would give Mr. Stern sole and permanent custody. (That does not mean that the existence of the contract and the circumstances under which it was entered may not be considered to the extent deemed relevant to the child's best interests.) With the surrogacy contract disposed of, the legal framework becomes a dispute between two couples over the custody of a child produced by the artificial insemination of one couple's wife by the other's husband. Under the Parentage Act the claims of the natural father and the natural mother are entitled to equal weight, i.e., one is not preferred over the other solely because he or she is the father or the mother. . . . The applicable rule given these circumstances is clear: the child's best interests determine custody. . . .

The circumstances of this custody dispute are unusual and they have provoked some unusual contentions. The Whiteheads claim that even if the child's best interests would be served by our awarding custody to the Sterns, we should not do so, since that will encourage surrogacy contracts—contracts claimed by the Whiteheads, and we agree, to be violative of important legislatively-stated public policies. Their position is that in order that surrogacy contracts be deterred, custody should remain in the surrogate mother unless she is unfit, regardless of the best interests of the child. We disagree. Our declaration that this surrogacy contract is unenforceable and illegal is sufficient to deter similar agreements. We need not sacrifice the child's interests in order to make that point sharper. . . .

There were eleven experts who testified concerning the child's best interests, either directly or in connection with matters related to that issue. Our reading of the record persuades us that the trial court's decision awarding custody to the Sterns (technically to Mr. Stern) should be affirmed since "its findings . . . could reasonably have been reached on sufficient credible evidence present in the record." . . .

Our custody conclusion is based on strongly persuasive testimony contrasting both the family life of the Whiteheads and the Sterns and the personalities and characters of the individuals. The stability of the Whitehead family life was doubtful at the time of trial. Their finances were in serious trouble . . . . Her inconsistent stories about various things engendered grave doubts about her ability to explain honestly and sensitively to Baby M—and at the right time—the nature of her origin. . . .

The Sterns have no other children, but all indications are that their household and their personalities promise a much more likely foundation for Melissa to grow and thrive. . . .

Based on all of this we have concluded, independent of the trial court's identical conclusion, that Melissa's best interests call for custody in the Sterns. . . .

VI.
VISITATION

The trial court's decision to terminate Mrs. Whitehead's parental rights precluded it from making any determination on visitation. Our reversal of the trial court's order, however, requires delineation of Mrs. Whitehead's rights to visitation. . . .

. . . .

We have decided that Mrs. Whitehead is entitled to visitation at some point, and that question is not open to the trial court on this remand. The trial court will determine what kind of visitation shall be granted to her, with or without conditions, and when and under what circumstances it should commence. . . .

CONCLUSION

This case affords some insight into a new reproductive arrangement: the artificial insemination of a surrogate mother. The unfortunate events that have unfolded illustrate that its unregulated use can bring suffering to all involved. . . .

We have found that our present laws do not permit the surrogacy contract used in this case. Nowhere, however, do we find any legal prohibition against surrogacy when the surrogate mother volunteers, without any payment, to act as a surrogate and is given the right to change her mind and to assert her parental rights. Moreover, the Legislature remains free to deal with this most sensitive issue as it sees fit, subject only to constitutional constraints. . . .

The judgment is affirmed in part, reversed in part, and remanded for further proceedings consistent with this opinion.

Discussion Questions

1. Do you agree with the court's implicit suggestion that the legislature may be a more appropriate forum for resolution of the ethical and social issues involved here? Why or why not?

2. Do you agree that "voluntary" surrogate parenting, under the terms the court describes in its conclusion, should be permissible?

3. Do you agree that the best interests of the child should prevail? Assuming that the parties agreed at the outset that the best interests of the child were that the Sterns should be considered its legal parents, why should Mrs. Whitehead be able to change that conclusion later? Is that not allowing her "best interests" to prevail merely because she has had a change of heart?

4. Could a court make a "best interests" determination in advance of the surrogacy procedure? On what basis would it make such a decision?

Davis v. Davis
842 S.W.2d 588 (Tenn. 1992)

[This case began as a divorce action in which the parties—appellee Junior Lewis Davis and his wife, Mary Sue Davis—agreed on all settlement terms except the disposition of seven frozen embryos that were the product of in vitro fertilization (IVF). Mrs. Davis had asked for custody of the embryos in order to become pregnant after the divorce; Mr. Davis refused to agree. The trial court held that the embryos were "human beings" from the point of conception, and it awarded custody to Mrs. Davis. The court of appeals reversed, holding that Mr. Davis had a constitutional right not to beget a child in this manner and that the state had no compelling interest to overrule either party's wishes.

Mrs. Davis then petitioned the Tennessee Supreme Court for review. Interestingly, during the appeal process she changed her mind about the embryos' disposition: she decided not to use them to become pregnant but wished to donate them to a childless couple. Both Mr. and Mrs. Davis had remarried by the time of the supreme court's decision.

The court begins its discussion by noting that the Davises had not signed any written agreement covering this eventuality, that there was no applicable Tennessee statute, and that no relevant case law could be found.]

One of the fundamental issues the inquiry poses is whether the preembryos in this case should be considered "persons" or "property" in the contemplation of the law. The Court of Appeals held, correctly, that they cannot be considered "persons" under Tennessee law . . . .

Nor do preembryos enjoy protection as "persons" under federal law. [The opinion cites *Roe v. Wade*, among other cases, for the proposition that the U.S. Constitution and other sources of federal law do not consider the unborn to be recognized "as persons in the whole sense."]

Left undisturbed, the trial court's ruling would have afforded preembryos the legal status of "persons" and vested them with legally cognizable interests separate from those of their progenitors. Such a decision would doubtless have had the effect of outlawing IVF programs in the state of Tennessee. But in setting aside the trial court's judgment, the Court of Appeals, at least by implication, may have swung too far in the opposite direction.

[The court here quotes favorably from the ethical standards of the American Fertility Society:]

[T]he preembryo deserves respect greater than that accorded to human tissue but not the respect accorded to actual persons. The preembryo is due greater respect than other human tissue because of its potential to become a person and because of its symbolic meaning for many people. Yet, it should not be treated as a person, because it has not yet developed the features of personhood, is not yet established as developmentally individual, and may never realize its biologic potential. * * *

. . . .

We conclude that preembryos are not, strictly speaking, either "persons" or "property," but occupy an interim category that entitles them to special respect because of their potential for human life. It follows that any interest that Mary Sue Davis and Junior Davis have in the preembryos in this case is not a true property interest. However, they do have an interest in the nature of ownership, to the extent that they have decision-making authority concerning disposition of the preembryos, within the scope of policy set by law.

. . . .

Although an understanding of the legal status of preembryos is necessary in order to determine the enforceability of agreements about their disposition, asking whether or not they constitute "property" is not an altogether helpful question. As the appellee points out in his brief, "[as] two or eight cell tiny lumps of complex protein, the embryos have no [intrinsic] value to either party." Their value lies in the "potential to become, after implantation, growth and birth, children." Thus, the essential dispute here is not where or how or how long to store the preembryos, but whether the parties will become parents. The Court of Appeals held in effect that they will become parents if they both agree to become parents. The Court did not say what will happen if they fail to agree. We conclude that the answer to this dilemma turns on the parties' exercise of their constitutional right to privacy.

The right to privacy is not specifically mentioned in either the federal or the Tennessee state constitution, and yet there can be little doubt about its grounding in the concept of liberty reflected in those two documents. . . .

. . . .

. . . Based on both the language and the development of our state constitution, we have no hesitation in drawing the conclusion that there is a right of individual privacy guaranteed under and protected by the liberty clauses of the Tennessee Declaration of Rights.

. . . .

Here, the specific individual freedom in dispute is the right to procreate. In terms of the Tennessee state constitution, we hold that the right of procreation is a vital part of an individual's right to privacy. Federal law is to the same effect.

. . . .

For the purposes of this litigation it is sufficient to note that, whatever its ultimate constitutional boundaries, the right of procreational autonomy is composed of two rights of equal significance—the right to procreate and the right to avoid procreation. Undoubtedly, both are subject to protections and limitations. . . .

The equivalence of and inherent tension between these two interests are nowhere more evident than in the context of in vitro fertilization. None of the concerns about a woman's bodily integrity that have previously precluded men from controlling abortion decisions is applicable here. We are not unmindful of the fact that the trauma (including both emotional stress and physical discomfort) to which women are subjected in the IVF process is more severe than is the impact of the procedure on men. In this sense, it is fair to say that women contribute more to the IVF process than men. Their experience, however, must be viewed in light of the joys of parenthood that is desired or the relative anguish of a lifetime of unwanted parenthood. As they stand on the brink of potential parenthood, Mary Sue Davis and Junior Lewis Davis must be seen as entirely equivalent gamete-providers.

It is further evident that, however far the protection of procreational autonomy extends, the existence of the right itself dictates that decisional authority rests in the gamete-providers alone, at least to the extent that their decisions have an impact upon their individual reproductive status. As discussed in Section V above, no other person or entity has an interest sufficient to permit interference with the gamete-providers' decision to continue or terminate the IVF process, because no one else bears the consequences of these decisions in the way that the gamete-providers do.

. . . .

The unique nature of this case requires us to note that the interests of these parties in parenthood are different in scope than the parental interest considered in other cases. Previously, courts have dealt with the childbearing and child-rearing aspects of parenthood. Abortion cases have dealt with gestational parenthood. In this case, the Court must deal with the question of genetic parenthood. We conclude, moreover, that an interest in avoiding genetic parenthood can be significant enough to trigger the protections afforded to all other aspects of parenthood. The technological fact that someone unknown to these parties could gestate these preembryos does not alter the fact that these parties, the gamete-providers, would become parents in that event, at least in the genetic sense. The profound impact this would have on them supports their right to sole decisional authority as to whether the process of attempting to gestate these preembryos should continue. This brings us directly to the question of how to resolve the dispute that arises when one party wishes to continue the IVF process and the other does not.

VII. Balancing the Parties' Interests

Resolving disputes over conflicting interests of constitutional import is a task familiar to the courts. One way of resolving these disputes is to consider the positions of the parties, the significance of their interests, and the relative burdens that will be imposed by differing resolutions. In this case, the issue centers on the two aspects of procreational autonomy—the right to procreate and the right to avoid procreation. We start by considering the burdens imposed on the parties by solutions that would have the effect of disallowing the exercise of individual procreational autonomy with respect to these particular preembryos.

Beginning with the burden imposed on Junior Davis, we note that the consequences are obvious. Any disposition which results in the gestation of the preembryos would impose unwanted parenthood on him, with all of its possible financial and psychological consequences. . . .

Balanced against Junior Davis's interest in avoiding parenthood is Mary Sue Davis's interest in donating the preembryos to another couple for implantation. Refusal to permit donation of the preembryos would impose on her the burden of knowing that the lengthy IVF procedures she underwent were futile, and that the preembryos to which she contributed genetic material would never become children. While this is not an insubstantial emotional burden, we can only conclude that Mary Sue Davis's interest in donation is not as significant as the interest Junior Davis has in avoiding parenthood. . . .

The case would be closer if Mary Sue Davis were seeking to use the preembryos herself, but only if she could not achieve parenthood by any other reasonable means. We recognize the trauma that Mary Sue has already experienced and the additional discomfort to which she would be subjected if she opts to attempt IVF again. Still, she would have a reasonable opportunity, through IVF, to try once again to achieve parenthood in all its aspects—genetic, gestational, bearing, and rearing. . . .

VIII. Conclusion

In summary, we hold that disputes involving the disposition of preembryos produced by in vitro fertilization should be resolved, first, by looking to the preferences of the progenitors. If their wishes cannot be ascertained, or if there is dispute, then their prior agreement concerning disposition should be carried out. If no prior agreement exists, then the relative interests of the parties in using or not using the preembryos must be weighed. Ordinarily, the party wishing to avoid procreation should prevail, assuming that the other party has a reasonable possibility of achieving parenthood by means other than use of the preembryos in question. If no other reasonable alternatives exist, then the argument in favor of using the preembryos to achieve pregnancy should be considered. However, if the party seeking control of the preembryos intends merely to donate them to another couple, the objecting party obviously has the greater interest and should prevail.

But the rule does not contemplate the creation of an automatic veto, and in affirming the judgment of the Court of Appeals, we would not wish to be interpreted as so holding.

For the reasons set out above, the judgment of the Court of Appeals is affirmed, in the appellee's favor. This ruling means that the Knoxville Fertility Clinic is free to follow its normal procedure in dealing with unused preembryos, as long as that procedure is not in conflict with this opinion. Costs on appeal will be taxed to the appellant.

Discussion Questions

1. How might these parties have avoided costly litigation?

2. The standard applied by courts when a child custody battle results between parents is the "best interests" test. Might that standard be applied in a custody fight regarding embryos?

Johnson v. State
602 So. 2d 1288 (Fla. 1992)

Harding, J.

We have [this case] for review . . . in which the Fifth District Court of Appeal certified the following question as one of great public importance:

WHETHER THE INGESTION OF A CONTROLLED SUBSTANCE BY A MOTHER WHO KNOWS THE SUBSTANCE WILL PASS TO HER CHILD AFTER BIRTH IS A VIOLATION OF FLORIDA LAW? [*sic*]

. . . [W]e answer the certified question in the negative.

The issue before the court is whether [the Florida law prohibiting the delivery of controlled substances to a minor] permits the criminal prosecution of a mother, who ingested a controlled substance prior to giving birth, for delivery of a controlled substance to the infant during the thirty to ninety seconds following the infant's birth, but before the umbilical cord is severed.

. . . .

The rules of statutory construction require courts to strictly construe criminal statutes, and that "when the language is susceptible to differing constructions, [the statute] shall be construed most favorably to the accused." . . . We find that the legislative history does not show a manifest intent to use the word "delivery" in the context of criminally prosecuting mothers for delivery of a controlled substance to a minor by way of the umbilical cord. This lack of legislative intent coupled with uncertainty that the term "delivery" applies to the facts of the instant case, compels this Court to construe the statute in favor of Johnson. . . .

[The court here quotes the full text of the dissenting opinion from the court below. In that opinion, it is disclosed that defendant Johnson was an abuser of crack cocaine and had given birth to two children while using the drug. The medical evidence tended to show that the drug could have been transmitted to the children after their birth but before the umbilical cords had been severed. However, after reviewing the legislative history of the statute under which the defendant was prosecuted, the lower court concluded that "the Legislature never intended for the general drug delivery statute to authorize prosecutions of those mothers who take illegal drugs close enough in time to childbirth that a doctor could testify that a tiny amount passed from mother to child in the few seconds before the umbilical cord was cut." The quotation from the lower court continues, as follows.]

There can be no doubt that drug abuse is one of the most serious problems confronting our society today. Of particular concern is the alarming rise in the number of babies born with cocaine in their systems as a result of cocaine use by pregnant women. Some experts estimate that as many as eleven percent of pregnant women have used an illegal drug during pregnancy, and of those women, seventy-five percent have used cocaine. Others estimate that 375,000 newborns per year are born to women who are users of illicit drugs.

It is well-established that the effects of cocaine use by a pregnant woman on her fetus and later on her newborn can be severe. On average, cocaine-exposed babies have lower birth weights, shorter body lengths at birth, and smaller head circumferences than normal infants. Cocaine use may also result in sudden infant death syndrome, neural-behavioral deficiencies as well as other medical problems and long-term developmental abnormalities. The basic problem of damaging the fetus by drug use during pregnancy should not be addressed piecemeal, however, by prosecuting users who deliver their babies close in time to use of drugs and ignoring those who simply use drugs during their pregnancy.

Florida could possibly have elected to make in utero transfers criminal. But it chose to deal with this problem in other ways. One way is to allow evidence of drug use by women as a ground for removal of the child to the custody of protective services, as was done in this case. Some states have responded to this crisis by charging women with child abuse and neglect.

However, prosecuting women for using drugs and "delivering" them to their newborns appears to be the least effective response to this crisis. Rather than face the possibility of prosecution, pregnant women who are substance abusers may simply avoid prenatal or medical care for fear of being detected. Yet the newborns of these women are, as a group, the most fragile and sick, and most in need of hospital neonatal care. A decision to deliver these babies "at-home" will have tragic and serious consequences.
. . .

. . . .

While unhealthy behavior cannot be condoned, to bring criminal charges against a pregnant woman for activities which may be harmful to her fetus is inappropriate. Such prosecution is counterproductive to the public interest as it may discourage a woman from seeking prenatal care or dissuade her from providing accurate information to health care providers out of fear of self-incrimination. This failure to seek proper care or to withhold vital infor-

mation concerning her health could increase the risks to herself and her baby.

Florida's Secretary of Health and Rehabilitative Services has also observed that potential prosecution under existing child abuse or drug use statutes already 'makes many potential reporters reluctant to identify women as substance abusers.' Prosecution of pregnant women for engaging in activities harmful to their fetuses or newborns may also unwittingly increase the incidence of abortion.

. . . .

In summary, I would hold that [the law in question] does not encompass "delivery" of an illegal drug derivative from womb to placenta to umbilical cord to newborn after a child's birth. If that is the intent of the Legislature, then this statute should be redrafted to clearly address the basic problem of passing illegal substances from mother to child in utero, not just in the birthing process.

[The Supreme Court of Florida then concludes the decision with the following.]

Since the Fifth District Court of Appeal's decision, several other courts have ruled on issues similar to ones presented in this case. At oral argument the State acknowledged that no other jurisdiction has upheld a conviction of a mother for delivery of a controlled substance to an infant through either the umbilical cord or an in utero transmission; nor has the State submitted any subsequent authority to reflect that this fact has changed. The Court declines the State's invitation to walk down a path that the law, public policy, reason and common sense forbid it to tread. Therefore, we quash the decision below, answer the certified question in the negative, and remand with directions that Johnson's two convictions be reversed.

It is so ordered.

Discussion Questions

1. Is there any deterrent value in applying criminal sanctions to a woman who violates criminal statutes and thus adversely affects her fetus?

2. Should a mother-to-be with known drug habits be imprisoned during the term of her pregnancy to protect the fetus?

3. The use of alcohol during pregnancy may result in fetal alcohol syndrome. How do we differentiate between the use of alcohol and cocaine during pregnancy? Is there a substantive difference?

12

Medical Records

The chapter on medical records demonstrates a basic tension: the conflict between a desire to know and the need to keep certain information confidential. Whenever someone (individuals, the government, insurance companies, etc.) seeks medical record information, the confidentiality of that information, gained in the context of the doctor-patient relationship, potentially conflicts with the public's asserted right to know.

The outcome of litigation regarding medical records thus affects the development of institutional policies regarding the maintenance and handling of medical records. Since medical records are primarily intended to guide physicians and other health care personnel in their treatment decisions, such hospital policies in turn directly affect the continuity of patient care. Thus, legal issues regarding medical records are not merely administrative, technical, or procedural matters; they influence the quality of service that health care institutions provide.

Much legal activity regarding medical records today is occurring with respect to the treatment of AIDS and testing for the HIV virus. The availability of confidential and anonymous testing for the HIV antibodies exemplifies the importance of the legal standards regarding medical record controversies and underscores their effect on diagnosis and treatment.

The cases in this chapter reflect a wide range of medical record issues. As always, the student is encouraged to look beneath the specific legalities involved and visualize the interpersonal relationships and human frailties involved in each situation.

Horne v. Patton
291 Ala. 701, 287 So. 2d 824 (1973)

Bloodworth, J.

Plaintiff Larry Horne comes here . . . assigning as error the trial court's ruling in sustaining defendant's demurrer to his complaint.

This case is alleged to have arisen out of the disclosure by Dr. Patton, defendant herein, to plaintiff's employer of certain information acquired in the course of a doctor-patient relationship between plaintiff Horne and defendant doctor, contrary to the expressed instructions of patient Horne. Plaintiff Horne's original complaint asserted that the alleged conduct constituted a breach of fiduciary duty and an invasion of the plaintiff's right of privacy. Demurrer to this complaint was sustained. Subsequently, three amended counts were filed and demurrer to these counts was also sustained. Plaintiff thereupon . . . filed this appeal.

. . . .

Count I of the amended complaint alleges in substance that defendant is a medical doctor, that plaintiff was a patient of defendant doctor for valuable consideration, that plaintiff instructed defendant doctor not to release any medical information regarding plaintiff to plaintiff's employer, and that defendant doctor proceeded to release full medical information to plaintiff's employer without plaintiff's authorization. Count I further alleges that the doctor-patient relationship between plaintiff and defendant was a confidential relationship which created a fiduciary duty from the defendant-doctor to the plaintiff patient, that the unauthorized release of said information breached said fiduciary duty, moreover that said disclosure violated the Hippocratic Oath which defendant had taken and therefore constitutes unprofessional conduct. Plaintiff avers that as a direct and proximate result of the release of said information, plaintiff was dismissed from his employment.

Count II alleges the same basic facts but avers that the release of said information was an unlawful and wrongful invasion of plaintiff's privacy.

Count III alleges, in substance, that plaintiff entered into a physician-patient contractual relationship for a consideration with the defendant, whereby through common custom and practice, impliedly, if not expressly, defendant agreed to keep confidential personal information given to him by his patient, that plaintiff believed the defendant would adhere to such an implied contract, with the usual responsibility of the medical profession and the traditional confidentiality of patient communications expressed in the Hippocratic Oath taken by the defendant. Count III goes on to allege that defendant breached said contract by releasing full medical information regarding the plaintiff to plaintiff's employer.

. . . .

Count I

Whether or not there is a confidential relationship between doctor and patient which imposes a duty on the doctor not to freely disclose information obtained from his patients in the course of treatment is a question of first impression in this state. The question has received only a limited consideration in other jurisdictions, and its resolution has been varied. Those states which have enacted a doctor-patient testimonial privilege statute have been almost uniform in allowing a cause of action for unauthorized disclosure.

Alabama, however, has not enacted such a privilege statute. In reviewing cases from other states which also do not have a doctor-patient testimonial privilege, the jurisdictions are split about evenly on this issue. After careful consideration of this issue, it appears that the sounder legal position recognizes at least a qualified duty on the part of a doctor not to reveal confidences obtained through the doctor-patient relationship.

[Here the court reviews decisions from various other jurisdictions, beginning with a New Jersey case that is quoted favorably, as follows:]

"... The benefits which inure to the relationship of physician-patient from the denial to a physician of any right to promiscuously disclose such information are self-evident. On the other hand, it is impossible to conceive of any countervailing benefits which would arise by according a physician the right to gossip about a patient's health.

"A patient should be entitled to freely disclose his symptoms and condition to his doctor in order to receive proper treatment without fear that those facts may become public property. Only thus can the purpose of the relationship be fulfilled. So here, when

the plaintiffs contracted with defendant for services to be performed for their infant child, he was under a general duty not to disclose frivolously the information received from them, or from an examination of the patient. . . .

. . . . "

. . . .

[A Pennsylvania decision] went one step farther and condemned a disclosure made prior to trial, even though the information disclosed would not have been privileged at trial due to Pennsylvania's lack of a doctor-patient testimonial privilege statute. The court observed:

"* * * We are of the opinion that the members of a profession, especially the medical profession, stand in a confidential or fiduciary capacity as to their patients. They owe their patients more than just medical care for which payment is expected; there is a duty of total care: that includes and comprehends a duty to aid the patient in litigation, to render reports when necessary and to attend court when needed. That further includes a duty to refuse affirmative assistance to the patient's antagonist in litigation. The doctor, of course, owes a duty to conscience to speak the truth; he need, however, speak only at the proper time. . . ."

[After reviewing other decisions, the court points out that the Alabama medical licensing statute provides penalties for "wilful betrayal of a professional secret," and it goes on to note that the Hippocratic Oath (which it calls the "established ethical code of the medical profession itself") contains a pledge to keep secret "Whatever in connection with my professional practice . . . I see or hear . . . which ought not to be spoken of abroad . . . ." Finally, the court points out that the American Medical Association's (AMA's) ethical principles reaffirm this pledge: "A physician may not reveal the confidences entrusted to him in the course of medical attendance, or the deficiencies he may observe in the character of patients, unless he is required to do so by law or unless it becomes necessary in order to protect the welfare of the individual or of the community."]

It is thus that it must be concluded that a medical doctor is under a general duty not to make extra-judicial disclosures of information acquired in the course of the doctor-patient relationship and that a breach of that duty will give rise to a cause of action. It is, of course, recognized that this duty is subject to exceptions prompted by the supervening interests of society, as well as the private interests of the patient himself. Whether or not the alleged disclosure by the defendant doctor in the instant case falls within such an exception, is not now an issue before this court.

The trial court erred in sustaining the demurrer to Count I.

Count II

The gravamen of Count II is that defendant's release to plaintiff's employer of information concerning plaintiff's health constituted an invasion of plaintiff's privacy.

This court has recognized the right of a person to be free from unwarranted publicity or unwarranted appropriation or exploitation of one's personality, publicization of one's private affairs with which the public has no legitimate concern, or the wrongful intrusion of one's private activities in such manner as to outrage or cause mental suffering, shame or humiliation to a person of ordinary sensibilities.

Whether or not unauthorized disclosure of a person's medical record constitutes an invasion of this right of privacy is likewise a question of first impression in Alabama. Looking to other jurisdictions which have considered this question, those courts have almost uniformly recognized such disclosure as a violation of the patient's right of privacy.

. . . .

Unauthorized disclosure of intimate details of a patient's health may amount to unwarranted publicization of one's private affairs with which the public has no legitimate concern such as to cause outrage, mental suffering, shame or humiliation to a person of ordinary sensibilities. Nor can it be said that an employer is necessarily a person who has a legitimate interest in knowing each and every detail of an employee's health. Certainly, there are many ailments about which a patient might consult his private physician which have no bearing or effect on one's employment. If the defendant doctor in the instant case had a legitimate reason for making this disclosure under the particular facts of this case, then this is a matter of defense.

The trial court erred in sustaining the demurrer to Count II.

Count III

The gravamen of Count III is that the alleged disclosure breached an implied contract to keep confidential all personal information given to defendant doctor by his patient. . . .

. . . .

We have not been cited to, nor have we found in our research, any case in which a cause of action for the breach of an implied contract of confidentiality on the part of the doctor has been rejected. Moreover, public knowledge of the ethical standards of the medical profession . . . may well be sufficient justification for reasonable expectation on a patient's part that the physician has promised to keep confidential all information given by the patient.

Again, of course, any confidentiality between patient and physician is subject to the exceptions already noted where the supervening interests of society or the private interests of the patient intervene. These are matters of defense.

The trial court erred in sustaining demurrer to Count III.

The judgment of the trial court is therefore due to be reversed and remanded.

Reversed and remanded.

Discussion Questions

1. What is the difference between *testimonial privilege* and *nontestimonial privilege*?

2. From the standpoint of the plaintiff, the violation of which kind of privilege would be more harmful?

3. Do you feel it is proper that the Hippocratic Oath and the AMA policy become the standard of care in this case?

4. What would be a legitimate reason for disclosing confidential information?

Estate of Berthiaume v. Pratt
365 A.2d 792 (Me. 1976)

Pomeroy, J.

The appellant, as administratrix, based her claim of right to damages on an alleged invasion of her late husband's "right to privacy" and on an alleged assault and battery of him. At the close of the evidence produced at trial, a justice of the Superior Court granted defendant's motion for a directed verdict.

Appellant's seasonable appeal brings the case to this court.

The appellee is a physician and surgeon practicing in Waterville, Maine. It was established at trial without contradiction that the deceased, Henry Berthiaume, was suffering from a cancer of his larynx. Appellee, an otolaryngologist, had treated him twice surgically. A laryngectomy was performed, and later, because of a tumor which had appeared in his neck, a radical neck dissection on one side was done. No complaint is made with respect to the surgical interventions.

During the period appellee was serving Mr. Berthiaume as a surgeon, many photographs of Berthiaume had been taken by appellee or under his direction. The jury was told that the sole use to which these photographs were to be put was to make the medical record [more complete] for the appellee's use. There is nothing in the case to suggest that the photographs were to be shown to students for teaching purposes or were to be used as illustrative photographs in any text books or papers. The only persons to whom the photographs were available were those members of appellee's staff and the appropriate hospital personnel who had duties to perform with respect to medical records.

Although at no time did the appellee receive any written consent for the taking of photographs from Berthiaume or any members of his family, it was appellee's testimony that Berthiaume had always consented to having such photographs made.

At all times material hereto Mr. Berthiaume was the patient of a physician other than appellee. Such other physician had referred the patient to appellee for surgery. On September 2, 1970, appellee saw the patient for the last time for the purpose of treatment or diagnosis. The incident which gave rise to this lawsuit occurred on September 23, 1970.

It was also on that day Mr. Berthiaume died.

Although appellee disputed the evidence appellant produced at trial in many material respects, the jury could have concluded from the evidence that shortly before Mr. Berthiaume died on the 23rd, the appellee and a nurse appeared in his hospital room. In the presence of Mrs. Berthiaume and a visitor of the patient in the next bed, either Dr. Pratt or the nurse, at his direction, raised the dying Mr. Berthiaume's head and placed some blue operating room toweling under his head and beside him on the bed. The appellee testified that this blue toweling was placed there for the purpose of obtaining a color contrast for the photographs which he proposed to take. He then proceeded to take several photographs of Mr. Berthiaume.

The jury could have concluded from the testimony that Mr. Berthiaume protested the taking of pictures by raising a clenched fist and moving his head from the camera's range. The appellee himself testified that before taking the pictures he had been told by Mrs. Berthiaume when he talked with her in the corridor before entering the room that she "didn't think that Henry wanted his picture taken."

It is the raising of the deceased's head in order to put the operating room towels under and around him that appellant claims was an assault and battery. It is the taking of the pictures of the dying Mr. Berthiaume that appellant claims constituted the actionable invasion of Mr. Berthiaume's right to privacy.

. . . .

By our decision in this case we join a majority of the jurisdictions in the country in recognizing a "right to privacy." We also declare it to be the rule in Maine that a violation of this legally protected right is an actionable tort.

Specifically in this case we rule an unauthorized intrusion upon a person's physical and mental solitude or seclusion is a tort for the commission of which money damages may be had.

The law of privacy addresses the invasion of four distinct interests of the individual. Each of the four different interests, taken as a whole, represent[s] an individual's right "to be let alone." These four kinds of invasion are:

(1) intrusion upon the plaintiff's physical and mental solitude or seclusion;
(2) public disclosure of private facts;
(3) publicity which places the plaintiff in a false light in the public eye;
(4) appropriation for the defendant's benefit or advantage of the plaintiff's name or likeness.

. . . .

In this case we are concerned only with a claimed intrusion upon the plaintiff's intestate's physical and mental solitude or seclusion. The jury had a right to conclude from the evidence that plaintiff's intestate was dying. It could have concluded he desired not to be photographed in his hospital bed in such condition and that he manifested such desire by his physical motions. The jury should have been instructed, if it found these facts, that the taking of pictures without dece-

dent's consent or over his objection was an invasion of his legally protected right to privacy, which invasion was as actionable tort for which money damages could be recovered.

Instead, a directed verdict for the defendant was entered, obviously premised on the presiding justice's announced incorrect conclusion that the taking of pictures without consent did not constitute an invasion of privacy and the further erroneous conclusion that no tort was committed in the absence of "proof they (the photographs) were published."

[The court proceeds to address the assault and battery argument, saying that it was erroneous for the trial court judge to conclude that consent to the touching was "implied from the existence of a physician-patient relationship." This conclusion, the court holds, was based on the assumption that the physician-patient relationship still existed when the photographs were taken, yet since Dr. Pratt came to Mr. Berthiaume's room solely to take photographs and not to treat him, the jury could have concluded that the relationship of physician and patient had ceased to exist before that time.]

We recognize the benefit to the science of medicine which comes from the making of photographs of the treatment and of medical abnormalities found in patients [*sic*]. However, we agree with the reasoning expressed [by a Pennsylvania judge, who said]:

" . . . [A]n individual has the right to decide whether that which is his shall be given to the public and not only to restrict and limit but also to withhold absolutely his talents, property, or other subjects of the right of privacy from all dissemination. The facial characteristics or peculiar caste of one's features, whether normal or distorted, belong to the individual and may not be reproduced without his permission. Even the photographer who is authorized to take a portrait is not justified in making or retaining additional copies for himself.
    . . . . "

Because there were unresolved, disputed questions of fact, which if decided by the factfinder in favor of the plaintiff, would have justified a verdict for plaintiff, it was reversible error to have directed a verdict for the defendant.

The entry must be:
Appeal sustained
New trial ordered.

Discussion Questions

1. The patient's right to confidentiality in the medical arena may call into play the legal theories of invasion of privacy, breach of contract, breach of confidential relationships, malpractice, and defamation. Were any legitimate medical purposes being served by the medical photographs at issue in this case?

2. As a health care executive, how could you have prevented this lawsuit?

Gilbert v. Medical Economics Co.
665 F.2d 305 (10th Cir. 1981)

McKay, J.

This is an appeal from the trial court's grant of summary judgment for defendants in a diversity case arising from defendants' alleged tortious invasion of plaintiff's privacy. On April 3, 1978, defendants published in the periodical *Medical Economics* an article entitled "Who Let This Doctor In The O.R.? The Story Of A Fatal Breakdown In Medical Policing." The article, a copy of which is contained in the record before us, outlines two incidents of alleged medical malpractice in which patients of plaintiff, an anesthesiologist, suffered fatal or severely disabling injuries in the operating room as a result of plaintiff's acts of alleged malpractice. The article indicates that in the case of the disabling injuries, plaintiff's insurer settled the ensuing malpractice action for $900,000. It notes further that in the case of the fatal injury, the patient's family was attempting to reach a settlement. Following a description of these incidents, the article suggests that they occurred because of "a collapse of self-policing by physicians and of disciplinary action by hospitals and regulatory agencies." To show the substantiality of this inadequate policing of medical personnel, the article discusses plaintiff's history of psychiatric and related personal problems. The article suggests (1) that there was a causal relationship between plaintiff's personal problems and the acts of alleged malpractice, (2) that plaintiff's lack of capacity to engage responsibly in the practice of medicine was or should have been known to the policing agents of the medical profession, and (3) that more intensive policing of medical personnel is needed. The article identified plaintiff by name and included her photograph.

On the basis of the pleadings and a copy of the article, the district court held a hearing on cross-motions for summary judgment. Defendants moved for summary judgment on the ground that the article contained only truthful factual statements or opinions relating to newsworthy matters and therefore was protected by the first amendment. Plaintiff conceded that no issues of fact were involved. She urged summary judgment on the theory that although the general theme of the article was newsworthy and therefore privileged, the defendants nevertheless had tortiously invaded her privacy by including in the article her name, photograph, and certain private facts about her life that were not privileged.

In granting summary judgment for the defendants, the trial court agreed that the general subject of the article was indeed newsworthy insofar as it dealt with the competency of licensed professionals. The court noted that the public has a legitimate concern with the fitness of professionals to hold the public trust that a professional license bestows. It further noted that the area of legitimate public concern extends far enough to encompass accounts of factors in the life of a li-censed professional that may impair that person's ability to perform competently. The court concluded that, where the general contents of an article are newsworthy, editors must be allowed a measure of discretion to determine how an article should be written and what details should be included. To question whether defendants should have omitted certain details from this particular article, the court believed, would amount to "editorial second-guessing" rather than legal analysis. The court therefore held that the entire article was protected by the first amendment.

I.

On appeal, plaintiff's first contention is that defendants tortiously invaded her privacy by publicly disclosing embarrassing private facts about her personal life. Colorado has recognized a common-law right to privacy. Defendants, however, raised the defense of first amendment privilege, and thus, we must turn to federal substantive law in this diversity case to determine the extent of defendants' federal constitutional defense.

The first amendment sometimes protects what would otherwise be an actionable invasion of privacy where a publication by the media is involved. This constitutional privilege clearly applies to the public disclosure of private facts, the invasion of privacy tort alleged in this action. The privilege extends to public figures, as well as to those private individuals "who have not sought publicity or consented to it, but through their own conduct or otherwise have become a legitimate subject of public interest." This privilege is not absolute, however, and as in other areas involving the media, the right of the individual to keep information private must be balanced against the right of the press to disseminate newsworthy information to the public. In attempting to strike an acceptable balance between these competing interests, liability may be imposed for publicizing matters concerning the private life of another "if the matter publicized is of a kind that (a) would be highly offensive to a reasonable person, and (b) is not of legitimate concern to the public."

. . . [T]he first amendment protects the publication of private facts that are "newsworthy," that is, of legitimate concern to the public. This standard has been accepted by other courts. In our view, this standard properly restricts liability for public disclosure of private facts to the extreme case, thereby providing the breathing space needed by the press to properly exercise effective editorial judgment. This standard provides a privilege for truthful publications that ceases to operate only when an editor abuses his broad discretion to publish matters that are of legitimate public interest.

Even where certain matters are clearly within the protected sphere of legitimate public interest, some private facts about an individual may lie outside that sphere. In *Virgil v. Time, Inc.* (1975), an action by a surfer based on publicity about his private affairs in an article about surfing, the Ninth

Circuit pointed out that "[t]he fact that [people] engage in an activity in which the public can be said to have a general interest does not render every aspect of their lives subject to public disclosure." Because each member of our society at some time engages in an activity that fairly could be characterized as a matter of legitimate public concern, to permit that activity to open the door to the exposure of any truthful secret about that person would render meaningless the tort of public disclosure of private facts. The first amendment does not require such a result. Therefore, to properly balance freedom of the press against the right of privacy, every private fact disclosed in an otherwise truthful, newsworthy publication must have some substantial relevance to a matter of legitimate public interest. When these conditions are satisfied, the facts in the publication and inferences reasonably drawn therefrom fall within the ambit of first amendment protection and are privileged.

Plaintiff maintains that the publishing of her photograph, name, and private facts about her psychiatric history and marital life adds nothing to the concededly newsworthy topic of policing failures in the medical profession. Plaintiff argues that any relationship between her psychiatric history and marital life and the incidents of alleged malpractice is purely speculative, that this information was not of legitimate public interest, and that defendants unjustifiably "appointed themselves judge, jury and executioner of [plaintiff]."

With respect to the publication of plaintiff's photograph and name, we find that these truthful representations are substantially relevant to a newsworthy topic because they strengthen the impact and credibility of the article. They obviate any impression that the problems raised in the article are remote or hypothetical, thus providing an aura of immediacy and even urgency that might not exist had plaintiff's name and photograph been suppressed. Similarly, we find the publication of plaintiff's psychiatric and marital problems to be substantially relevant to the newsworthy topic. While it is true that these subjects would fall outside the first amendment privilege in the absence of either independent newsworthiness or any substantial nexus with a newsworthy topic, here they are connected to the newsworthy topic by the rational inference that plaintiff's personal problems were the underlying cause of the acts of alleged malpractice.

Plaintiff claims that the drawing of such inferences is not within the protected scope of editorial discretion unless a public tribunal first declares such an inference to be legally established. We conclude, however, that a rule forbidding editors from drawing inferences from truthful newsworthy facts would result in a far too restrictive and wholly unjustifiable construction of the first amendment privilege. If the press is to have the generous breathing space that courts have accorded it thus far, editors must have freedom to make reasonable judgments and to draw one inference where others also reasonably could be drawn. This is precisely the editorial discretion contemplated by the privilege. Because the inferences of causation drawn in this case are not, as a matter

of law, so purely conjectural that no reasonable editor could draw them other than through guesswork and speculation, we hold that defendants did not abuse their editorial discretion in this case.

Since we have concluded that the inference of causation properly could be drawn in the exercise of reasonable editorial discretion, we find that plaintiff's name, photograph, and psychiatric and marital problems, are substantially relevant to the newsworthy topic of policing the medical profession. If plaintiff's psychiatric and marital problems plausibly contributed to her commission of medical malpractice, then the publication of these facts together with her name and photograph serves the legitimate public interest of warning potential future patients, as well as surgeons and hospitals, of the risks they might encounter in being treated by or in employing the plaintiff. This is particularly crucial where, as here, potential patients and colleagues may not otherwise receive notice of these risks. Clearly, under these circumstances the public has a very strong and immediate legitimate interest, and the first amendment protects the media's right to reveal this information.

We must ourselves apply the law to the facts in this case. Every relevant fact is set forth in the article itself, a copy of which is before us. There are no issues of fact that turn on demeanor evidence or other evidence of witness credibility. The parties agree that all the facts are undisputed. Although application of the newsworthiness standard to undisputed facts may well present a jury question in some cases, here objective and reasonable minds cannot differ in finding the article in question to be privileged in its entirety, thus precluding liability for public disclosure of private facts. . . .

. . . .

AFFIRMED.

Discussion Questions

1. The duty to maintain confidentiality and the torts of defamation and invasion of privacy come into conflict with the First Amendment when publication by the media is involved. When the person subjected to media attention is a public figure, the standards may be different than when a private individual is involved. How would you distinguish between a public figure and a private individual?

2. Assuming that you can make that distinction accurately enough, how do you decide what is newsworthy information and what is merely tending toward gossip? What are the tests for making the distinction between newsworthy information and nonnewsworthy information?

3. How does this court view the publication of the physician's photograph, name, psychiatric history, and marital life? In which category does it put that information?

4. Does it matter to you how accurate the published information is? If it is completely accurate but subjects a private

individual to public scorn, should truth be a defense? Suppose a piece of investigative journalism contains some errors but is generally rather accurate and as a result a public figure has to resign his or her position; should the errors enable the individual to sue the journalists or the publication? Would it matter if they were innocent errors rather than known falsehoods? Does it matter whether the journalists were out to get the individual?

Thurman v. Crawford
652 S.W.2d 240 (Mo. Ct. App. 1983)

Crandall, J.

Appellant, Gary Thurman, appeals from the trial court's order sustaining respondents' . . . motion for summary judgment. We affirm.

Appellant received medical treatment at St. Louis University Hospital . . . for injuries sustained in an automobile accident. In preparation of his claim for damages arising out of the automobile accident, appellant executed a medical authorization for his attorney to copy his medical records at St. Louis University Hospital. The medical authorization [is shown in Exhibit A on page 150].

On December 30, 1981, an employee of the copying service employed by appellant's attorney went to St. Louis University Hospital and gave the authorization to the hospital records clerk, Zatie Crawford. St. Louis University Hospital policy requires that the medical authorization must be signed by the patient and must be dated no more than ninety days prior to the request for the records. Ms. Crawford refused access to the records based on her determination that the medical authorization did not meet hospital policy because the date on the form had been altered. Despite subsequent telephone conversations between Ms. Crawford and appellant's attorney and the attorney's secretary, Ms. Crawford refused access to the records unless a "properly" dated medical authorization was presented.

Appellant filed suit against respondents for refusing access to his medical records. Respondents' motion for summary judgment was sustained and this appeal ensues.

In reviewing the granting of a motion for summary judgment, we view the record in the light most favorable to the party against whom the motion for summary judgment was filed and against whom the judgment was rendered and accord that party the benefit of every doubt.

Respondents do not contest appellant's common law right to inspect his records. Certainly this right extends to appellant's agent. Respondent hospital contends[, however,] that it may restrict the release of their patients' records to insure the privacy of privileged matter.

. . . Since the hospital has the duty to protect its patients from the unauthorized release of privileged information, we hold that the hospital may take reasonable precautions to check the credentials and authority of persons seeking access to that information.

Appellant argues that the trial court's order granting respondents' motion for summary judgment was inappropriate. Respondents cannot deny appellant access to his medical records. Unreasonable restriction of access to medical records can be tantamount to a refusal to release the records. Generally, the question of reasonableness is a question of fact for the jury rather than a question of law for the court. However, in this case, respondent Crawford was presented with a medical authorization which was altered on its face and which failed to comply with hospital policy. This, coupled with Ms. Crawford's willingness to release the records if presented with a properly dated authorization, did, as a matter of law, constitute a reasonable refusal to release the records. The trial court, therefore, properly granted summary judgment.

The trial court's order granting summary judgment in favor of respondents is affirmed.

REINHARD and CRIST, JJ., concur.

Discussion Questions

1. What additional information would you like to know that the opinion does not tell you? How would that information be significant?

2. What standard is used by an appellate court in deciding a case like this?

3. Are you persuaded that the form shown in Exhibit A was, in fact, altered? If so, was the alteration significant? Does it matter how significant the alteration was?

4. How could this matter have been resolved without litigation?

EXHIBIT "A"

Refused by hospital on 12-30-81
John Stephenson

LAW OFFICES OF

NEWMAN & BRONSON
1015 LOCUST STREET, SUITE 728
ST. LOUIS, MISSOURI 63101
TELEPHONE (314) 231-4600

PATIENT'S AUTHORIZATION FOR RELEASE OF MEDICAL AND/OR HOSPITAL RECORDS

TO: Doctor/Hospital *Firmin Desloge Hospital*
                          1325 So. Grand

RE: Patient: *Gary Thurman*
        Address: *316 Cameron*
        DOB:

You are hereby authorized to furnish to the law offices of NEWMAN & BRONSON, or to their representative, MARKELL & ASSOCIATES, INC., who has my authority to copy records pertaining to me which are in your possession.

All prior authorizations executed by me are hereby revoked.

This authorization does not extend to any other attorney or copy service. Therefore, any release of my records to any company or individual other than NEWMAN & BRONSON, my attorneys and MARKELL & ASSOCIATES, INC., their representative, will be considered a violation of my confidential privilege and subject to civil action.

_____
Patient (or adult with authority to act for minor). If patient is deceased - legal representative.

Subscribed and sworn to before me this *12th* day of *November*, 198*0*.

_____
Notary Public

My term expires: *August 10, 1982*

Doe v. Goldman
No. 79-0313-MA (D. Mass. May 20, 1980) (unreported)

Mazzone, J.

This is a civil rights action under 42 U.S.C. § 1983 for damages stemming from the alleged deprivation of the plaintiffs' constitutional rights as parents. The claim is based on the wrongful withholding of medical records and information concerning the treatment of their daughter during voluntary commitment at the Massachusetts Mental Health Center from 1972 to 1973. In a prior action in state court, the plaintiff, John Doe, sued the Commissioner of Mental Health and another defendant named here for failure to produce his daughter's records pursuant to [a Massachusetts statute] which provides for access by attorneys who have obtained patient consent. In that case, the defendants refused to furnish records or any other written reports to the plaintiff, even though he was representing his daughter in a trust management suit and had obtained permission from the daughter on forms supplied by the department. The reason for refusing access after consent had been obtained was that the plaintiff's parental interest overrode his interest as an attorney and that it was therefore necessary "to protect the welfare of the patients and the relationship between patients and families." The Supreme Judicial Court held that since the plaintiff was legitimately acting as the child's attorney, the Commissioner had no discretion under the law to withhold records after lawful consent had been obtained. No damages were found, however, and because there was a legitimate issue over the ability of a minor to consent, the Court conditioned the father's access to the procurement of a new consent by his daughter, who has since reached the age of majority and no longer has contact with her parents. Constitutional issues were expressly reserved.

In this case, the plaintiffs claim that the failure to receive the records when requested, coupled with the defendants' refusal to provide any substantive reports about their daughter's treatment, prevented essential decision-making about the health and welfare of the child after her release, and, as a consequence, led to the breakdown of their relationship. The claim of entitlement is grounded primarily upon the concept of parental rights.

The case is now before the Court on the defendants' motion to dismiss. In this context, all averments are taken as admitted, and we must construe the complaint in the light most favorable to the plaintiff. Though overly long and repetitious the complaint does raise important questions about the scope of parental rights and the power of the state to intervene in the mental health area.

The Standard for Liability under 42 U.S.C. § 1983

As officials in a state hospital, the defendants are entitled to a qualified immunity against suits for damages. Whether immunity extends in this action depends on if defendants knew or reasonably should have known that the actions taken within the sphere of official responsibility would violate the Constitutional rights of the plaintiff or if there was malicious intention to cause a deprivation of Constitutional rights or other injury. The policy is to encourage good faith fulfillment of official responsibilities and to insure that discretion will be exercised without undue timidity. Taking the second part of the test first, immunity will be forfeited if there is a subjective intent to injure, regardless of the nature of the rights recognized at the time. Beyond the bare allegations in the pleadings, however, there is nothing in the complaint which, if proven, could establish intent in the tortious sense required under this standard. The most that could be said is that defendants erred in not following their counsel's advice that the plaintiff as an attorney could obtain records despite his parental status. In view of the strict wording of the statute, however, we believe this decision fell within administrative discretion which the immunity doctrine is designed to protect.

Recovery under Section 1983 is therefore possible only under the first part of the test, which subjects an official to liability if at the time of his conduct, the actions violated settled, indisputable law even if he acted in good faith. The hospital administrators, as a result, cannot be charged with foreseeing later developments in constitutional theories affecting their responsibilities.

The claim to mental health records and reports is based on a very generalized concept. While parental rights have been fostered in many areas of child care, however, in the field of mental health the proper allocation of responsibility between parent, child, and state has been examined only recently, and with ambiguous results. An inspection of the current state of the law is helpful in determining the strength of the complaint.

The Scope of Parental Rights

It has long been recognized that parental authority over minor children is a right encompassed within the ambit of liberty protected by the Due Process Clause of the 14th Amendment. As the Supreme Court states in *Stanley v. Illinois*, (1972), "the private interest * * * of a man in the children he has sired and raised undeniably warrants deference, and, absent a powerful countervailing interest * * * protection."

It is not enough to say that the right exists to prove its applicability in all circumstances, however, for like all constitutional rights, parental authority is not beyond regulation. Although it is protected against unreasonable interference, countervailing interests both of the state and child may compel intrusion on the parental role. Thus, under its parens patriae power, the state may assume authority where the health or welfare of the child is at stake. Similarly, controls imposed on the child for societal or parental benefit may be prohibited if they abridge the child's fundamental rights. In recent years, for example, the protections of the Bill of

Rights, particularly the right of privacy, have been invoked to strike down unjustified restrictions on a minor's right to an abortion or to access to contraceptives.

The interests of the state, child, and the parent intertwine and conflict to an equal degree in the mental health field. To the child, even in the voluntary commitment setting, confinement and treatment represent a substantial infringement on interests in liberty and reputation. In the context of this case, the privacy interest is equally as strong as the desire for proper care and confinement. The parent, conversely, would like to assert a paramount interest in the "care and nurture" of the child. For its part, the state has a legitimate interest under its parens patriae power to provide care for the emotionally disturbed, and to protect its patients' privacy. In voluntary commitment cases, the state's interest may be subrogated to some degree to the child's, but the duty to protect becomes preeminent when the child's welfare is threatened.

No subject in this field can be more fraught with conflicting rights and obligations than the control and dissemination of information about patients. The unrestricted right which plaintiffs demand strikes at the very balance of responsibilities on which our present mental health care system rests. During the time of the incidents presented here, we can find no suggestion that a right to such information existed or was ever recognized. While recent Supreme Court cases do indicate that in the future parental authority may require more adequate recognition in the areas of mental health care, no clearly established theory has been expanded which, by implication, proves the existence of a heretofore unsuspected "right" to information.

The *Parham* case is most pertinent, since it examines the parents' role in mental health treatment. The issue was whether voluntary commitment constituted an invasion of the child's liberty interest so as to require an adversary hearing prior to commitment. In rejecting this notion, the Court carefully balanced parental rights against the independent state interest in an efficient system fostering the legitimate needs of its patients. To the parents the Court explicitly delegated the primary responsibility for mental health treatment of minors, concluding that the right to seek and follow medical advice for their children requires that they retain "a substantial, if not the dominant role * * * " in the voluntary commitment setting. However, the power of commitment is not "absolute and unreviewable," and the decision to commit was thus made contingent on a neutral screening process in which the independent judgment of the physician assumes a pivotal role.

The *Bellotti* case reached a similar result in an equally critical area of health care, holding that while a state could legitimately choose to foster parental involvement in a medical decision, a minor's right to an abortion could not be predicated on parental consent.

As the most recent expositions on parental rights, *Parham* and *Bellotti* provide no basis for determining that the mechanism regulating access to confidential information in mental hospitals should be disturbed on constitutional grounds. Parental consent and involvement in decisions by minors is important to their well being and may ultimately be preferred. This is indeed commensurate with common law understanding that parental consent to medical treatment, absent emergency or threat of harm, is usually required. At the same time, the cases make clear, where a critical interest of the child arises, the parental role must be tailored appropriately, either to preserve exercise of a fundamental right or to insure that the best interests of the child are adequately protected. In this context, several lower courts have recently struck down statutory provisions requiring even notice to parents before their children undergo abortions, construing the requirement as unduly burdening the minor's fundamental right. We do not suggest that a demand for psychiatric reports rises to this level of infringement, but the little decisional law existing on access to actual mental health records, the nub of the dispute here, does indicate that privacy interests and the need to insure a stable atmosphere for treatment support restrictions on information, even to the patients themselves.

Access to Mental Health Records

The issue of access to mental health files has most often arisen in the context of a patient's or former patient's claim for copies under state law. On the statutory level, these claims have failed because, as in the majority of states, former patient access to medical records without resort to litigation is the exception rather than the rule. In Massachusetts mental health records are specifically exempted from the direct access law for general hospital records.

The rationale for these laws is compelling and can be applied to a generalized claim for detailed written reports, as asserted here. Information can be misconstrued and thus affect the recovery and well-being of the patient. The records often contain information and personal observations from third parties, such as relatives, which are entirely confidential. In addition, the records can properly be considered the property of the physician and the hospital, and not of the patient.

In constitutional terms, this lack of entitlement under state law deprives plaintiffs of any possible claim to a property interest under the Due Process Clause, since the establishment of such an interest is the result of state and not of constitutional law. While the Supreme Judicial Court held that the plaintiff may be entitled to records as an attorney, such a decision does not mandate finding an unrestricted direct claim to the records, as is sought in this action. Moreover, entitlement as a parent, accompanied by consent of the child, was an issue expressly reserved by the Court.

Other constitutional grounds for access have been reviewed elsewhere and rejected. There can be no claim to deprivation of liberty because neither the plaintiffs nor their daughter have, to any degree, been "stigmatized" by the non-disclosure. Though not advanced here, claims under the First and Fourth Amendments also merit little attention. We are thus left with the concept of parental rights which, although substantial, does not warrant a wholesale invasion of the rights of both the minor child and her physicians. To so hold here would not only overcome the substantial policy reasons for maintaining confidentiality of these records, but would also contravene the intention of the Commonwealth. As the Supreme Judicial Court noted, [the statute in question] "was intended to protect patients from the potentially detrimental impact of disclosure of records to third parties." No clear constitutional policy has yet been established which would diminish this interest in favor of parents.

There are other sound reasons for not placing a constitutional imprimatur on the demand for patient information where the rights of others are involved. For some time, for example, courts have recognized that unrestricted access to confidential family records in the adoption field would represent an undue infringement on parental privacy rights not warranted by the public interest or the interests of the child seeking the records. Thus, the limitation of access based on a valid state interest in protecting the rights of others is not an unconstitutional exercise.

. . . .

Conclusion

For the foregoing reasons, the plaintiffs have failed to establish a settled, indisputable right to the information and records demanded in the complaint. In the particular area of access to psychiatric files, decisional and statutory law dictate that confidential records remain secret except to the extent permitted by law. Parental rights have not yet expanded to foreclose state assertion of the child's interest in privacy, which protects as well the interests of physicians and other third parties who have taken part in the treatment process. . . .

In accordance with the above, the defendants' motion to dismiss is granted.

Discussion Questions

1. What are the precise issues and procedural history of this case? Based on the decision, does a future plaintiff like Mr. "Doe" have a right of access or does he not?

2. Should patients have a right to review their own records? Does that right differ depending on whether the patient is competent or incompetent?

3. What constitutes patient consent to access medical records?

4. In whom does the property interest in medical records reside?

Fox v. Cohen
84 Ill. App. 3d. 744, 406 N.E.2d 178 (1980)

Downing, J.

Plaintiff, Mary Lou Fox, appeals the dismissal of her second amended complaint. Plaintiff, as administrator of the estate of Donald R. Fox, filed a wrongful death action in the circuit court of Cook County. Count I of her second amended complaint alleged that certain acts of medical malpractice by defendant, Dr. Sheldon Cohen, caused the death of her decedent and prayed for $500,000 in damages. Count II of this complaint alleged, hypothetically and in the alternative, that Alexian Brothers Medical Center and its employees, Helen Lottman and Linda Lukaski, had negligently lost, destroyed, or misplaced EKG [electrocardiogram] tracings and reports relating to the decedent, and that the medical center and its named employees had a duty to exercise reasonable care in the custody, safekeeping, and maintenance of records relative to patient care. Count III alleged, hypothetically and in the alternative, that William Shields, an administrator, and nurses Lottman and Lukaski, all employees of Alexian Brothers Medical Center, conspired with defendant Cohen, a staff member of the medical center, to and did hide, lose, or secrete EKG tracings relative to the decedent. Both counts II and III alleged that the actions of the defendants deprived plaintiff of vital evidence necessary to sustain her burden of proof against defendant Cohen under count I, resulting in the loss of plaintiff's cause of action, and prayed for damages in the amount of $500,000.

Prior to the filing of the second amended complaint and pursuant to court order, defendant Cohen filed an affidavit in which he stated that "no records [were] in his possession or control, including, *inter alia*, EKG tracings or analysis, emergency room records, notes or other written documents."

Defendants, Alexian Brothers Medical Center, Helen Lottman, and William Shields, filed a motion to dismiss counts II and III on the grounds that they failed to state a cause of action; failed to allege grounds upon which tort relief could be granted; were barred by the two-year statute of limitations; and, in the alternative, were improperly joined with count I. Defendant Cohen filed a motion to dismiss count III on these same grounds.

The trial court granted defendants' motions and dismissed counts II and III of plaintiff's second amended complaint. As to count II the court stated that defendants owed no duty to the plaintiff to maintain certain medical records pertaining to the decedent. Absent such a duty, the trial court stated that the conspiracy as alleged in count III could not be proven; that joinder of counts II and III was therefore improper; and that because of these findings plaintiff's request for leave to amend was denied. The court found no reason to delay enforcement or appeal of this order. Plaintiff filed a timely notice of appeal from this order.

I.

A.

On appeal, we are concerned only with whether counts II and III stated a valid cause of action in negligence. In order to state a cause of action founded upon negligence, plaintiff must plead the existence of a duty owed by the defendant to plaintiff, a breach of that duty, and an injury proximately resulting from the breach. The trial court dismissed count II on the basis that plaintiff failed to allege a duty. Count II was directed only against the hospital and its employees and not against the defendant doctor. The basis of the trial court's order requires this court to initially consider whether a hospital has a duty to maintain medical records on its patients.

Defendants argue that there is no common law or statutory authority for imposing such a duty on a hospital. . . .

. . . .

In determining the standard of conduct here, we look to pertinent legislative enactments, administrative regulations, and standards set forth by the American Hospital Association. The Hospital Licensing Act empowers the Illinois Department of Public Health to adopt rules, regulations, standards, and statements of policy needed to implement, interpret, or make specific the provisions and purposes of the Act.

Pursuant to its rule-making power, the Department of Public Health has promulgated certain licensing requirements. [A portion] of the licensing requirements, in pertinent part, provides:

"For each patient there shall be an adequate, accurate, timely, and complete medical record. Minimum requirements for medical record contents are as follows: * * * physical examination report; * * * diagnostic and therapeutic reports on laboratory test results, * * * and any other diagnostic or therapeutic procedure performed; * * *."

[Another portion] of the licensing requirements provides that "[a]ll original medical records or photographs of such records shall be preserved in accordance with a hospital policy based on American Hospital Association recommendations and legal opinion."

According to a statement prepared by the American Hospital Association's committee on medical records and the American Medical Record Association's planning and bylaws committee . . . :

"The primary purpose of the medical record is to document the source of the patient's illness and the treatment he receives. Although the medical record is kept for the benefit of the patient, the physician, and the health care institution, it is the property of the health care institution with other interests recognized by law."

The statement goes on to say:

"The length of time medical records should be retained will vary depending upon the purposes for which the record is being kept. In formulating a record-retention policy, a health care institution must be guided by its own clinical, scientific and audit needs and the possibility of future patient litigation."

The Association, taking into consideration that the period of retention would be affected by the type of legal action pursued and the statute of limitations applicable to that action as established by the laws of different States, recommended that complete patient medical records in health care institutions be retained for 10 years after the most recent patient care usage.

The introduction of the Record Retention Guide for Illinois Hospitals published by the Illinois Hospital Association provides, "[a]n Illinois health care institution in formulating a record retention policy must be guided by its own needs * * *, *the possibility of future patient litigation* and state and federal laws." (Emphasis added.) The Guide recommends that medical records and EKG tracings be retained for 10 to 22 years.

The *Accreditation Manual for Hospitals*, published by the Joint Commission on Accreditation of Hospitals provides that "[t]he hospital shall maintain such facilities and services as are adequate to provide medical records that are accurately documented, readily accessible and can be easily used for retrieving and compiling information." The purposes of the medical record as stated in the manual include, among others, to furnish documentary evidence of the course of the patient's illness and treatment during each hospital stay; to serve as a basis for review, study, and evaluation of the care rendered to the patient; and to assist in protecting the legal interests of the patient, hospital, and responsible practitioner.

The regulations require that a hospital keep a complete and accurate medical record on each patient. The purposes of this requirement are manifold, each relating to the betterment and protection of the patient as well as the hospital. It is clear that the regulations and recommendations set forth above contemplate the possibility of future patient litigation based upon treatment or care rendered. In view of the increasing number of medical malpractice actions being filed and in order to safeguard the patient's interest as well as the hospital's interest in such litigation, we think it necessary that reasonable care be used to maintain complete and accurate medical records. The authorities advocate that it is both desirable and feasible that a hospital assume the responsibility of keeping such records. By finding that a hospital does owe a duty to its patients to use reasonable care in maintaining medical records, we need not resolve such questions as how long or in what specific manner such medical records must be maintained. Those questions are reserved for the trier of fact in its determination as to what is reasonable under the facts of each case.

The conspiracy alleged in court III of the complaint is merely an aggravation of the wrongful acts alleged in count

II. In a civil case, the wrongful acts alleged to have been done in pursuance of a conspiracy, and not the fact of the conspiracy itself, is the gist of the action for damages. Thus, the viability of count III depends upon whether the allegations of count II state a cause of action.

The existence of a legal duty fulfills only one of the elements necessary for stating a valid cause of action in negligence. Another necessary element is that an injury proximately occurred from a breach of that duty. The injury must be actual; the threat of future harm not yet realized is not enough.

Counts II and III allege that the hospital's breach of its duty caused plaintiff to lose her malpractice action against the defendant doctor as alleged in count I of the complaint. However, plaintiff has not yet sustained any injury. The medical malpractice claim under count I is still pending. Plaintiff's theory of recovery in counts II and III is based upon the notion that she will sometime in the future lose her malpractice action because of the absence of an EKG tracing. Such a notion at this point in time is contingent on the unheard proof and result in the malpractice action. That plaintiff will lose her malpractice action because of a missing EKG is, as of now, purely speculative and uncertain. Liability cannot be predicted upon surmise or conjecture as to the cause of the injury. Plaintiff's action under counts II and III is premature.

Based upon the foregoing, we affirm the judgment of the circuit court of Cook County dismissing counts II and III of plaintiff's complaint. . . .

Discussion Questions

1. Medical records are essential evidence in malpractice actions. What inferences can be drawn from falsification, the concealment of information, or premature disposition of medical records? How could the defendants counter such inferences?

2. The trial court found that defendants "owed no duty to the plaintiff to maintain [the] medical records" in question. The appellate court finds "that a hospital *does* owe a duty to its patients to use reasonable care in maintaining medical records" (emphasis added), but it nevertheless affirms the trial court's ruling. Why is this so?

3. Why are Counts II and III premature? Has not the plaintiff already suffered injury because the pursuit of her malpractice litigation has been hampered and the chances of success have thereby been diminished?

4. Suppose the decedent's entire medical record and all related materials had been negligently and prematurely destroyed and that the plaintiff was therefore effectively unable to bring the malpractice action at all. Do you suppose there would be a cause of action for the negligent destruction of the records?

Doe v. American Red Cross Blood Servs., S.C. Region

125 F.R.D. 646 (D. S.C. 1989)

Hamilton, J.

In these companion cases the plaintiffs, Jane Doe and her husband John Doe, contend that Jane Doe contracted the human immunodeficiency virus ("HIV"), which causes the deadly acquired immune deficiency syndrome ("AIDS"), from a unit of blood collected and processed by the defendant, American Red Cross Blood Services, S.C. Region ("Red Cross"). The matter is presently before the court on plaintiffs' motion to compel Red Cross to identify the HIV positive donor whose blood was transfused into Jane Doe during an operation on January 9, 1985. Plaintiffs have moved, in the alternative, for an Order compelling the Red Cross to subpoena the blood donor to a "veiled" deposition, at which the donor, whose identity would remain confidential, would be questioned by plaintiffs' counsel regarding Red Cross' alleged negligence in accepting his blood.

[The contaminated unit of blood was transfused during Jane Doe's surgery in January 1985. This lawsuit was filed alleging, among other things not relevant here, that the Red Cross was negligent in not excluding the unidentified man who donated the blood in question.]

The donor visited the Red Cross on July 25, 1984. He read the standard pamphlet entitled "What You Should Know About Giving Blood." The pamphlet described various illnesses that can be transmitted by blood transfusions (including AIDS and hepatitis), listed categories of persons who should not donate blood, and—quoting the Code of Federal Regulations (CFR)—specifically stated that "persons with a past history of viral hepatitis" were permanently disqualified from donating. The donor then responded "No" to each of 20 questions on a health history questionnaire, but in a standard interview with a Red Cross "health history nurse" he admitted that he had tested positive for something he called the "Australian antibody."

Being unsure of this term, the nurse declined to allow the man to donate blood pending consultation with Red Cross officials. Those persons reviewed the case and sought additional information from the prospective donor; he confirmed that he was antibody-positive but stated that he had never had any clinical symptoms of hepatitis. The Red Cross ultimately decided that this last piece of information was determinative, and the man was allowed to donate.

The plaintiffs contend that unless it was a false positive test or was due to immunization, "a past history of viral hepatitis" includes testing positive for the hepatitis antibody. Therefore, plaintiffs contend that the Red Cross was negligent in not disqualifying the donor. The Red Cross argues that, consistent with the accepted standards of blood banks in

July of 1984, the absence of clinical symptoms made the man an acceptable donor.

The court points out that the case will turn largely on expert testimony concerning the meaning of "a past history of viral hepatitis" in the context of the CFR provision. The plaintiffs, however, urge that the donor's testimony about the Red Cross employees' screening procedures will also be necessary to their case; they have filed a motion to compel identification of the donor or for a "veiled" deposition in which he could be questioned without unduly revealing his identity. The Red Cross objects, arguing that to do so would violate the donor's privacy and would not be likely to provide significant, relevant information.

After reviewing the arguments of counsel and the sparse but emerging case law, the court, avoiding the constitutional question raised by Red Cross, determines that the donor's interest in privacy and society's interest in preserving the integrity of the nation's voluntary blood programs outweigh the plaintiffs' interest in deposing the donor in this case.]

Red Cross first contends that permitting plaintiffs to discover the donor would violate his right to privacy embodied in the South Carolina and United States Constitutions. Under the South Carolina Constitution, the donor has the right to be secure in his person, home, papers, and effects from "unreasonable invasions of privacy." The United States Constitution likewise has been held to embody the right to privacy. [In a 1977 case, the U.S. Supreme] Court indicated that the right to privacy encompassed "the individual interest in avoiding disclosure of personal matters." . . . But the donor's right to privacy under either Constitution is not absolute. In determining whether the donor's identification deserves constitutional protection, the court would have to weigh the donor's interest in privacy against the State's interests in allowing discovery. . . . Because this court finds that the Federal Rules of Civil Procedure adequately protect the donor's privacy interests in this case, the court need not engage in a constitutional analysis. In so holding, the court is mindful of its duty to avoid addressing constitutional questions where possible. . . .

The Federal Rules of Civil Procedure allow for discovery of any matter, not privileged, that is relevant to the subject matter of the action. Although broad in their scope, the rules of discovery are not without limitation. As Rule 26(b)(1) indicates, irrelevant or privileged matters are not discoverable. Moreover, the rules limit the discovery of relevant, nonprivileged matters where there is good cause to protect a party or person from annoyance, embarrassment, oppression, or undue burden or expense. In determining whether information sought should be protected under Rule 26(c), the court must balance the competing interests that would be served by granting or denying discovery. . . .

Red Cross argues that the donor's identity is "privileged" under several South Carolina statutes and administrative regulations. [South Carolina law] provides that: "When a person is identified, [by a state, district, county, or municipal health official] as being infected with human immunodeficiency virus (HIV), the virus which causes acquired immune deficiency syndrome (AIDS), his known sexual contacts or intravenous drug user contacts, or both, must be notified but the identity of the donor infected must not be revealed." [Another provision] requires that a laboratory that performs a positive test for a sexually transmittable disease report the case to the Department of Health and Environmental Control ("DHEC"), and [another] requires that DHEC and its agents keep all information and records relating to such cases "strictly confidential." [A provision] even prevents DHEC from disclosing such information under subpoena, except in certain circumstances. Finally, [a regulation] provides that: "All information and reports concerning persons infected with venereal diseases shall be inaccessible to the public except insofar as publicity may attend the performance of the duties imposed by these regulations and by the laws of the State."

These laws evidence a clear intent on the part of South Carolina legislators and administrators to prevent DHEC and its agents from disclosing the identification of victims of sexually-transmitted diseases. These measures serve not only the victim's interest in privacy, but they also serve the State's important interest in encouraging victims to seek help voluntarily and to give honest responses to screening questions. But these laws, by their own terms, are directed at DHEC—not at the courts. Therefore, they do not, individually or collectively, render the identity of the donor absolutely "privileged" within the context of a negligence action against a blood bank.

Unlike the absolute nature of a privilege, Rule 26(c) determinations fall within the sound discretion of the trial court. . . . In assessing plaintiffs' motion to compel in light of Rule 26(c), the court must balance the donor's interest in privacy and society's interest in maintaining the confidentiality of volunteer blood donors against the plaintiffs' interest in questioning the donor. The court begins its analysis with an examination of the donor's interest in privacy.

Plaintiffs have indicated that if this court permitted them to take a "veiled" deposition of the donor, they would like to question him, among other things, about the intimate details of his health history and how he believes that he became infected with the virus that causes AIDS. On the contrary, the Red Cross, like other blood banks, gave the donor written assurance that his identity and medical history would remain confidential. . . .

The court must also take into account the ramifications of possible disclosure of the donor's identification to persons outside this litigation. The public has reacted to AIDS with hysteria. Law review articles addressing this issue indicate that AIDS, or even the suspicion of AIDS, leads to discrimination in employment, education, housing, and even medical treatment. . . .

Turning to society's interest, the goal of nonprofit blood banks such as the Red Cross is to ensure the safety and adequacy of the nation's blood supply. Because the blood of volunteer donors is less likely to be contaminated with infectious diseases than that of paid donors, the federal government has encouraged the promotion of an all volunteer blood donation system. The testimony of blood banking experts in this and other cases indicates that the assurance of confidentiality is absolutely essential to maintain a volunteer blood donation system that can meet society's demands. . . .

The erosion of confidentiality may not only affect the quantity of the blood supply, it could well affect its safety. This is because the safety of the blood supply depends largely on donors' willingness to provide accurate and detailed histories of private and sometimes sensitive medical information, and some donors may be reluctant to supply accurate information out of fear that personal aspects of their lives may be disclosed to persons not connected to the donation process. . . .

. . . .

In sum, assurances of confidentiality play a central role in maintaining a healthy and adequate blood supply. Permitting discovery of blood donors necessarily undermines the blood banks' assurances in that regard. If enough courts permit discovery of donors, blood banks, for purposes of ensuring that the consent of their donors is informed, will have to warn donors that they may be subject to questioning by litigants should their blood contaminate the recipient. Such a warning is likely to cause even the most civic-minded individual to think twice before voluntarily donating his blood to help another.

The interests outlined above must be balanced against the plaintiffs' important interest in discovering information relevant to their claims against Red Cross. The court is satisfied, however, that this interest has been adequately accommodated by the information already provided to them during discovery.

As mentioned earlier, the only substantive issue left in this case is whether Red Cross was negligent for not permanently disqualifying the donor based upon the health history he gave while attempting to give blood on July 25, 1984. Red Cross has provided plaintiffs with all of the documentation it possesses which is relevant to this issue. Plaintiffs, for instance, have the donor's health history questionnaires, his donor evaluation card, and a copy of the pamphlet "What You Should Know About Giving Blood," which donor acknowledged by his signature that he read and understood. In addition, Red Cross has identified the nurses who reviewed and evaluated the donor's health history.

. . . Plaintiffs argue . . . that Red Cross employees were negligent for accepting the donor's blood without confirming that he had tested positive because of vaccination or immunization or because his test was false positive. As mentioned earlier, however, the issue of whether the donor should have been deferred permanently based upon his answer to Question 1.1 is one that will turn largely on expert testimony of what constitutes a past history of viral hepatitis . . . and evidence of how the blood banking community treated like do-

nors in July of 1984. The court fails to appreciate how the donor's testimony can add anything meaningful to this charge of negligence.

Plaintiffs argue that they should be permitted to ask the donor whether he possibly meant Australian antigen when he said Australian antibody and whether the Red Cross made sure that he had not confused the two terms. The court cannot agree. Even plaintiffs concede that blood banks are entitled to rely on the honesty and accuracy of responses by prospective donors unless it has reason to doubt a particular response. In this case, the donor used the term Australian antibody not only with Nurse MacKay, but repeated it in a subsequent conversation with Nurse White. Moreover, the donor said he had worked as a medical technician in the past, which makes it likely that he, certainly more than the average person, appreciated the difference between a positive test for the Australian antibody and a positive test for the Australian antigen. After balancing what plaintiffs realistically stand to gain from questioning the donor against the countervailing interests in favor of denying discovery, the court is constrained to deny plaintiffs' motion to discover the donor.

Significantly, in those few cases where courts permitted discovery of HIV infected donors, the plaintiffs' interest in questioning the donor was far greater than the plaintiffs' interest in questioning the donor in this case. . . .

. . . While the suggestion that disclosure of identities will serve to deter high-risk donors from donating is no doubt true, it will likely go much further and discourage numerous healthy individuals from donating their blood. . . . This is especially true with the spread of AIDS into the heterosexual community. As mentioned earlier, leaders of the blood banking community agree that disclosure of the names of individuals whose blood injures another will act as a serious deterrent to voluntary donations by even the most civic-minded of individuals. . . .

. . . .

In sum, Red Cross' health history questionnaire, by admission of plaintiffs' own experts, met the prevailing standard of care and the donor answered all but one of the potentially disqualifying questions in the negative. From notes on the donor's health history questionnaire and donor evaluation card, the parties and the court have a very reliable idea why he answered "no" to Question 1.1, and his further testimony on that question will most likely add nothing to plaintiffs' charge of negligence. Red Cross' pamphlet "What You Should Know About Giving Blood," which the donor indicated by his signature that he read and understood, likewise met the prevailing standard of care for self-exclusion policies. In light of this, the court believes that exposing the donor to questioning will have only marginal utility in advancing plaintiffs' case against Red Cross. Therefore, the court finds that the plaintiffs' interest in discovering the donor is far outweighed by the donor's interest in privacy and society's interest in maintaining the integrity of the nation's volunteer blood programs. . . .

Discussion Questions

1. Do you agree with the balance the court struck in this case? What arguments are persuasive to you? How might you argue the opposite viewpoint?

2. What legal theories protect the confidentiality of medical information, and when might those theories conflict with an alleged duty to disclose information?

3. Assuming that the duty to disclose might sometimes outweigh the duty to maintain confidentiality, under what circumstances is AIDS a sufficiently compelling situation to justify disclosure?

13

Liability of the Health Care Institution

Recall that—according to Oliver Wendell Holmes—"the life of the law has not been logic; it has been experience."[1] The evolution of the health care institution's legal status is a case in point.

Holmes served as either a state or a federal judge for 50 years (from 1882 until 1932). When he was first appointed to the bench, the hospital was a far different institution than it was when he retired, and more different still than it is today. More an almshouse than anything else, the post–Civil War hospital was mostly a place where society kept the sick poor away from those more "respectable" people who could pay to have medical care delivered in their homes by private physicians.

Because these early hospitals were, in fact, charitable organizations and because like other charities they subsisted on unpaid labor (often members of religious orders) and the financial contributions of private donors, the courts made them immune from tort liability. The doctrine can be traced at least as far back as a decision of the Supreme Judicial Court of Massachusetts in 1876. And in the landmark *Schloendorff* decision, Justice Cardozo of New York's highest court reaffirmed the doctrine in the following words:

Certain principles of law governing the rights and duties of hospitals, when maintained as charitable institutions have, after much discussion, become no longer doubtful. It is the settled rule that such a hospital is not liable for the negligence of its physicians and nurses in the treatment of patients. This exemption has been placed upon two grounds. The first is that of implied waiver. It is said that one who accepts the benefit of a charity enters into a relation which exempts one's benefactor from liability for the negligence of his servants in administering the charity. The hospital re-

mains exempt, though the patient makes some payment to help defray the cost of board. Such a payment is regarded as a contribution to the income of the hospital, to be devoted, like its other funds[,] to the maintenance of the charity. The second ground of the exemption is the relation subsisting between a hospital and the physicians who serve it. It is said that this relation is not one of master and servant [employer-employee], but that the physician occupies the position, so to speak[,] of an independent contractor, following a separate calling, liable, of course, for his own wrongs to the patient whom he undertakes to serve, but involving the hospital in no liability, if due care has been taken in his selection. On one or the other, and often on both of these grounds, a hospital has been held immune from liability to patients for the malpractice of its physicians. *Schloendorff v. Society of New York Hospital*, 211 N.Y. 125, 128–129, 105 N.E. 92, 93 (1914).

The situation Justice Cardozo describes lasted about another 40 years, but by the 1950s,

A hospital was no longer an almshouse. Insurance became available to cover costs of defense and to pay judgments resulting from personal injury litigation. The understanding grew that nonprofit enterprises should be treated in the same manner as profit-making companies so far as third-party liability claims were concerned. (Southwick, 156)

This feeling intensified in the 1970s and 1980s for at least two reasons. First, private health insurance plans, Medicare and Medicaid, and other third-party payers became the source of the vast majority of most hospitals' revenues. Philanthropy was virtually a forgotten item on hospital balance sheets.

Second, in an attempt to control the health care portions of their budgets, federal and state governments encouraged hospitals to engage in free-market competition. As advertising, marketing, and similar business techniques became

---

1. O. Holmes, *The Common Law* 1 (1881).

more common in the health care setting, the public and the courts began to view hospitals as simply another industry. Any remaining chance of once again applying charitable immunity to health care institutions was completely destroyed.

Following the death of charitable immunity, then, it was open season on hospitals. *Respondeat superior* cases began to flood in, followed by claims of direct corporate negligence of the hospital entity. Thus, in a period of about 25 years (roughly from 1945 to 1970), health care organizations fell from a position of smug immunity to being the target of multimillion-dollar lawsuits.

This change surprised and angered many health care professionals. It should not have. The life of the law is experience, and experience shows that at the same time charitable immunity was dying, the hospital was evolving from a modest "mom and pop" operation—a doctor's workshop—to a multilayered corporate conglomerate that is both horizontally and vertically integrated, has consolidated financial statements with tens of millions of dollars in revenues and expenses, makes available the highest possible treatment technologies, and uses the latest marketing and communications strategies for its greatest competitive advantage.

Thus, the evolution of hospital liability is a Holmesian metaphor: as it learns from experience, the law adapts to meet the changing needs of society.

In this chapter we examine the current state of the law regarding the liability of health care organizations and the professionals who make them run.

Johnson v. Misericordia Community Hosp.
99 Wis. 2d 708, 301 N.W.2d 156 (1981)

Coffey, J.

[This case involves negligent surgery performed on Mr. Johnson by a Dr. Salinsky at Misericordia hospital in July 1975. Because of undisputed negligence by the doctor, the plaintiff has "a permanent paralytic condition of his right thigh muscles with resultant atrophy and weakness and loss of function." The doctor settled before trial, but the hospital disputed allegations that it was negligent. The court of appeals affirmed a verdict in favor of the plaintiff.

The Misericordia Community Hospital had previously been a religiously affiliated hospital but was sold to a private group of physicians who first operated it as a nursing home but subsequently reinstituted acute care services there. At the time of the incidents complained of, it had never been accredited by the Joint Commission on Accreditation of Hospitals (JCAH).]

On March 5, 1973, shortly after Misericordia Community Hospital returned to the status of a general hospital, Dr. Salinsky applied for orthopedic privileges on the medical staff. In his application, Salinsky stated that he was on the active medical staff of [other hospitals and that] his privi-

leges at other hospitals had never "been suspended, diminished, revoked, or not renewed." In another part of the application form, he failed to answer any of the questions pertaining to his malpractice insurance, i.e., carrier, policy number, amount of coverage, expiration date, [and] agent, and represented that he had requested privileges only for those surgical procedures in which he was qualified by certification.

In addition to requiring the above information, the application provided that significant misstatements or omissions would be a cause for denial of appointment. Also, in the application, Salinsky authorized Misericordia to contact his malpractice carriers, past and present, and all the hospitals that he had previously been associated with, for the purpose of obtaining any information bearing on his professional competence, as well as his moral and ethical qualifications for staff membership. [The application also contained language releasing the hospital for any liability as a result of doing a background check on the applicant.]

Mrs. Jane Bekos, Misericordia's medical staff coordinator (appointed April of 1973) testifying from the hospital records, noted that Salinsky's appointment to the medical staff was recommended by the then hospital administrator, David A. Scott, Sr., on June 22, 1973. Salinsky's appointment and requested orthopedic privileges, according to the hospital records, were not marked approved until August 8, 1973. This approval of his appointment was endorsed by Salinsky himself. Such approval would, according to accepted medical administrative procedure, not be signed by the applicant but by the chief of the respective medical section. Additionally, the record establishes that Salinsky was elevated to the position of Chief of Staff shortly after he joined the medical staff. However, the court record and the hospital records are devoid of any information concerning the procedure utilized by the Misericordia authorities in approving either Salinsky's appointment to the staff with orthopedic privileges or his elevation to the position of Chief of Staff.

Mrs. Bekos testified that although her hospital administrative duties entailed obtaining all the information available regarding an applicant from the hospitals and doctors referred to in the application for medical staff privileges, she failed to contact any of the references in Salinsky's case. In her testimony she attempted to justify her failure to investigate Salinsky's application because she believed he had been a member of the medical staff prior to her employment in April of 1973, even though his application was not marked approved until some four months later on August 8, 1973. Further, Mrs. Bekos stated that an examination of the Misericordia records reflected that at no time was an investigation made by anyone of any of the statements recited in his application.

. . . .

At trial, the representatives of two Milwaukee hospitals . . . gave testimony concerning the accepted procedure for evaluating applicants for medical staff privileges. Briefly, they stated that the hospital's governing body, i.e., the board of directors or board of trustees, has the ultimate responsibility in granting or denying staff privileges. However, the governing board delegates the responsibility of evaluating the professional qualifications of an applicant for clinical privileges to the medical staff. The credentials committee (or committee of the whole) conducts an investigation of the applying physician's or surgeon's education, training, health, ethics and experience through contacts with his peers in the specialty in which he is seeking privileges, as well as the references listed in his application to determine the veracity of his statements and to solicit comments dealing with the applicant's credentials. Once [this has been done, a recommendation is relayed] to the governing body, which . . . has the final appointing authority.

The record demonstrates that had [such an investigation been conducted, Misericordia] would have found, contrary to [Dr. Salinsky's] representations, that he had in fact experienced denial and restriction of his privileges, as well as never having been granted privileges at the very same hospitals he listed in his application. This information was readily available to Misericordia, and a review of Salinsky's associations with various Milwaukee orthopedic surgeons and hospital personnel would have revealed that they considered Salinsky's competence as an orthopedic surgeon *suspect*, and viewed it with a great deal of concern.

[The court summarizes some of Dr. Salinsky's professional history. At one hospital his request for expanded orthopedic privileges was denied after being on the staff for a year and a half. At another, his privileges were temporarily suspended and subsequently limited after a report of "continued flagrant bad practices." At a third, his initial application for privileges was flatly denied. The court adds, "The testimony at trial established many other discrepancies in Salinsky's Misericordia application," and it points out that experts in the field testified that, in their opinion, a prudent hospital would not have granted Salinsky's application under these circumstances.]

The jury found that the hospital was negligent in granting orthopedic surgical privileges to Dr. Salinsky and thus apportioned eighty percent of the causal negligence to Misericordia. Damages were awarded in the sum of $315,000 for past and future personal injuries and $90,000 for past and future impairment of earning capacity. . . .

Issues

1. Does a hospital owe a duty to its patients to use due care in the selection of its medical staff and the granting of specialized surgical (orthopedic) privileges?

2. What is the standard of care that a hospital must exercise in the discharge of this duty to its patients[,] and did Misericordia fail to exercise that standard of care in this case?

At the outset, it must be noted that Dr. Salinsky was an independent contractor, not an employee of Misericordia,

and that the plaintiff is not claiming that Misericordia is vicariously liable for the negligence of Dr. Salinsky under the theory of *respondeat superior*. Rather, Johnson's claim is premised on the alleged duty of care owed by the hospital directly to its patients.

. . . "The concept of duty in Wisconsin, as it relates to negligence cases, is irrevocably interwoven with foreseeability. Foreseeability is a fundamental element of negligence." In [a prior case,] this court set the standard for determining when a duty arises:

"A defendant's duty is established when it can be said that it was foreseeable that his act or omission to act may cause harm to someone. A party is negligent when he commits an act when some harm to someone is foreseeable. Once negligence is established, the defendant is liable for unforeseeable consequences as well as foreseeable ones. In addition, he is liable to unforeseeable plaintiffs." (emphasis supplied [by the court]).

Further, we defined the term "duty" as it relates to the law of negligence:

"The duty of any person is the obligation of due care to refrain from any act which will cause foreseeable harm to others even though the nature of that harm and the identity of the harmed person or harmed interest is unknown at the time of the act."

. . .

Thus, the issue of whether Misericordia should be held to a duty of due care in the granting of medical staff privileges depends upon whether it is foreseeable that a hospital's failure to properly investigate and verify the accuracy of an applicant's statements dealing with his training, experience and qualifications as well as to weigh and pass judgment on the applicant would present an unreasonable risk of harm to its patients. The failure of a hospital to scrutinize the credentials of its medical staff applicants could foreseeably result in the appointment of unqualified physicians and surgeons to its staff. Thus, the granting of staff privileges to these doctors would undoubtedly create an unreasonable risk of harm or injury to their patients. Therefore, the failure to investigate a medical staff applicant's qualifications for the privileges requested gives rise to a foreseeable risk of unreasonable harm and we hold that a hospital has a duty to exercise due care in the selection of its medical staff.

Our holding herein is in accord with the public's perception of the modern day medical scientific research center with its computed axial tomography (CAT-scan), radio nucleide imaging thermography, microsurgery, etc., formerly known as a general hospital. The public is indeed entitled to expect quality care and treatment while a patient in our highly technical and medically computed hospital complexes. The concept that a hospital does not undertake to treat patients, does not undertake to act through its doctors and nurses, but only procures them to act solely upon their own responsibility, no longer reflects the fact. . . . [T]he person who avails himself of our modern "hospital facilities" . . . expects that the hospital staff will do all it reasonably can to cure him and does not anticipate that its nurses, doctors and other employees will be acting solely on their own responsibility.

Further, our holding is supported by the decisions of a number of courts from other jurisdictions. These cases hold that a hospital has a direct and independent responsibility to its patients, over and above that of the physicians and surgeons practicing therein, to take reasonable steps to (1) insure that its medical staff is qualified for the privileges granted and/or (2) to evaluate the care provided.

[The court here embarks on a lengthy discussion of similar cases from various other states. It particularly points out the leading case of *Darling v. Charleston Community Memorial Hosp.* in which the Supreme Court of Illinois found a direct duty flowing from hospital to patient regarding the qualifications of members of the medical staff. The *Johnson* court favorably quotes from the *Darling* opinion, including the following passage: "The Standards for Hospital Accreditation, the state licensing regulations and the defendant's bylaws demonstrate that the medical profession and other responsible authorities regard it as both desirable and feasible that a hospital assume certain responsibilities for the care of the patient."]

There was credible evidence to the effect that a hospital, exercising ordinary care, [would have known of the deficiencies in Dr. Salinsky's qualifications and] would not have appointed Salinsky to its medical staff. . . .

This court has held "* * * a jury's finding of negligence * * * will not be set aside when there is any credible evidence that under any reasonable view supports the verdict. * * *" Thus, the jury's finding of negligence on the part of Misericordia must be upheld [because] the testimony of [the expert witnesses] constituted credible evidence which reasonably supports this finding.

In summary, we hold that a hospital owes a duty to its patients to exercise reasonable care in the selection of its medical staff and in granting specialized privileges. The final appointing authority resides in the hospital's governing body, although it must rely on the medical staff and in particular the credentials committee (or committee of the whole) to investigate and evaluate an applicant's qualifications for the requested privileges. However, this delegation of the responsibility to investigate and evaluate the professional competence of applicants for clinical privileges does not relieve the governing body of its duty to appoint only qualified physicians and surgeons to its medical staff and periodically monitor and review their competency. The credentials committee (or committee of the whole) must investigate the qualifications of applicants. [Paragraph break added by this editor.]

The facts of this case demonstrate that a hospital should, at a minimum, require completion of the application and verify the accuracy of the applicant's statements, especially in regard to his medical education, training and experience. Additionally, it should: (1) solicit information from the applicant's peers, including those not referenced in his application, who are knowledgeable about his education, training, experience, health, competence and ethical character; (2) determine if the applicant is currently licensed to practice in this state and if his licensure or registration has been or is currently being challenged; and (3) inquire whether the applicant has been involved in any adverse malpractice action and whether he has experienced a loss of medical organization membership or medical privileges or membership at any other hospital. The investigating committee must also evaluate the information gained through its inquiries and make a reasonable judgment as to the approval or denial of each application for staff privileges. The hospital will be charged with gaining and evaluating the knowledge that would have been acquired had it exercised ordinary care in investigating its medical staff applicants and the hospital's failure to exercise that degree of care, skill and judgment that is exercised by the average hospital in approving an applicant's request for privileges is negligence. This is not to say that hospitals are *insurers* of the competence of their medical staff, for a hospital will not be negligent if it exercises the noted standard of care in selecting its staff.

The decision of the Court of Appeals is affirmed.

Discussion Questions

1. How is this case an example of the adaptability of the law in response to the needs of society? Do you agree with the court's rationale in stating its conclusions?

2. What would have been the implications of the opposite result?

3. At one point, the court discusses a "public perception of the modern day medical scientific research center . . . formerly known as a general hospital." What evidence is there that this is the public's perception? Do you agree that the public perceives the hospital in this manner, or that it should?

4. What is the significance of the fact that the hospital was not accredited by the JCAH? Since it was not accredited, why are the accreditation standards referred to in the opinion, and are they relevant?

5. What difference does it make that Dr. Salinsky was an independent contractor rather than an employee?

6. Does this decision mean that a hospital is going to be liable for every incident of malpractice committed by its staff physicians? Why or why not?

Norton v. Argonaut Ins. Co.
144 So. 2d 249 (La. Ct. App. 1962)

Landry, J.

Plaintiffs herein, Glynace H. Norton and his wife, Anne Graves Norton, instituted this wrongful death action to recover damages for the accidental demise of their infant daughter, Robyn Bernice Norton, three months of age, who, on January 2, 1960, died in Baton Rouge General Hospital, of an overdose of the drug digitalis administered by injection. Named defendants herein are Argonaut Insurance Company, liability insurer of the Baton Rouge General Hospital; Mrs. Florence Evans, the Registered Nurse who administered the fatal hypodermic; and Aetna Casualty & Surety Company, liability insurer of Dr. John B. Stotler, the attending physician who issued the order for the medication administered by Mrs. Evans. A lengthy trial by jury in the court below resulted in judgment in solido against all defendants in favor of plaintiff, Glynace H. Norton, in the sum of $10,807.35 (including funeral and burial expenses in the sum of $807.35) and in favor of Anne Graves Norton in the amount of $13,000.00. All defendants have appealed and plaintiffs have answered the appeals praying that the awards be increased.

[Shortly after her birth, the Norton baby was diagnosed as having congenital heart disease and was placed on Lanoxin (a form of digitalis) to strengthen her heart and reduce the pulse rate. She was discharged from the hospital at two and one-half months of age, and her mother administered the medication at home by using a medicine dropper. The child was readmitted about two weeks later, on December 29, 1959, by her pediatrician, Dr. Bombet.]

On this occasion [Dr. Bombet] issued admission orders on the infant to be placed in the child's hospital chart or record. Included in his admission orders were instructions regarding medication, diet, etc., and the notation that special medication was being administered by the mother. In this connection it appears that Mrs. Norton preferred to continue administration of the daily maintenance dose of the lanoxin herself since she had been performing this function since the child's initial admission to the hospital on December 15th. Dr. Bombet noted in the hospital admission orders of December 29, 1959, that special medication was being given by the mother to thusly advise the hospital staff and employees that some medication was being administered the child other than that which he placed on the order sheet and would, therefore, be administered by the hospital nursing staff.

On January 2, 1960 (Saturday) Dr. Stotler examined the Norton baby at approximately noon while in the course of making his rounds in the hospital. As a result of this examination he concluded that the child needed an increase in the daily maintenance dose of lanoxin and instructed Mrs. Norton, who was present in the room, to increase the daily dose of the lanoxin for that day only to 3 c.cs. instead of the usual 2.5 c.cs. Following this instruction to Mrs. Norton, Dr. Stotler went to the nurse's station in the hospital pediatric unit floor to check the hospital chart or record on the Norton infant and noted on the Doctor's Order Sheet contained therein certain instructions among which only the following is pertinent to the issues involved herein: "Give 3.0 cc lanoxin today for 1 dose only".

Dr. Stotler's entry of the foregoing order for medication constitutes the basis of plaintiff's claim against Aetna as the professional liability insurer of Dr. Stotler. It is frankly conceded by Aetna that unless Dr. Stotler indicated on the order sheet that he had instructed the patient's mother to increase the daily maintenance dose of lanoxin to 3.0 c.cs. and administer the medication, his entry of the aforesaid prescription on the order sheet would indicate that the nursing staff of the hospital was to give the medication prescribed. It is further conceded that under such circumstances the child was subjected to the possibility of being administered a second dose of lanoxin. The possibility thus presented is exactly what occurred in the instant case. A member of the nursing staff noting Dr. Stotler's orders to administer the 3 c.cs. of lanoxin for 1 dose only administered 3 c.cs. of lanoxin in its injectible form instead of the elixir form which Dr. Stotler intended. The importance of this difference in the form of the medication has hereinbefore been shown. It is readily conceded by all concerned that the 3 c.cs. of lanoxin administered the baby by hypodermic was a lethal overdose and was in fact the cause of the infant's demise.

. . . .

The date of the tragedy with which we are here concerned, namely, January 2, 1960, was a Saturday. The nurse in charge of the pediatric unit, Miss Joan Walsh, a Registered Nurse, was absent from the hospital because it was her day off. The pediatric unit was in charge of Miss Barbara Jean Sipes, a Registered Nurse, who was assisted by a nurse's aid. Mrs. Florence Evans, Assistant Director of Nursing Service was the Senior Nurse on duty at the hospital at the time and in such capacity, exercised complete supervision and control of all nurses. Her duties were primarily administrative and supervisory. However, the rules of the institution required that when necessary she render assistance to the nurses on duty and perform routine nursing services. In addition, in the course of checking the operation of the numerous departments and units of the hospital (making the rounds, as it is referred to) Mrs. Evans went to the pediatric unit sometime after the lunch hour and discovered that the only Registered Nurse on duty, Miss Sipes, was quite busy with an emergency patient brought to the hospital and being attended by a Dr. Ruiz. Observing that the pediatric unit was in need of additional nurses under the circumstances shown, Mrs. Evans summoned a senior student nurse, Miss Meadows, to the pediatric unit from another department and Mrs. Evans herself remained in the unit for a time. In checking the charts of the patients on the unit, Mrs. Evans noted the order which

Dr. Stotler had that day previously entered on the chart of the Norton baby including the prescription for 3 c.cs. of Lanoxin for one dose only.

The evidence discloses that although Mrs. Evans is a registered nurse with many years experience it also appears that for the past several years her employment as a nurse has been principally in an administrative or supervisory capacity. It further appears that although Lanoxin in elixir preparation (in which form it can only be administered orally) had been available for a number of years, Mrs. Evans was not aware that the drug was manufactured in solution to be given orally. Because she had not practiced nursing as such for the past few years her knowledge of and familiarity with the drug in question was limited to the medicine as an injectible to be given only by hypodermic needle.

Noting that Dr. Stotler had ordered 3 c.cs. Lanoxin be given the Norton infant in one dose for that day only and knowing that it was the duty of the nursing staff to administer the medication, Mrs. Evans made inquiry and learning that the prescribed drug had not been administered decided to give the medication herself. She at no time considered administration of the drug other than by injection since by her own admission she was not then aware that Lanoxin came in elixir form. However, despite her limited knowledge of the drug, her training and womanly intuition warned her that 3 c.cs. of Lanoxin given by injection to a 3 month old infant appeared to be a rather large dose. She discussed the matter very briefly with the student nurse, Miss Meadows, and inquired of the Registered Nurse, Miss Sipes, whether or not the child had previously received Lanoxin. Mrs. Evans then examined the patient's hospital chart and found nothing therein which indicated the child had been receiving Lanoxin while in the hospital. In this regard, however, her testimony is vigorously disputed by defendant Aetna. Considering administration of the drug only by hypodermic needle, Mrs. Evans, accompanied by the Student Nurse, Miss Meadows, went to the medicine room of the pediatric unit and obtained two ampules of Lanoxin each containing 2 c.cs. of the drug in its injectible form. While pondering the advisability of thusly administering what she considered to be a large dose, Mrs. Evans noted that Dr. Beskin, one of the consultants on the child's case, had entered the pediatric ward so Mrs. Evans consulted him about the matter and was advised that if Dr. Stotler prescribed 3 c.cs. he meant 3 c.cs. Still not certain about the matter Mrs. Evans also discussed the subject with Dr. Ruiz and was informed by him in effect that although the dose was the maximum dose that if the doctor had prescribed that amount she could give it. The foregoing inquiry having satisfied Mrs. Evans' suspicions about the matter, Mrs. Evans then obtained a syringe, extracted 3 c.cs. of the medicine from the two ampules and injected one-half thereof into each buttock of the child. Following the injection Mrs. Evans noted on the chart that she administered the drug intramuscularly at 1:30 P.M. The injections upset the baby causing her

to cry. Mrs. Norton then requested a hot water bottle to place on the baby's buttocks to alleviate the pain occasioned by the injections and was advised that such could not be obtained without the orders of the attending physician. Mrs. Norton then called Dr. Stotler and in the course of the conversation mentioned that the child had received additional medication by injection. Dr. Stotler immediately called the nurses' station of the pediatric unit and upon learning of the administration of the lethal dose of injectible Lanoxin issued emergency orders and summoned Doctors Bombet and Beskin. Despite all emergency measures, including opening the child's chest and massaging her heart, the infant died at 2:45 P.M., approximately one hour and 15 minutes following the fatal injection.

. . . .

The rule applicable in the instant case is well stated in the following language [of an earlier Louisiana case]:

"(1) A physician, surgeon or dentist, according to the jurisprudence of this court and of the Louisiana Courts of Appeal, is not required to exercise the highest degree of skill and care possible. As a general rule it is his duty to exercise the degree of skill ordinarily employed, under similar circumstances, by the members of his profession in good standing in the same community or locality, and to use reasonable care and diligence, alone with his best judgment, in the application of his skill to the case.["]

From the foregoing resume of the testimony appearing in the record of this case it is manifest that Dr. Stotler was negligent in failing to denote the intended route of administration and failing to indicate that the medication prescribed had already been given or was to be given by the patient's mother. It is conceded by counsel for Dr. Stotler that the doctor's oversight in this regard exposed the child to the distinct possibility of being given a double oral dose of the medicine. Although it is by no means certain from the evidence that a second dose of oral Lanoxin would have proven fatal, Dr. Stotler's own testimony does make it clear that in all probability it would have produced nausea. In this regard his testimony is to the effect that even if the strength of two oral doses were sufficient to produce death in all probability death would not result for the reason that nausea produced by overdosing would have most probably induced the child to vomit the second dose thereby saving her life.

The contention that Dr. Stotler followed the practice and custom usually engaged in by similar practitioners in the community is clearly refuted and contradicted by the evidence of record herein. Of the four medical experts who testified herein only Dr. Stotler testified in effect that it was the customary and usual practice to write a prescription in the manner shown. The testimony of Drs. Beskin, Bombet and Ruiz falls far short of corroborating Dr. Stotler in this important aspect. The testimony of Dr. Stotler's colleagues was clearly to the effect that the better practice is to specify the route of administration intended. . . . In view of the foregoing, we hold that the act acknowledged by Dr. Stotler does not relieve him from liability to plaintiffs herein on the ground that it accorded with that degree of skill and care employed, under similar circumstances, by other members of his profession in good standing in the community. We find and hold that the record before us fails to establish that physicians in good standing in the community follow the procedure adopted by defendant herein but rather the contrary is shown.

Pretermitting the issue of charitable immunity (with which we are not herein concerned in view of the fact that the suit is against the insurer of the hospital in the instant case) it is the settled jurisprudence of this state that a hospital is responsible for the negligence of its employees including, inter alia, nurses and attendants under the doctrine of respondeat superior.

In the case at bar it is not disputed that Mrs. Evans was not only an employee of the hospital but that on the day in question she was in charge of the entire institution as the senior employee on duty at the time.

Although there have been instances in our jurisprudence wherein the alleged negligence of nurses has been made the basis of an action for damages for personal injuries resulting therefrom, we are not aware of any prior decision which fixes the responsibility or duty of care owed by nurses to patients under their care or treatment. The general rule, however, seems to be to extend to nurses the same rules which govern the duty and liability of physicians in the performance of professional services. Thus . . . we find the rule stated as follows:

"* * * The same rules that govern the duty and liability of physicians and surgeons in the performance of professional services are applicable to practitioners of the kindred branches of the healing profession, such as dentists, and, likewise, are applicable to practitioners such as drugless healers, oculists, and manipulators of X-ray machines and other machines or devices.

The foregoing rule appears to be well founded and we see no valid reason why it should not be adopted as the law of this state. Tested in the light of the rule hereinabove enunciated the negligence of Mrs. Evans is patent upon the face of the record. We readily agree with the statement of Dr. Ruiz that a nurse who is unfamiliar with the fact that the drug in question is prepared in oral form for administration to infants by mouth is not properly and adequately trained for duty in a pediatric ward. As laudable as her intentions are conceded to have been on the occasion in question, her unfamiliarity with the drug was a contributing factor in the child's death. In this regard we are of the opinion that she was negligent in attempting to administer a drug with which she was not familiar. While we concede that a nurse does not have the same degree of knowledge regarding drugs as is possessed by members of the medical profession, nevertheless, common sense dictates that no nurse should attempt to administer a drug under the circumstances shown in the case at bar. Not only was Mrs. Evans unfamiliar with the medicine in ques-

tion but she also violated what has been shown to be the rule generally practiced by the members of the nursing profession in the community and which rule, we might add, strikes us as being most reasonable and prudent, namely, the practice of calling the prescribing physician when in doubt about an order for medication. True, Mrs. Evans attempted to verify the order by inquiring of Doctors Beskin and Ruiz but evidently there was a complete lack of communication with these individuals. The record leaves no doubt but that neither Doctor Beskin nor Doctor Ruiz was made aware of just what Mrs. Evans intended to administer. Dr. Beskin was of the impression she referred to oral Lanoxin and Dr. Ruiz was of the impression she intended only 1 cubic centimeter of the injectible. For obvious reasons we believe it the duty of a nurse when in doubt about an order for medication to make absolutely certain what the doctor intended both as to dosage and route. In the case at bar the evidence leaves not the slightest doubt that whereas nurses in the locality do at times consult any available physician, it appears equally certain that all of the nurses who testified herein agree that the better practice (and the one which they follow) is to consult the prescribing physician when in doubt about an order for medication. With regard to nurses consulting any available physician when in doubt about an order for medication, the testimony of Drs. Beskin and Ruiz indicates clearly that in their experience such inquiries are generally restricted solely to interpretation of the doctor's handwriting and are not usually related to dosage or route. Having elected to deviate from the general and better practice of consulting the physician who ordered the medication in question, Mrs. Evans was under the duty and obligation of making herself understood beyond the possibility of error. This she did not do as has herein previously been shown. It appears reasonably clear that had she consulted Dr. Stotler and advised him of her intention to administer the 3 c.cs. of Lanoxin hypodermically he would have warned her of the danger and this tragic accident would not have occurred.

Aetna's defense predicated on the ground that because the negligence of the nurse was so inconceivable, gross and unpredictable as to constitute an independent intervening cause thereby relieving its insured of liability is without merit under the facts of the instant case.

The evidence in the case at bar leaves not the slightest doubt that when Dr. Stotler entered the order for the medication on the chart, it was the duty of the hospital nursing staff to administer it. Dr. Stotler frankly concedes this important fact and for that reason acknowledged that he should have indicated on the chart that the medication had been given or was to given by the mother, otherwise some nurse on the pediatric unit would give it as was required of the hospital staff. Not only was there a duty on the part of Dr. Stotler to make this clear so as to prevent duplication of the medication but also he was under the obligation of specifying or in some manner indicating the route considering the drug is prepared in two forms in which dosage is measured in cubic centimeters. In dealing with modern drugs, especially of the type with which we are herein concerned, it is the duty of the prescribing physician who knows that the prescribed medication will be administered by a nurse or third party, to make certain as to the lines of communication between himself and the party whom he knows will ultimately execute his orders. Any failure in such communication which may prove fatal or injurious to the patient must be charged to the prescribing physician who has full knowledge of the drug and its effects upon the human system. The duty of communication between physician and nurse is more important when we consider that the nurse who administers the medication is not held to the same degree of knowledge with respect thereto as the prescribing physician. It, therefore, becomes the duty of the physician to make his intentions clear and unmistakable. If, as the record shows, Dr. Stotler had ordered Elixir Lanoxin, or specified the route to be oral, it would have clearly informed all nurses of his intention to administer the medication by mouth. Instead, however, he wrote his order in an uncertain, confusing manner considering that the drug in question comes in oral and injectible form and that in both forms dosage is prescribed in terms of cubic centimeters.

It is settled jurisprudence of this state that where the negligence of two persons combines to produce injury to a third, the parties at fault are liable in solido to the injured plaintiff.

. . . .

We believe the awards allotted to plaintiffs herein are excessive in view of the prior jurisprudence. As was recently stated by this court, awards made in similar cases for personal injuries are so considered that within the limits prescribed by the facts of each individual case, a degree of uniformity will be maintained so that recoveries will not be out of all proportion with one another. While we concede the foregoing principle was stated in a case involving personal injuries to an adult the rationale of the rule is equally applicable in wrongful death cases.

. . . .

We are not herein concerned with the loss of an only child by a couple incapable of producing additional offspring due to the age factor or other causes. The record reveals Mr. Norton's age to be 40 years but is silent as to the age of Mrs. Norton. Fortunately for plaintiffs herein they are blessed with three remaining healthy, normal children upon whom they may lavish some of the affection which they unquestionably would have extended the deceased infant. Insofar as the present record is concerned it may well be that they are capable of having additional children although we concede this latter observation to be purely conjectural. At least their inability to have additional children is not shown in the record. We readily acknowledge that the remaining children cannot compensate for the loss of little Robyn—only render plaintiffs' loss less tragic and their grief more consolable.

. . . [W]e conclude that the awards should be reduced to the sum of $5,000.00 for plaintiff Glynace H. Norton and $5,000.00 for plaintiff Anne Graves Norton. In addition, plaintiff Glynace H. Norton is, of course, entitled to special damages in the sum of $807.35 awarded by the lower court.

It is common knowledge that attachment to a child becomes progressively more intense and pronounced with the passage of time. Human experience teaches that the loss of an infant three months of age while calculated to cause profound grief to a parent is not so keenly or acutely felt nor is such loss likely to produce sorrow of such duration or intensity as the loss of an older child to whom the parents have had time to become more attached.

For the reasons hereinabove assigned, the judgment of the trial court is hereby amended and judgment rendered herein in favor of plaintiff Glynace H. Norton in the sum of Five Thousand Eight Hundred Seven and 45/100 ($5,807.45) Dollars, and in favor of plaintiff Ann Graves Norton in the sum of Five Thousand and 00/100 ($5,000.00) Dollars, against defendants Argonaut Insurance Company, Mrs. Florence Evans and Aetna Casualty & Surety Company, in solido, together with legal interest thereon at the rate of five per cent per annum from date of judicial demand, until paid, said defendants to pay all costs of these proceedings.

Amended and affirmed.

Discussion Questions

1. What are the precise issues involved in this case?

2. What is the relationship between the standards of nursing practice and the vicarious liability of the hospital?

3. How does the role of the prescribing physician enter into the liability picture? Was the hospital liable for Dr. Stotler's prescribing practices?

4. What lessons does *Norton* teach to health care administration?

5. Is the reasoning of the court regarding reducing the amount of damages awarded persuasive?

Jackson v. Power
743 P.2d 1376 (Alaska 1987)

Burke, J.

This case presents an issue of first impression in this state, concerning health care delivery in hospital emergency rooms. The question that we must resolve is whether a hospital may be held vicariously liable for negligent health care rendered by an emergency room physician who is not an employee of the hospital, but is, instead, an independent contractor. We hold that the hospital in this case had a non-delegable duty to provide non-negligent physician care in its emergency room and, therefore, may be liable.

I

On the evening of May 22, 1981, sixteen year old Brett Jackson was seriously injured when he fell from a cliff. Jackson was airlifted to Fairbanks Memorial Hospital (FMH). Shortly after midnight, he was received in the hospital's emergency room.

Jackson was examined by respondent John Power, M.D., one of two emergency room physicians on duty at the time. Dr. Power's examination revealed multiple lacerations and abrasions of the patient's face and scalp, multiple contusions and lacerations of the lumbar area, several broken vertebrae and gastric distension, suggesting possible internal injuries. Dr. Power ordered several tests, but did not order certain procedures that could have been used to ascertain whether there had been damage to the patient's kidneys. Jackson had, in fact, suffered damage to the renal arteries and veins which supply blood to and remove blood from the kidneys. This damage, undetected for approximately 9 to 10 hours after Jackson's arrival at FMH, ultimately caused Jackson to lose both of his kidneys.

II

Jackson and his mother, Linda Estrada . . . filed suit. In their complaint they alleged negligence in the diagnosis, care and treatment Jackson received at FMH. Jackson moved for partial summary judgment seeking to hold FMH vicariously liable as a matter of law for the care rendered by Dr. Power. In support of his motion, Jackson advanced three separate theories: (1) enterprise liability; (2) apparent authority; and (3) non-delegable duty.

After briefing and argument, the superior court held, as a matter of law, that FMH could not be held liable under an enterprise liability theory, and the genuine issues of material fact precluded summary judgment on the two remaining theories. We subsequently granted Jackson's petition for review of the court's ruling.

III

Initially, it is important to clarify the exact issue that we have been asked to resolve. Jackson has conceded, for purposes of this appeal, that Dr. Power was not an employee of FMH, but an independent contractor employed by respondent Emergency Room, Inc. (ERI), and that ERI and FMH are separate legal entities. Traditional rules of *respondeat superior* are, therefore, inapposite. Jackson also makes no claim that FMH was itself negligent in its selection, retention, or supervision of Dr. Power. Consequently, we have no occasion to consider the doctrine of corporate negligence.[1] Jackson asks us to resolve only whether a hospital should be vicariously liable, as a matter of public policy, for the negligence or malpractice[2] of an independent contractor/physician, committed while treating a patient in the hospital's emergency room, under theories of (1) enterprise liability; (2) apparent authority; or (3) non-delegable duty.

IV

As previously noted, this case presented this court with an issue of first impression.

The generally accepted rule is that, where an employment relationship exists between the physician and the hospital, the hospital will be liable, under the traditional rule of *respondeat superior*, for any negligence or malpractice which results in injury to a hospital patient. Conversely no liability attaches to the hospital when the physician is an independent contractor.

Jackson conceded that Dr. Power was an independent contractor; however, he asserts that Alaska's law of *respondeat superior* mandates a result different than that which would be reached under the general rule. Jackson argues that our decision in *Fruit v. Schreiner* (1972), establishes that the law of "vicarious legal responsibility" in Alaska is "enterprise liability." Thus, he contends, if the enterprise impacts society and the negligent act occurred during an activity performed for the benefit or in the interest of the enterprise, the enterprise is liable.

Jackson's argument proves unpersuasive. First, Jackson's interpretation of *Fruit* is flawed. A close reading of the case shows that we did not view "enterprise liability" as a separate theory of liability or a distinct cause of action. Rather, enterprise liability was seen as one of two widely accepted theories used by courts to justify imposition of vicarious liability in an established employer/employee context. As was noted in *Fruit*:

[T]he "enterprise" theory * * * finds liability whenever the enterprise of the employer would have benefited by the context of the act of the *employee* but for the unfortunate injury.

* * * *

The rule of *respondeat superior* however, * * * is *limited* to requiring an enterprise to bear the loss incurred as a result of the *employee's* negligence. The acts of the *employee* need be so con-

---

1. The doctrine of corporate negligence holds that a hospital owes an independent duty to its patients to use reasonable care to insure that physicians granted hospital privileges are competent, and to supervise the medical treatment provided by members of its medical staff.
2. Jackson has yet to prove that any negligence or malpractice did in fact occur. In order to resolve the issue presented here, however, we must assume negligence. We, of course, express no opinion as to the actual merits of Jackson's claim.

nected to his employment as to justify requiring that the employer bear that loss.

Additionally, our decisions since *Fruit* show that we have applied the theory of *respondeat superior* only in an employer/employee context, unless one of the well established exceptions to that rule exists. Jackson's theory presents no such exception.

Finally, the cases from other jurisdictions cited by Jackson provide little support for this theory; those cases deal only with theories of apparent agency or corporate negligence. Moreover, although at least two courts appear to have implicitly indicated a willingness to recognize a theory of enterprise liability, to date, no court has explicitly embraced that concept.[3]

In short, Jackson's theory of enterprise liability is not yet the law in Alaska.

V

Jackson next argues that the trial court erred in holding that genuine issues of material fact prevented it from granting summary judgment on his theory of apparent authority.

Although we have recognized the doctrine of apparent authority in other contexts, this is the first time we have been asked to apply this doctrine to a hospital–independent contractor/physician relationship.

Cases from other jurisdictions show a strong trend toward liability against hospitals that permit or encourage patients to believe that independent contractor/physicians are, in fact, authorized agents of the hospitals. These courts have held hospitals vicariously liable under a doctrine labeled either "ostensible" or "apparent" agency or "agency by estoppel." Although courts and commentators often use these terms interchangeably, they are not theoretically identical.

The "ostensible" or "apparent" agency theory is based on Section 429 of the Restatement (Second) of Torts (1965), which provides:

One who employs an independent contractor to perform services for another which are accepted in the reasonable belief that the services are being rendered by the employer or by his servants, is subject to liability for physical harm caused by the negligence of the contractor in supplying such services, to the same extent as though the employer were supplying them himself or by his servants.

Two factors are relevant to a finding of ostensible agency: (1) whether the pertinent looks to the institution, rather than the individual physician, for care; and (2) whether the hospital "holds out" the physician as its employee.

"Agency by estoppel," in contrast, is predicated on the arguably stricter standard of the Restatement (Second) of Agency § 267 (1958). Section 267 provides:

One who represents that another is his servant or agent and thereby causes a third person justifiably to rely upon the care or skill of such apparent agent is subject to liability to the third person for harm caused by the lack of care or skill of the one appearing to be a servant or other agent as if he were such.

Under this theory, there must be actual reliance upon the representations of the principal by the person injured.

Thus, theoretically, there need be no causal relationship between the principal's conduct and the plaintiff's reliance to warrant a conclusion of ostensible agency; such a causal relationship and such a change of position, however, is the essence of estoppel to deny agency.

Jackson, in essence, asks us to adopt a rule of ostensible agency. FMH, on the other hand, requests that we . . . refuse to apply this doctrine in the hospital-physician context or, alternatively, that we adopt a rule which is essentially estoppel by agency. Although we find nothing antithetical about applying the doctrine of apparent authority to a hospital–independent contractor/physician relationship, we perceive no reason to adopt a special rule in this area. We believe that traditional rules of apparent authority provide sufficient guidelines.

In *City of Delta Junction*, we defined the doctrine of apparent authority in Alaska as follows:

Apparent authority to do an action is created as to third persons by written or spoken word or any other conduct of the principal which, reasonably interpreted, causes the third person to believe that the principal consents to have the act done on his behalf by the person purporting to act for him.

We went on to emphasize that it is the *principal's* conduct that gives rise to his liability and not the conduct of the alleged agent; "one dealing with an alleged agent must prove that the principal was responsible for the appearance of authority, by doing something or permitting the alleged agent to do something that led others, including the plaintiff, to believe that the agent had the authority he purported to have."

Relying on *City of Delta Junction*, the trial court held that existing factual disputes required Jackson to submit his apparent authority theory to the jury. When reviewing the denial of a motion for summary judgment, we must determine whether genuine issues of material fact exist, and if not, whether the moving party is entitled to judgment as a matter of law. In reaching this decision we must draw all reasonable inferences in favor of the non-moving party and against the movant.

---

3. Some commentators have suggested an enterprise tort doctrine as a basis for imposing liability for an tort occurring as a part of the hospital enterprise. *See* Southwick, *Hospital Liability: Two Theories Have Been Merged*, 4 J. Leg. Med. 1 (1983).

Drawing all reasonable inferences in the light most favorable to FMH, the record shows the following: at the time of Jackson's accident, FMH was the only civilian hospital north of Anchorage providing emergency room services in Alaska. Two road signs in Fairbanks note the location of the hospital. However, neither of these signs specifically refer to the existence of emergency room services. The signs were not constructed or situated by FMH. In fact, FMH does no advertising at all.

From the time of its establishment in 1972, FMH has never staffed its emergency room with its own physician employees, but has always relied upon local physicians to provide the service. Prior to the formation of ERI in 1977, FMH's emergency room was serviced by three local clinics, each providing one physician on a nightly basis. After 1977, ERI provided one physician on a nightly basis who worked a 14-hour graveyard shift (6:00 p.m. to 8:00 a.m.). While on duty in the emergency room, the ERI physician was "in charge" and no FMH personnel were responsible for either scheduling or monitoring the emergency room physicians. No contractual arrangement existed between FMH and ERI for the provision of emergency room physicians.

In apparent non–life threatening situations the first person an incoming patient sees at the emergency room is the admission clerk. Immediately adjacent to the clerk's desk is a sign which indicated that physicians from ERI were working in the emergency room. Although the exact state of Jackson's awareness is not entirely clear, there is evidence suggesting that he was admitted in a conscious state. Neither Jackson nor his mother selected FMH as the place of treatment nor Dr. Power as Jackson's physician.

From the above, a jury could conclude that FMH held itself out as providing emergency care services to the public. A jury could also find that Jackson reasonably believed that Dr. Power was employed by the hospital to deliver emergency room service. It is also possible, however, that a jury could find to the contrary.

Unless the evidence allows but one inference, the question of apparent authority is one of fact for the jury. In the case at bar, the record is not susceptible to a single inference. Thus, the trial court properly denied summary judgment on this issue.

VI

Jackson's final point is that the trial court erred in refusing to rule, as a matter of law, that FMH, as a general acute care hospital, has a non-delegable duty to provide non-negligent physician care in its emergency room. In essence, Jackson's position is that when a hospital undertakes to operate an emergency room as an integral part of its health care enterprise, public policy dictates that it not be allowed to insulate itself from liability by shunting that responsibility onto another.

. . . .

The hospital regulatory scheme and the purpose underlying it (to "provide for the development, establishment, and enforcement of standards for the care and treatment of hospital patients that promote safe and adequate treatment"), along with the statutory definition of a hospital (an institution devoted primarily to providing diagnosis, treatment or care to individuals), manifests the legislature's recognition that it is the hospital as an institution which bears ultimate responsibility for complying with the mandate of the law. It is the hospital that is required to ensure compliance with the regulations and thus, relevant to the instant case, it is the hospital that bears final accountability for the provision of physicians for emergency room care. We, therefore, hold that a general acute care hospital's duty to provide physicians for emergency room care is non-delegable. Thus, a hospital such as FMH may not shield itself from liability by claiming that it is not responsible for the results of negligently performed health care when the law imposes a duty on the hospital to provide that health care.

We are persuaded that the circumstances under which emergency care is provided in a modern hospital mandates the rule we adopt today. Not only is this rule consonant with the public perception of the hospital as a multifaceted health care facility responsible for the quality of medical care and treatment rendered, it also treats tort liability in the medical arena in a manner that is consistent with the commercialization of American medicine. Finally, we simply cannot fathom why liability should depend upon the technical employment status of the emergency room physician who treats the patient. It is the hospital's duty to provide the physician, which it may do through any means at its disposal. The means employed, however, will not change the fact that the hospital will be responsible for the care rendered by physicians it has a duty to provide.

This holding is necessarily limited. We do not change the standard of care with which a physician must comply, nor do we extend the duty which we find non-delegable beyond its natural scope. Our holding does not extend to situations where the patient is treated by his or her own doctor in an emergency room provided for the convenience of the doctor. Such situations are beyond the scope of the duty assumed by an acute care hospital. Rather our holding is limited to those situations where a patient comes to the hospital, as an institution, seeking emergency room services and is treated by a physician provided by the hospital. In such situations, the hospital shall be vicariously liable for damages proximately caused by a physician's negligence or malpractice.

In the instant case, Jackson came to FMH as an institution seeking emergency room services. Dr. Power was a physician FMH has a non-delegable duty to provide. FMH is, therefore, vicariously liable as a matter of law for any negligence or malpractice that Dr. Power may have committed. Accordingly, the trial court's ruling on this issue must be reversed. Jackson is entitled to partial summary judgment on the issue of FMH's vicarious liability.

VII

For the reasons outlined above, the trial court's denial of summary judgment on Jackson's theories of enterprise liability and apparent authority are AFFIRMED. However because we hold that FMH has a non-delegable duty to provide non-negligent physician care in its emergency room, the trial court's denial of summary judgment on the theory of non-delegable duty, is REVERSED and REMANDED with instructions to enter partial summary judgment on the issue of FMH vicarious liability in favor of Jackson.

AFFIRMED in part; REVERSED in part; and REMANDED.

Discussion Questions

1. What does *inapposite* mean? Can you explain its significance in section III of the opinion?

2. Do you understand what the enterprise liability theory is?

3. Can you explain the difference between *ostensible agency* (also known as *apparent agency*) and *agency by estoppel*? Which one applies to this case, and why?

4. Jackson lost the argument about his motion for summary judgment on the theory of apparent agency. What, therefore, is the status of that legal principle in Alaska following this case? Is it a viable concept or not?

5. Does the result of this case make good public policy? For example, if a hospital contracts with an organization such as ERI to provide emergency room physicians and if the contract includes a provision to the effect that the hospital has no control over the physicians and ERI alone may choose, credential, schedule, and supervise the services of those physicians, is it fair to hold the hospital liable? Is such a "no control" provision valid? Should it determine the outcome of the case?

6. What is the hospital's remedy for ERI's or the physicians' negligence? How can the hospital control the actions of such physicians?

7. What do you suppose happened when this case went back to the trial court for further proceedings?

Schleier v. Kaiser Found. Health Plan of the Mid-Atlantic States, Inc.
876 F.2d 174 (D.C. Cir. 1989)

PER CURIAM:

Kaiser Foundation Health Plan of the Mid-Atlantic States, Inc. [hereinafter Kaiser] appeals from a judgment entered on a jury verdict in favor of Ingeborg Schleier [hereinafter Schleier], as Personal Representative of the Estate of Shedd H. Smith, her husband. Schleier brought this action under the District of Columbia survival statute claiming that Kaiser physicians negligently failed to diagnose and treat Smith's latent coronary artery disease which caused his death on June 20, 1983.

The case was submitted to the jury on Schleier's negligence claim and the jury returned a $825,000 lump-sum verdict in her favor. Kaiser now appeals raising several issues. For the reasons herein stated we hold that it was reversible error not to instruct the jury, as defendant requested, that any award to plaintiff would not be subject to income taxation; we therefore reverse the judgment in part and remand for a new trial on damages.

I. BACKGROUND

At the time of his death, Shedd Smith was a 48-year-old urban planner for the General Services Administration in Washington, D.C. Kaiser is a health maintenance organization that provides health care to federal government employees. Smith was a paid Kaiser subscriber.

Smith was first treated at a Kaiser Clinic for abdominal pain in March 1983. On May 6, 1983, Smith spoke with a Kaiser advice nurse and complained of continual stomach pain. Six days later Smith called Kaiser again, this time because of a forty-five minute episode of severe chest pain radiating into his left shoulder. Smith was sent to the Fairfax Hospital Emergency Room where an electrocardiogram (EKG) was performed and interpreted as having non-specific S-T wave changes. Although the tests were inconclusive as to whether Smith had suffered a heart attack, a Kaiser physician admitted Smith to Fairfax Hospital Coronary Care Unit. The next day, Dr. Sherber, a cardiologist who was an outside consultant and not a Kaiser physician, was brought in to examine Smith.

Sherber's initial conclusion, after reviewing the information then available, was that it was unlikely that Smith had suffered a heart attack. However, he scheduled additional tests. Sherber found Smith's MUGA test [which measures the heart's contractility and pumping ability] was normal but his stress EKG was abnormal. Nevertheless, Sherber thought it unlikely that Smith had coronary heart disease, and did not recommend further cardiac testing, nor did he restrict any of

Smith's activities. The results of the stress EKG were then sent to Kaiser to be placed in Smith's medical chart.

During the four nights following his MUGA test, Smith complained to a Kaiser physician of profuse night sweats. After reviewing Smith's medical chart, which had not yet been updated to include his abnormal stress EKG, a Kaiser physician told Smith that the night sweats were not cardiac related. Smith did not suffer any other symptoms until June 19, 1983, when he began to sweat heavily and became exhausted after mowing his lawn and doing some housework. The next day his condition deteriorated. He began to vomit and was in a very weak and tired condition.

Schleier, concerned about her husband's state, called the Kaiser advice nurse who responded that Smith would have to sweat out his condition. After making this phone call, Schleier returned to her husband and found him gasping for air. She called the rescue squad but before it arrived Smith had stopped breathing despite her attempts to resuscitate him. Smith died in the ambulance en route to the Fairfax Hospital Emergency Room.

Kaiser raises several issues on appeal including the court's denial of Kaiser's motion to transfer the case to the Eastern District of Virginia, as well as the trial court's decision denying Kaiser's motion for a judgment notwithstanding the verdict. Kaiser also claims that it was not adequately shown that it breached its contractual duty to provide adequate health care, nor was it shown that Kaiser was liable for Sherber's negligence. Kaiser asserts that the jury could not properly determine Smith's lost future earnings, because it was not given sufficient guidance on Smith's employment history, his life expectancy, inflation or discounting to present value. Finally, Kaiser contends that the jury was not adequately instructed that any amounts awarded as damages would not be subject to income taxation.

II. DISCUSSION

A. *Motion to Transfer*

[The court dismisses the appellant's arguments that the case should have been transferred to another district.]

B. *Kaiser's Liability for its Independent Contractor's Negligence*

Next we examine Kaiser's appeal of the court's denial of Kaiser's motions for a directed verdict. When considering the denial of a motion for a directed verdict, we must look at all the evidence in the light most favorable to the non-movant and resolve all conflicts in the evidence in the non-movant's favor. Bearing that standard in mind, we find insubstantial Kaiser's contention that it is not vicariously liable for the negligence of Sherber, its consulting physician, because he is an independent contractor.

To determine whether the requisite "master-servant" relationship exists between an employer and an independent contractor for the purpose at hand, i.e., ascertaining whether the employer is liable for the independent contractor's negligence, the District of Columbia considers five factors: "(1) the selection and engagement of the servant, (2) the payment of wages, (3) the power to discharge, (4) the power to control the servant's conduct, (5) and whether the work is part of the regular business of the employer. Standing alone, none of these indicia, excepting (4), seem controlling. * * *" An application of those factors to the instant case supports the conclusion that Kaiser is liable for Sherber's negligence. Sherber was brought in as a consultant by a Kaiser physician, so it cannot be gainsaid that Kaiser selected and engaged him. The record does not reveal who paid Sherber, so that point is inconclusive. It does, however, appear as though Kaiser could discharge Sherber from the Smith case, but as Sherber is an independent physician, this factor does not carry the same weight as it might if Sherber had no other source of income. As to the fourth and most important factor, Kaiser had some ability to control Sherber's behavior in that he answered to Smith's primary caretaker, a Kaiser doctor. Finally, as Kaiser provided health care and Sherber was performing health care (albeit negligently) we may safely conclude that Sherber's actions fell within the ambit of Kaiser's regular business. It might be said that because Kaiser had eliminated cardiology from its coverage, the actions of Sherber, a cardiologist, do not fall within Kaiser's regular business offerings, but we think such an argument circumvents the intention of this final factor—to shield an employer from liability for the actions of an employee who was acting outside his field of expertise (for example, a doctor who negligently fixes a car)—and so we consider Sherber's actions to fall within the scope of Kaiser's regular business. . . . [W]e thus conclude, liability for Sherber's negligence attaches to Kaiser.

Although the District of Columbia has not explicitly opined on the question of when an independent contractor is an apparent or ostensible agent, we may draw added support from *Haven v. Randolph*, which declared that a "hospital is liable for the acts of a physician only if he is employed by the hospital and/or acts as agent for the hospital." The district court held that sufficient evidence was presented to the jury to support the finding that Kaiser was liable for Sherber's acts under the theory that he was an apparent or ostensible agent. The *Haven* court stated that the doctrine of *respondeat superior* is not applied when "a physician * * * acts upon his own initiative, and in the exercise of his own judgment and skill, without direction or control of an employer, * * * and [when] there is negligence in the treatment of a patient on the part of a physician who is not the servant or employee of the hospital, and who is pursuing an independent calling." By implication, the *Haven* court would apply *respondeat supe-*

rior here, where Sherber acted neither on his own initiative nor independently of the Kaiser physician. To the contrary, Sherber only made recommendations to the Kaiser doctor.

The *Haven* case seems to be the only decision on point applying D.C. law, but there is a sensibly-reasoned Maryland case which supports finding Sherber to be Kaiser's agent. In [that case], the hospital was held to be responsible for its emergency room doctors even though they were independent contractors because patients who came to the emergency room reasonably expected—and were not disabused of the notion—that the doctors in the emergency room were hospital employees. In the instant case, Sherber was brought in by Kaiser to examine Smith who had every reason to believe that Sherber was Kaiser's agent.

Having thus satisfied ourselves of Kaiser's liability for Sherber's negligent treatment of Smith, we need not tarry over Kaiser's contention that no showing was made that it breached its contractual duty of care to Smith. The record is replete with such evidence.

[Reversed.]

Discussion Questions

1. How, if at all, does the liability of an HMO differ from that of a physician in a group practice or from that of a solo physician?

2. Is the *Schleier* situation any different than any other case in which one physician calls another for a consultation? If so, how?

3. Could the concept of apparent or ostensible agency be applied to these facts to hold Kaiser liable?

14

Medical Staff Appointments and Privileges

The hospital's relationship with its medical staff is not always harmonious. Clearly the hospital exists to serve the needs of its physicians, for a hospital, after all, is not licensed to practice medicine, and without physicians to treat patients, the hospital has no reason to survive. On the other hand, the medical staff probably creates more difficulties for administration than any other single cohort of the organization.

Physicians as a group have occasionally been known to be difficult to deal with, and they may view health care administrators as a necessary (or even unnecessary) inconvenience to their autonomy and professional responsibilities. At the same time, a loyal and supportive medical staff can be an administrator's most effective tool for creating a smoothly running organization. Thus, legal disputes with the organized medical staff or any one or more of its members should be avoided if at all possible because they are difficult, disruptive, expensive, and frustrating cases to pursue.

The following cases exemplify some of the challenges presented by medical staff relations. As the students consider these materials, they must carefully distinguish between (1) the general principles of the common law of negligence (Chapters 3 and 13); (2) the standards of the federal and state antitrust laws (Chapters 6 and 7); and (3) other statutory principles (e.g., the Health Care Quality Improvement Act of 1986, discussed in the comments at the beginning of Chapter 15 and in *Mahmoodian v. United Hosp. Center, Inc.* below). Each of these areas of law can apply to medical staff relations, and each can be a quagmire for the unwary.

Greisman v. Newcomb Hosp.
40 N.J. 389, 192 A.2d 817 (1963)

Jacobs, J.

[The plaintiff was a doctor of osteopathy (DO) who had been granted an unrestricted license to practice medicine and surgery in the state of New Jersey. He was the only osteopath in the metropolitan Vineland, New Jersey, area, which was said to have a population of about 100,000 people, and Newcomb Hospital was the only hospital in the area. Newcomb was a private, not-for-profit corporation.

Despite being requested to do so, Newcomb refused to permit Dr. Greisman to apply for admission to its medical staff. It rested this decision on a provision in the hospital bylaws that said applicants must be graduates of an AMA-approved medical school and must be members of the county medical society. Dr. Greisman's application to the county medical society had never been acted on, and he was not a graduate of a proper school since the AMA approved no schools of osteopathy.

By the time the case came to this court, the AHA and JCAH had changed their policies and begun to approve of hospitals having DOs on their staffs; the AMA adopted a statement of policy allowing DOs "where it was determined locally that they practice on the same scientific principles as those adhered to by the American Medical Association"; and the state medical society in New Jersey also dropped its opposition.

Given this background, the court dealt with the issues as follows.]

The defendants contend that the Newcomb Hospital is a private rather than a public hospital, that it may in its discretion exclude physicians from its medical staff, and that no legal ground exists for judicial interference with its refusal to consider the plaintiff's application for membership. . . .

Broad judicial expressions may, of course, be found to the effect that hospitals such as Newcomb are private in nature and that their staff admission policies are entirely discretionary. They are private in the sense that they are nongovernmental but they are hardly private in other senses. Newcomb is a nonprofit organization dedicated by its certificate of incorporation to the vital public use of serving the sick and injured, its funds are in good measure received from public sources and through public solicitation, and its tax benefits are received because of its nonprofit and non-private aspects. It constitutes a virtual monopoly in the area in which it functions and it is in no position to claim immunity from public supervision and control because of its allegedly private nature. Indeed, in the development of the law, activities much less public than the hospital activities of Newcomb, have commonly been subjected to judicial (as well as legislative) supervision and control to the extent necessary to satisfy the felt needs of the times.

During the course of history, judges have often applied the common law so as to regulate private businesses and professions for the common good; perhaps the most notable illustration is the duty of serving all comers on reasonable terms which was imposed by the common law on innkeepers, carriers, farriers and the like. In the *Messenger* case Chief Justice Beasley, speaking for the former Supreme Court, noted that a railroad, though a private corporation, is engaged in a "public employment," that it "owes a duty to the community," and that under considerations of public policy it must be held under obligation to serve without discrimination. On appeal, Justice Bedle, speaking for the Court of Errors and Appeals, expressed the view that although railroad corporations are private, they hold their property "as a quasi-public trust," and that as trustees they must conduct their operations in such manner so as to insure to every member of the community the equal enjoyment of the means of transportation.

Implemented by specific legislation, the supervision of private businesses and professions for the public good has gone far beyond the early common law fields. . . .

Consistent with the historic precedents in the common law and its valued principle of growth, and independent of any specific implementing legislation, this court in *Falcone v. Middlesex Co. Medical Soc.* recently exercised its judicial function to strike down an arbitrary membership requirement of a nonprofit organization engaged in activity of public concern. There the Middlesex County Medical Society sought to exclude Dr. Falcone from membership because, though fully licensed and otherwise qualified, he could not fulfill its requirement of four years of study at a medical college approved by the American Medical Association—most of his

study was at the Philadelphia College of Osteopathy. The [trial court] found the requirement to be contrary to the public policy of our State and entered judgment directing that the Society admit him to full membership. On appeal, its judgment was sustained in an opinion which, after pointing out that the Society had virtually monopolistic power to preclude Dr. Falcone from successfully continuing his practice and to restrict his patients in their freedom of choice of physicians, held that public policy dictated that this power was not to remain unbridled but was to "be viewed judicially as a fiduciary power to be exercised in reasonable and lawful manner for the advancement of the interests of the medical profession and the public generally." . . .

In *Falcone*, the Society had taken the position that it was a private organization whose admissions policy was immune from judicial disturbance. In response, it was pointed out that the Society was not a voluntary membership association in which the public had little or no concern but was, rather, an association in which the public was vitally concerned and which was engaged in activities directly affecting the health and welfare of the people. In the course of its opinion, the court expressed the following thoughts which are particularly pertinent in view of the comparable position of the defendants here:

"The persistent movement of the common law towards satisfying the needs of the times is soundly marked by gradualness. Its step by step process affords the light of continual experience to guide its future course. When courts originally declined to scrutinize admission practices of membership associations they were dealing with social clubs, religious organizations and fraternal associations. Here the policies against judicial intervention were strong and there were no significant countervailing policies. When the courts were later called upon to deal with trade and professional associations exercising virtually monopolistic control, different factors were involved. The intimate personal relationships which pervaded the social, religious and fraternal organizations were hardly in evidence and the individual's opportunity of earning a livelihood and serving society in his chosen trade or profession appeared as the controlling policy consideration. Here there have been persuasive indications, as noted earlier in this opinion, that in a case presenting sufficiently compelling factual and policy considerations, judicial relief will be available to compel admission to membership; we are entirely satisfied, as was Judge Vogel in the Law Division, that Dr. Falcone has presented such a case."

In essence, *Falcone* declared, on strong policy grounds, that the Medical Society's authority to pass on membership applications by licensed physicians is a power which is fiduciary in nature, to be exercised accordingly, and it held that, under the evidence presented, Dr. Falcone was entitled to admission despite the Society's requirement of four years' study at a school approved by the American Medical Association. It is evident that, though we are here concerned with a hospital rather than a medical society, similar policy considerations apply with equal strength and call for, [*sic*] a declaration that the hospital's power to pass on staff membership applications is a fiduciary power, and a holding that Dr. Greisman is entitled to have his application evaluated on its own individual merits without regard to the bylaw requirement rejected by the Law Division. His personal and professional qualifications are not in dispute here, he lives in Vineland, has an office in Newfield in the Vineland metropolitan area, has an unrestricted license to practice medicine and surgery, and is engaged in the general practice of medicine. All he seeks, at this juncture, is simply permission to file his application for membership on the courtesy staff of the Newcomb Hospital and have it considered to the end that, if he is passed on favorably in accordance with the hospital's valid bylaws, he and his patients, as such, will have hospital facilities when needed.

The Newcomb Hospital is the only hospital in the Vineland metropolitan area and it is publicly dedicated, primarily to the care of the sick and injured of Vineland and its vicinity and, thereafter to the care of such other persons as may be accommodated. Doctors need hospital facilities and a physician practicing in the metropolitan Vineland area will understandably seek them at the Newcomb Hospital. Furthermore, every patient of his will want the Newcomb Hospital facilities to be readily available. It hardly suffices to say that the patient could enter the hospital under the care of a member of the existing staff, for his personal physician would have no opportunity of participating in his treatment; nor does it suffice to say that there are other hospitals outside the metropolitan Vineland area, for they may be too distant or unsuitable to his needs and desires. All this indicates very pointedly that, while the managing officials may have discretionary powers in the selection of the medical staff, those powers are deeply imbedded in public aspects, and are rightly viewed, for policy reasons entirely comparable to those expressed in *Falcone*, as fiduciary powers to be exercised reasonably and for the public good.

It must be borne in mind that we are not asked to pass on a discretionary exercise of judgment but only on the validity of the bylaw requirement. Therefore, we need not concern ourselves with any of the larger issues relating to discretionary limits or the general lengths to which a hospital may go in conditioning staff admissions on the approval of outside bodies. Viewed realistically, our proper concern here is whether the hospital had the right to exclude consideration of the plaintiff, solely because he was a doctor of osteopathy and had not been admitted, because of his osteopathic schooling, to his County Medical Society. In the light of *Falcone* and its aftermath and the discrediting of the notion that doctors of osteopathy are merely cultists and may not safely be permitted to associate with doctors of medicine, it is clear to us that it had no such right. In this day there should be no hesitancy in rejecting as arbitrary, the stand that a doctor of osteopathy, though fully licensed by State authority and reputably engaged in the general practice of medicine and as the local

school and plant physician, is nonetheless automatically, and without individual evaluation, to be considered unfit for staff membership at the only available hospital in the rather populous metropolitan area where he resides and practices. The public interest and considerations of fairness and justness point unerringly away from the hospital's position and we agree fully with the Law Division's judgment rejecting it.

Hospital officials are properly vested with large measures of managing discretion and to the extent that they exert their efforts toward the elevation of hospital standards and higher medical care, they will receive broad judicial support. But they must never lose sight of the fact that the hospitals are operated not for private ends but for the benefit of the public, and that their existence is for the purpose of faithfully furnishing facilities to the members of the medical profession in aid of their service to the public. They must recognize that their powers, particularly those relating to the selection of staff members, are powers in trust which are always to be dealt with as such. While reasonable and constructive exercises of judgment should be honored, courts would indeed be remiss if they declined to intervene where, as here, the powers were invoked at the threshold to preclude an application for staff membership, not because of any lack of individual merit, but for a reason unrelated to sound hospital standards and not in furtherance of the common good.

Affirmed.

Discussion Questions

1. What is the traditional judicial view applicable to the appointment of a private fee-for-service physician to the medical staff of a nonprofit private hospital?

2. Why did the New Jersey Supreme Court in *Greisman* depart from this traditional rule? Explain the rationale of the New Jersey approach. Have other states followed New Jersey's view?

3. As a hospital administrator, how should you handle applications for appointment from licensed podiatrists, psychologists, and other allied health care practitioners?

Moore v. Board of Trustees of Carson-Tahoe Hosp.
88 Nev. 207, 495 P.2d 605 (1972)

Mowbray, J.

The appellant, George L. Moore, is a doctor of medicine and is licensed to practice in the State of Nevada. He also enjoyed medical staff privileges at the Carson-Tahoe Hospital until they were terminated on February 19, 1970, by action of the Hospital Board of Trustees. Doctor Moore filed a petition in the district court seeking a writ of mandate in an effort to force the Board to restore his medical staff privileges. The district judge denied his request and hence this appeal.

The issues presented for our consideration may be summarized under two headings: (1) is the action of a governing board of a public hospital arbitrary, capricious, and unreasonable when it terminates the medical staff privileges of a physician on the grounds of unprofessional conduct, where the acts constituting the conduct complained of are not expressly defined and prohibited on the bylaws, rules, and regulations promulgated by the hospital? (2) is there sufficient evidence in this case to support the findings of the Board?

1. Doctor Moore was charged with 12 alleged acts of unprofessional conduct, and he was found guilty of Charges Nos. 7 and 11 of the complaint. Those charges read as follows:

"7. On or about July 26, 1969, you attempted to administer to an O.B. patient, ready to deliver a baby, a spinal anesthetic without benefit of sterile technique in that you prepared the medication, performed a minimal skin preparation and placed your fingers on the spinal needle, all without wearing sterile gloves. Additionally, you attempted the spinal puncture several times, all attempts being unsuccessful."

"11. On or about July 28, 1969, you had a meeting with the Chief of Staff, Doctor Thomas Hines, and Doctor William King, at approximately 7:30 a.m. in the morning, after which Doctor Hines, with the concurrence of Doctor King, canceled certain surgery you had scheduled on the basis that you were in no condition physically or mentally to perform surgery."

2. The Carson-Tahoe Hospital is a public hospital and is governed by the provision of [Nevada law]:

"The board of hospital trustees shall make and adopt such bylaws, rules and regulations for its own guidance and for the government of the hospital, and such rules and regulations governing the admission of physicians to the staff, as may be deemed expedient for the economic and equitable conduct thereof, not inconsistent with [Nevada statutes] or the ordinances of the city or town wherein such hospital is located."

. . . .

"The board of hospital trustees shall have the power:

"* * *

"4. To control the admission of physicians, surgeons and interns to the staff by promulgating appropriate rules, regulations and standards governing such appointments."

The Hospital Board of Trustees, as the governing body of the institution, promulgated bylaws, rules, and regulations designed to govern the medical staff of the Hospital. [Nevada law] provides:

"1. The board of hospital trustees shall organize a staff of physicians composed of every regular practicing physician in the county in which the hospital is located who meets the standards fixed by the rules and regulations laid down by the board of hospital trustees."

The delegated power to establish admission standards for medical staff members impliedly includes the power to continue to regulate membership after admission. It is axiomatic under the rule of statutory construction that a power conferred by statute necessarily carries with it the power to make it effective and complete.

Article 4, Section 5, of the Hospital's "By-Laws, Rules & Regulations Governing the Medical Staff" provides in part that any Medical Staff member "who is guilty of unprofessional conduct may have his privileges reviewed[,] altered or rescinded by the Board of Trustees on recommendation of the Medical Staff." Doctor Moore was formally charged by a complaint that set forth with specificity in 12 counts the acts with which he was charged. He was present with counsel at all stages of the proceedings and was afforded the right of cross-examination of witnesses and the right to call witnesses in his own behalf. There is no procedural due process challenge presented in this case. Rather, Doctor Moore complains that he was denied substantive due process because the acts of which he was found guilty (numbered paragraphs 7 and 11 of the complaint) were not specifically proscribed in the Hospital's "By-Laws, Rules & Regulations Governing the Medical Staff," and therefore they cannot constitute a predicate for the Board's conclusion that he was guilty of unprofessional conduct. We do not agree.

In [a 1962 case, a Florida] court held that the governing body of the hospital should be permitted certain discretion under the broad standard "[for] the good of the hospital or the patients therein," and that such words were essentially the same in meaning, when used in such context, as those used in other instances to authorize suspension for "unprofessional conduct." The court ruled that the particular bylaw provision set an objective standard upon which a board could act and by which a physician would have sufficient notice to guide him in his conduct. The court said:

"* * * There is at least equal difficulty in precise definition of professional fitness for staff membership in any given institution * * *[.] Detailed description of prohibited conduct is concededly impossible, perhaps even undesirable in view of rapidly shifting standards of medical excellence and the fact that a human life may be and quite often is involved in the ultimate decision of the board."

The Oregon Supreme Court, in a case involving a revocation of a physician's license to practice medicine, said:

" * * * [T]he variety of forms which unprofessional conduct may take makes it infeasible to attempt to specify in a statute or regulation all of the acts which come within the meaning of the term. The fact that it is impossible to catalogue all of the types of professional misconduct is the very reason for setting up the statutory standard in broad terms and delegating to the board the function of evaluating the conduct in each case. . . ."

If the standard "unprofessional conduct" is sufficiently objective in the case of a revocation of a physician's license to practice, it should be a sufficiently objective standard to guide a hospital board in acting upon the revocation of a physician's medical staff privileges in a community hospital.

Today, in response to demands of the public, the hospital is becoming a community health center. The purpose of the community hospital is to provide patient care of the highest possible quality. To implement this duty of providing competent medical care to the patients, it is the responsibility of the institution to create a workable system whereby the medical staff of the hospital continually reviews and evaluates the quality of care being rendered within the institution. The staff must be organized with a proper structure to carry out the role delegated to it by the governing body. All powers of the medical staff flow from the board of trustees, and the staff must be held accountable for its control of quality. The concept of corporate responsibility for the quality of medical care was forcibly advanced in *Darling v. Charleston Community Memorial Hospital*, wherein the Illinois Supreme Court held that hospitals and their governing bodies may be held liable for injuries resulting from imprudent or careless supervision of members of their medical staffs. The role of the hospital vis-a-vis the community is changing rapidly. The hospital's role is no longer limited to the furnishing of physical facilities and equipment where a physician treats his private patients and practices his profession in his own individualized manner.

The right to enjoy medical staff privileges in a community hospital is not an absolute right, but rather is subject to the reasonable rules and regulations of the hospital. Licensing, *per se*, furnishes no continuing control with respect to a physician's professional competence and therefore does not assure the public of quality patient care. The protection of the public must come from some other authority, and that in this case is the Hospital Board of Trustees. The Board, of course, may not act arbitrarily or unreasonably in such cases. The Board's actions must also be predicated upon a reasonable standard.

In [an Illinois case], the court ruled that the recommendation of the medical staff executive committee, based on the observations of its members of another physician's work, established a sufficient standard upon which to act in the granting of medical staff privileges. In the present case, Dorothy Haman, a nurse anesthetist, testified regarding Doctor Moore's unsuccessful attempts to administer the spinal anesthetic. She also testified regarding the procedure normally utilized. Dr. Thomas Hines testified that the procedure used by Doctor Moore substantially deviated from the accepted practice. Doctor King likewise testified. These three witnesses established the objective standard for administering spinal anesthetics. Doctor Moore failed to establish any other standard. Rather, he admitted deviating from the standard procedure but felt that he was justified in doing so. Doctors

Hines and King testified that Doctor Moore was in no physical or mental condition to perform surgery that he had scheduled on the morning of July 28, 1969. Doctor Hines, in conference with Doctor Moore, so advised him, and it was agreed that the scheduled surgery be canceled. No physician should perform surgery when he is not physically or mentally fit to do so.

After reviewing the record, it is clear that the Board did not act arbitrarily in this case, or without a standard to guide it, and that the record does contain sufficient evidence to support the charge of violation of the standard of professional care required in such cases. Therefore, the judgment of the district court is affirmed.

ZENOFF, C.J., and BATJER, J., concur.

THOMPSON, Justice, with whom GUNDERSON, Justice, agrees, dissenting:

Doctor Moore, a Board certified physician and surgeon . . . is licensed to practice in Nevada . . . [and] was excluded from staff privileges for [two occasions of] "unprofessional conduct"[. On one occasion,] the spinal anesthetic was administered without damage to the patient. [On the other occasion,] Dr. Moore acquiesced in the postponement of the scheduled surgery and successfully performed the operation at a later time.

1. . . . One searches [hospital bylaws and policies] in vain for a description of "unprofessional conduct" even in general terms. Herein lies the difficulty with the instant matter. A hospital should not be permitted to adopt standards for the exclusion of doctors which are so vague and ambiguous as to provide a substantial danger of arbitrary discrimination in their application.

Our legislature has defined "unprofessional conduct" for the guidance of the Board of Medical Examiners in exercising its disciplinary powers. A definition was deemed essential in order to guard against discriminatory action by the Board of Medical Examiners. A suitable definition is equally essential to protect a hospital staff member from arbitrary conduct by a Board of Hospital Trustees of a public hospital. Absent that definition, the Board is clothed with almost unlimited power, susceptible of abuse.

2. The acts for which Dr. Moore was expelled from the staff point to the need for a definition of "unprofessional conduct." His acquiescence in the request not to perform scheduled surgery was an act of compliance rather than an act of disobedience. And, the administration of an anesthetic without sterile gloves can be no more than an isolated instance of negligence which did not result in injury or damage. Such an isolated act without injury can not [*sic*] be a reasonable basis for revocation of staff privileges, for if it is, and if enforced equally and without discrimination, medical staffs will disappear entirely. Every professional [person] errs from time to time.

3. The Board is concerned with its liability to third persons for the misconduct of its staff members. [Citing *Darling*.] This is a legitimate concern, but it possesses no relevance to the case at hand. Neither of the instances relied upon by the Board to justify the expulsion of Dr. Moore could possibly result in Board liability to others. Consequently, this concern of the Board points to the arbitrariness of its action rather than to a reason for sustaining it. . . .

Discussion Questions

1. Read *Moore* and *Greisman* together and consider the differing approaches to the subject exemplified by the opinions. Can the two decisions be reconciled?

2. The opinion does not specify what it was that may have caused the physician to be in "no condition" to perform surgery. Do you think that the court's conclusion (that "it is clear that the board did not act arbitrarily") can be supported without that information?

3. What, in your opinion, would amount to unprofessional conduct? A single driving while intoxicated incident? Spouse or child abuse? An obnoxious personality? Disruptive behavior? Charging excessive fees?

4. Who should decide what amounts to unprofessional conduct? In that regard, do you find the majority opinion or the dissent more persuasive? Why?

Modaber v. Culpeper Memorial Hosp., Inc.
674 F.2d 1023 (4th Cir. 1982)

Russell, J.

Plaintiff, a physician specializing in obstetrics and gynecology, brought this [civil rights] action against a private nonprofit hospital, charging that its revocation of his clinical staff privileges deprived him of a valuable property right without affording him procedural due process under the Fourteenth Amendment. The district court dismissed the complaint for failure to state a claim, finding that the revocation was not "state action" and thus not subject to the Fourteenth Amendment. We affirm.

[The defendant hospital was the only hospital within 30 miles and was built with Hill-Burton funds. The plaintiff had held staff privileges there for four years until they were revoked for alleged incompetence.] Plaintiff has contended . . . that the withdrawal of his privileges was attributable to the state because defendant received Hill-Burton Act funds, accepted Medicare and Medicaid patients, and was required by statute to report the withdrawal to state medical licensing authorities. We disagree.

To determine whether or not defendant's termination of plaintiff's privileges is "state action", we must inquire "whether there is a sufficiently close nexus between the State and the challenged action of the regulated entity that the action of the latter may fairly be treated as that of the State itself." [Citing *Jackson v. Metropolitan Edison Co.*, in Chapter 1.] In holding that a privately-owned utility's termination of service is not "state action", the Court in *Jackson* makes it clear that state involvement without state responsibility cannot establish this nexus. A state becomes responsible for a private party's act if the private party acts (1) in an exclusively state capacity, (2) for the state's direct benefit, or (3) at the state's specific behest. It acts in an exclusively state capacity when it "exercises powers traditionally exclusively reserved to the state"; for the state's direct benefit when it shares the rewards and responsibilities of a private venture with the state; and at the state's specific behest when it does a particular act which the state has directed or encouraged. . . . We must examine plaintiff's contentions in this context.

. . . We have held in decisions prior to *Jackson* that a recipient hospital's action is state action because the hospital implements the Act's congressional purpose of providing health care. [Citing *Simkins*, among other cases.] We implicitly recognized in [another recent case] the possible inconsistency of these past decisions with *Jackson*, but did not reach the issue because the state criminal abortion statute involved in that case provided support independent of Hill-Burton for finding the recipient hospital's abortion policy to be state action.

The case before us squarely presents the question reserved in [that recent case]. We find that our former position that the mere receipt of Hill-Burton Act funds makes the recipient's every act state action is inconsistent with *Jackson*, which is controlling on us. Recipient hospitals undoubtedly "operate as integral parts of comprehensive joint or intermeshing state and federal plans or programs designed to effect proper allocation of available medical and hospital services for the best possible promotion and maintenance of public health." [Quoting from *Simkins*.] But the mere fact that the hospitals implement a governmental program does not establish the nexus which *Jackson* requires. The recipients do not act in an exclusively state capacity. Although health care is certainly an "essential public service", it does not involve the "exercise by a private entity of powers traditionally exclusively reserved to the State." . . . Although the hospitals are within a legislative design to better public health and are subject to extensive regulation, they remain solely responsible for providing the service and solely entitled to the profits therefrom. Finally, the Act does not require states to direct or encourage the procedure for making staff privileges decisions which was employed in this case. Although it prescribes that states compel recipients to make personnel decisions on a merit basis , it does not specify the method used here. At most, it declares that states must approve the policies which recipient hospitals adopt. Mere state approval is not "state action."

As for plaintiff's second contention, we have indicated in previous decisions that acceptance of patients receiving Medicare and Medicaid benefits does not make the accepting hospitals actions attributable to the state. . . . The Supreme Court's decision in *Jackson* does not affect this position. As these benefits are paid to the patients and not the hospitals, they have even less of a relationship to the challenged action than do Hill-Burton Act funds.

Plaintiff's final contention is likewise without merit. The state statutes do not authorize state officials to make privileges decision, or to set forth directions governing the outcome of such decisions, or attach consequences to their results. They simply require that revocations be reported, and confer immunity from civil liability upon the persons making the report. Absent evidence of authority to revoke a license, the mere duty to report the revocation of privileges does not involve the "exercise by a private entity of powers traditionally exclusively reserved to the State."

Nor do plaintiff's contentions, taken together, form a whole which is greater than the sum of its parts. The staff privileges decisions of a hospital which receives Hill-Burton Act funds, accepts Medicare and Medicaid patients[,] and reports privileges revocations to state medical licensing authorities do not constitute "state action." As state action is an essential prerequisite to obtaining relief under [the civil rights laws], the district court's decision dismissing plaintiff's claims should be affirmed. Accordingly, the judgment of the district court is

AFFIRMED.

Discussion Questions

1. What is the difference in the analysis between *Simkins v. Moses H. Cone Memorial Hosp.* (found in Chapter 8) and *Modaber*? What are the key factors?

2. Could you develop a rationale that would achieve the same result in *Modaber* without having to overrule *Simkins*?

3. What is the relationship between these last two cases and between each of them and *Jackson v. Metropolitan Edison Co.* (in Chapter 1)? Can you chart the holdings and rationales and interpret them as being consistent with each other?

4. What is the state's responsibility for the public health? If there were no private hospitals, would it be the state's responsibility to provide hospital facilities? What difference would your answer to that question make in the analysis of either *Simkins* or *Modaber*?

Leach v. Jefferson Parish Hosp. Dist. No. 2
870 F.2d 300 (5th Cir. 1989)

Gee, J.

Facts

In December 1986, East Jefferson General Hospital summarily suspended the physician privileges of the appellant, Dr. Richard E. Leach. The physician's suspension was upheld after a hearing before the Executive Committee of the Medical Staff and an appeal to the hospital's Board of Directors. The trial court found these actions were taken in accordance with hospital Medical Staff Bylaws.

In March 1987, after Dr. Leach allegedly continued disruptive behavior despite his suspension, the hospital's Chief of Staff, Dr. Herbert W. Marks, asked the Louisiana State Board of Medical Examiners to invoke the Louisiana Medical Practitioner's Act to determine the appellant's fitness and ability to practice medicine.

Dr. Leach asked the Medical Executive Committee to lift his summary suspension on May 19, 1987. Dr. Marks responded that the Bylaws failed to provide for review after the suspension had been affirmed by the hospital's Board of Directors. About a week later, Dr. Leach sought an outline of the procedures for again becoming an active staff member from the defendant, Peter J. Betts, who was the President and Chief Executive Officer of the hospital. The request for information was referred to the Medical Executive Committee, which informed Dr. Leach of the hospital's long-standing policy of requiring a one year moratorium for reapplication to staff membership.

The Medical Executive Committee considered the moratorium an appropriate length of time for a disciplined physician to resolve his problems. Although the By-laws do not stipulate such a moratorium, the East Jefferson Medical Staff's Credentials Committee Handbook recommends reapplication only after a period of at least one year. Mr. Betts thus informed Dr. Leach that he could reapply on February 19, 1988, which was one year after the hospital Board affirmed his summary suspension.

Dr. Leach was also informed that the Medical Staff only accepts applications from physicians with licenses not encumbered by the Louisiana State Board of Medical Examiners. The State Board informed Dr. Leach in August 1987, that it would not restrict his license to practice medicine. Dr. Leach then sought reinstatement and the hospital's Medical Executive Committee decided to allow him to reapply in advance of the one year moratorium since the Louisiana State Board indicated he was solving his problem.

Instead of reapplying, however, Dr. Leach filed this lawsuit. The only issue was whether Dr. Leach was deprived of the due process and equal protection of the laws guaranteed by the Constitution. The trial court granted the defendant's motion for summary judgment, determining that there were no genuine issues of material fact. We affirm.

Analysis

The appellant first argues that the hospital failed to follow its established rules and regulations. The trial court found, however, that the hospital reasonably followed its own rules in summarily suspending the appellant, and we agree. The hospital's Bylaws provided no guidance for reapplication after summary suspension, but the Committee Handbook delineated the policy of recommending a one year moratorium. The hospital clearly has a duty to protect patients and ensure their competent treatment. In addition, we note that courts are not the best fora for determining the competence of medical practitioners. As we have stated,

No court should substitute its evaluation of such matters for that of the Hospital Board. It is the Board, not the court, which is charged with the responsibility of providing a competent staff of doctors. * * * The court is charged with a narrow responsibility of assuring that the qualifications imposed by the Board are reasonably related to the operation of the hospital and fairly administered.

We agree with the trial court's finding that the measures employed by the hospital were reasonable. The appellant's argument that the hospital failed to follow its own rules and regulations is not supported by the record. In the one instance in which the hospital deviated from its stated policy, namely by shortening the length of the appellant's moratorium when it received evidence he was addressing his problems, it did so for his benefit. We find the appellant's argument of a due process violation unpersuasive and affirm the trial court's summary judgment on this issue.

The appellant also argues that the hospital rules and regulations were themselves inadequate to protect his constitutional interests. The argument must be evaluated in light of the United States Supreme Court's test for determining the sufficiency of procedures in safeguarding due process rights. In *Mathews v. Eldridge* (1976), the Court stated that due process requires considering the following factors: First, the private interest that will be affected by the official action; second, the risk of an erroneous deprivation of such interest through the procedures used, and the probable value, if any, of additional or substitute procedural safeguards; and finally, the Government's interest, including the function involved and the fiscal and administrative burdens that the additional or substitute procedural requirement would entail.

The first *Mathews* factor requires consideration of the private interest that will be affected. The private interest of Dr. Leach was his medical privilege. This was, of course, a very important interest; but Dr. Leach was at liberty to practice medicine at other hospitals. In addition, Dr. Leach was

permitted to reapply after a one year moratorium, a period of time that was later reduced by five months.

The second *Mathews* factor weighs the risk of wrongful deprivation from the procedures used against the probable value of other safeguards. As the trial court found, Dr. Leach was allowed to present any evidence he chose to bring forth, both at the hearing before the Executive Committee and the appeal before the hospital's Board. The record is devoid of any evidence that the appellant ever requested a delay in the proceedings. Nor is there any evidence that the Board acted unfairly to the appellant. The one year moratorium for reapplication was in fact shortened when the State Board informed the hospital, more than two months after the moratorium was imposed, that Dr. Leach was addressing his problems. In light of these circumstances, we are unable to say that the hospital failed to provide further necessary safeguards to protect the appellant's interests.

Finally, the hospital clearly has an interest in providing quality medical care to its patients. If a physician is disruptive or has personal problems, the hospital has a duty to intervene. When the moratorium was imposed, both the Medical Executive Committee and the hospital Board had agreed that summary suspension was necessary. The procedural safeguards were adequate to ensure that the appellant's constitutional rights were protected.

On balance, the *Mathews* factors convince us that the hospital's duty to maintain quality health care for its patients decisively outweighs the burden on the appellant of reapplying for staff privileges. The procedures provided a "meaningful hedge against erroneous action," and due process requirements of notice and an opportunity to be heard were met.

The appellant was not deprived of his constitutional rights to due process or equal protection when the hospital interpreted his summary suspension as permanent revocation and imposed the one year moratorium on reapplying for staff privileges. We therefore find the trial court properly granted the appellee's motion for summary judgment and the ruling is
AFFIRMED.

Discussion Questions

1. Recall the dissent in *Moore*, above. Do you believe the author of that opinion would dissent in this case as well? Why?

2. What were the "disruptive" actions involved here? Why does the court not describe them in detail?

3. Do you agree with the way the court has viewed its role in relation to the hospital's decision? Should the court have been more active in reexamining the merits of that decision? Why or why not?

Mahmoodian v. United Hosp. Center, Inc.
404 S.E.2d 750 (W.Va. 1991)

McHugh, J.

This appeal involves the revocation of a physician's staff appointment privileges as a member of the medical staff of a private hospital. The issues include whether such a revocation is subject to judicial review and, if so, the scope of that review, as well as whether such a revocation may be premised exclusively upon disruptive behavior of a competent physician which may affect adversely the quality of patient care at the hospital. We conclude that the Circuit Court of Harrison County improperly granted a permanent injunction against the revocation of medical staff appointment privileges in this case and, accordingly, we reverse, for the reasons stated in this opinion.

I.
PROCEDURAL HISTORY

[Plaintiff, Saeed Mahmoodian, M.D., is an obstetrician-gynecologist who has held medical staff privileges at United Hospital Center (UHC), Clarksburg, West Virginia, for 18 years. He has no privileges at any other hospital. UHC is a private, not-for-profit hospital not owned or operated by any governmental entity.

Doctor Mahmoodian's staff privileges were investigated by the medical staff beginning in February 1988, because of "disruptive and unprofessional behavior," some of which is described later in the opinion. Doctor Mahmoodian was informed in writing of the charges brought against him, was given an opportunity to testify and present other evidence to an investigative committee of physicians, and was represented by an attorney. The investigative committee unanimously recommended revocation of privileges, and the medical staff executive committee unanimously concurred.

At the doctor's request, an ad hoc hearing committee reconsidered the evidence and held additional hearings. Doctor Mahmoodian participated and was represented by counsel. This committee concurred in the prior actions. Doctor Mahmoodian then sent a written response to the charges to the entire UHC medical staff, which voted 32 to 17 (the OB/GYNs abstaining) to recommend to the board of directors that his privileges be revoked. Less severe action was not recommended because the doctor had been reprimanded once before, because his privileges had been suspended for a year on another occasion, and because he refused to accept any responsibility for the problems in the obstetrics department.

An appellate committee of the hospital board reviewed the matter, with Doctor Mahmoodian and his attorney present. It thereafter affirmed the medical staff decision and notified the doctor in writing of the decision. Doctor Mah-moodian then filed suit to obtain an injunction against revocation of his privileges. The trial court found in favor of UHC but granted an injunction pending appeal.]

. . . This Court is the seventh body to hear this matter (after the investigative committee, the medical staff executive committee, the hearing committee, the full medical staff, the appellate review committee of the hospital's board of directors and the circuit court).

II.
SCOPE OF JUDICIAL REVIEW

A. *The Law*

The threshold question in this case is whether the revocation of a physician's medical staff appointment privileges at a private hospital is subject to judicial review and, if so, what is the scope of that review.

. . . .

Utilizing breach of contract principles, most courts explicitly addressing the issue presented here have held, and we hereby hold, that the decision of a private hospital to revoke, suspend, restrict or to refuse to renew the staff appointment or clinical privileges of a medical staff member is subject to limited judicial review to ensure that there was substantial compliance with the hospital's medical staff bylaws governing such a decision, as well as to ensure that the medical staff bylaws afford basic notice and fair hearing procedures, including an impartial tribunal.

The judicial reluctance to review the medical staffing decisions of private hospitals, by way of injunction, declaratory judgment or otherwise, reflects the general unwillingness of courts to substitute their judgment on the merits for the professional judgment of medical and hospital officials with superior qualifications to make such decisions. Furthermore, a private hospital's actions do not constitute state action and, therefore, are not subject to scrutiny for compliance with procedural "due process," which is constitutionally required when there is state action. However, there are basic, common-law procedural protections which must be accorded a medical staff member by a private hospital in a disciplinary proceeding which could seriously affect his or her ability to practice medicine. Such basic procedural protections include notice of the charges and a fair hearing before an impartial tribunal. If a private hospital's medical staff bylaws provide these basic procedural protections, and if the bylaws' procedures are followed substantially in the particular disciplinary proceeding, a court usually will not interfere with the medical peers' recommendation and the hospital's exercise of discretion on the merits.

In this regard the fact that individuals conducting good-faith health care peer review are statutorily immunized from civil liability for damages evinces a public policy encouraging health care professionals to monitor the competency and professional conduct of their peers in order to safeguard and improve the quality of patient care. While these peer review immunity statutes do not foreclose judicial review in proceedings seeking injunctive or declaratory relief, it is evident that the intent of these statutes was not to disturb, but to reinforce, the preexisting reluctance of courts to substitute their judgment on the merits for that of health care professionals and of the governing bodies of hospitals in an area within their expertise.

. . . .

. . . Underlying the limited scope of judicial review of health care peer review decisions is an awareness that courts should allow hospitals, as long as they proceed fairly, to run their own business. That awareness is tempered by the recognition that physicians need hospital medical staff appointment privileges and clinical privileges to serve their patients; therefore, hospitals must treat physicians fairly in making decisions about those privileges.

B. *Fairness of Hearing Procedures Here*

Dr. Mahmoodian claims that UHC in one aspect did not comply substantially with the bylaws of its medical staff and in another aspect did not provide a fair procedure for revocation of his staff appointment privileges. This Court disagrees.

Dr. Mahmoodian contends that it was an unfair procedure to allow members of the investigative committee to testify before the hearing committee as to their interpretation of what other persons had said before the investigative committee. Dr. Mahmoodian argues that this procedure, over his objection at the time, denied him his right to confront and cross-examine these other persons not appearing as witnesses at the evidentiary hearing before the hearing committee.

Dr. Mahmoodian was not denied his right to cross-examine those persons who were witnesses at the evidentiary hearing. The medical staff and the hospital lacked the power to subpoena persons to be witnesses. The hearsay testimony in question certainly was not the only evidence before the hearing committee; there was substantial evidence supporting the charges of disruptive conduct by Dr. Mahmoodian and supporting the finding that such conduct was creating a work environment detrimental to the quality of patient care. On the critical question of whether Dr. Mahmoodian's disruptive conduct could threaten the care of obstetrical patients at the hospital, Dr. Mahmoodian had full opportunity at the evidentiary hearing to cross-examine the members of the investigative committee whose opinions it was that Dr. Mahmoodian's conduct put obstetrical patients at risk. In addition, prior to the evidentiary hearing, Dr. Mahmoodian had access to the written materials relied upon by the medical staff executive committee, and Dr. Mahmoodian had the opportunity at the evidentiary hearing to rebut the adverse evidence. The record indicates that he was thoroughly prepared to rebut all of the adverse evidence at the evidentiary hear-

ing. It is interesting to note in this regard that Dr. Mahmoodian utilized the same form of evidence about which he complains, by submitting a few favorable letters from third parties who were not witnesses at the evidentiary hearing.

The procedure in question was reasonable for peer review. The procedure here certainly complied with the medical staff bylaws, which authorized an evidentiary hearing without strict adherence to evidentiary rules applicable to civil or criminal trials in courts of law. Also, each of the procedural rights afforded Dr. Mahmoodian would satisfy the hearing standards established by the Federal Health Care Quality Improvement Act of 1986.

As found by the trial court, there was substantial compliance with the hospital's medical staff bylaws in this case, and we believe that those bylaws afforded Dr. Mahmoodian basic notice and fair hearing procedures.

III.
BYLAWS ON DISRUPTIVE CONDUCT

Dr. Mahmoodian challenges the revocation of his medical staff appointment privileges upon the basis of his disruptive conduct. He asserts: (1) that the medical staff bylaws are vague on this point; (2) that disruptive conduct of a medical staff member does not constitute a legally sufficient ground for revoking or otherwise affecting adversely a medical staff member's staff appointment privileges at a hospital, unless there is a "substantial" and "specific" threat to patient care from that conduct; and (3) that there was insufficient evidence supporting the hospital's decision to revoke his staff appointment privileges. This Court disagrees with each of these assertions.

A. *Vagueness of Disruptive Conduct Bylaws*

The pertinent part of section 7.01 of UHC's medical staff bylaws provides:

> Whenever the activities or professional conduct of any practitioner with clinical privileges are considered to be lower than the standards or aims of the medical staff or to be disruptive to the operations of the hospital or if any such practitioner is exercising or intending to exercise unauthorized clinical privileges, corrective action against such practitioner may be requested[.]

In addition, section 3.02 of UHC's medical staff bylaws provides, in relevant part, that one of the qualifications for membership is "an ability to work with others" so as to assure the medical staff and the hospital's governing board "that any patient treated by [the physician in question] will be given a high quality of medical care[.]"

Consistent with the authorities elsewhere, this Court holds that a private or a public hospital, regardless of the breadth of discretion that is extended to it, may revoke or otherwise affect adversely the staff appointment or clinical privileges of a medical staff member only if, as an element of basic notice, the medical staff bylaws provide a reasonably definite standard proscribing the conduct upon which the revocation or other adverse action is based.

. . . .

Accordingly, we believe . . . the medical staff bylaws in this case set forth a reasonably definite standard of professional conduct for purposes of basic notice to medical staff members as to what behavior is and is not expected of them. Moreover, in this particular case, given Dr. Mahmoodian's history as far back as 1974 of seven other "corrective actions" by the medical staff for similarly disruptive behavior, his assertion that he did not know what constituted such behavior is implausible.

B. *Disruptive Conduct as Ground for Revocation*

In making medical staffing decisions a private or a public hospital may consider factors in addition to technical medical skills or medical competence. In fact, a hospital may establish, and a court should sustain, a standard for granting or maintaining medical staff appointment or clinical privileges if that standard is rationally related to the delivery of quality health care to patients as a whole. Thus, a hospital has the right, indeed the duty, to ensure that those persons who are appointed to its medical staff meet certain standards of professional competence and professional conduct, so long as there is a reasonable nexus between those standards and the hospital's mission of providing overall quality patient care.

. . . .

As a specific type of unprofessional conduct, behavior "disruptive to the operations of the hospital" or, stated another way, an inability to work with other health care personnel at the hospital, is a matter of legitimate concern to a hospital in making medical staffing decisions. Consequently, virtually all of the courts addressing the issue have held, and this Court hereby holds, that a hospital may adopt and enforce a medical staff bylaw providing that the disruptive conduct of a physician, in the sense of his or her inability to work in harmony with other health care personnel at the hospital, is a ground for denying, suspending, restricting, refusing to renew or revoking the staff appointment or clinical privileges of the offending physician, when such inability may have an adverse impact upon overall patient care at the hospital. . . .

Several [other] courts have emphasized that one of the principal reasons for upholding a "disruptive conduct" bylaw of a hospital's medical staff is that quality patient care in a hospital setting requires "team work" and compatibility between physicians, nurses and other health care personnel.

. . . .

Virtually all of the other courts, however, which have specified the degree of likelihood that overall patient care

will be threatened have upheld the right of a hospital to act whenever the physician's disruptive conduct, in the expert opinion of the hospital authorities, "may" or "could" affect adversely overall patient care. This majority view is consistent with the Federal Health Care Quality Improvement Act of 1986, which addresses peer review activity based upon the competence or professional conduct of a physician which "affects or could affect adversely the health or welfare of a patient or patients[.]" We believe the formulation of most courts is reasonable, although we do observe that the potential effect on patient care may not be presumed but must be shown by the evidence. As even the New Jersey courts have recognized, though, a hospital need not wait for a disruptive physician to harm a patient before revoking a medical staff member's privileges.

The mere fact that a physician is irascible, however, or that he or she generally annoys other physicians, nurses or administrators does not constitute sufficient cause for termination of his or her hospital privileges. Likewise, a physician should not be removed from medical staff membership merely because he or she has criticized hospital practices or other health care personnel at the hospital. On the other hand, a physician may be so disruptive as to throw the hospital, or a segment of it, into turmoil and to prevent it from functioning effectively. So substantial a disruption reasonably could lead the hospital authorities to find that overall patient care may be threatened, thereby constituting good cause for termination of the physician's hospital privileges.

In the present case the pertinent bylaws are quoted at the outset of section III.A. of this opinion, *supra*. Section 3.02 of UHC's medical staff bylaws explicitly links (1) the ability to work with others and (2) its effect on patient care at the hospital. Reading section 7.01 of the bylaws in the same fashion, that is, as requiring a showing that the professional conduct is so "disruptive to the operations of the hospital" that it may have an adverse impact upon overall patient care at the hospital, this Court concludes that these two bylaws are substantively reasonable.

C. *Sufficiency of the Evidence*

Dr. Mahmoodian finally argues that there was insufficient evidence to support UHC's decision to revoke his staff appointment privileges.

While some courts refuse to review the sufficiency of the evidence to support a private hospital's decision adversely affecting a medical staff member's hospital privileges, and while the expertise of the medical peers and the discretion of the governing body of a private (or a public) hospital with respect to medical staffing decisions are entitled to judicial deference, an inherent element of "fair hearing procedures" is a requirement of sufficient evidence to support the hospital's decision, a matter to be determined by a court in a proceeding seeking injunctive or declaratory relief.

Other courts have stated in various terms the amount of evidence necessary upon judicial review to support a private hospital's decision affecting adversely a medical staff member's hospital privileges. Regardless of the phraseology of these courts, the prevailing standard for judicial review of the findings of a private hospital in these decisions affecting medical staff members' privileges appears to be either an arbitrary and capricious (or abuse of discretion) standard or a substantial evidence standard.

Consistent with these authorities, this Court holds that the decision of a private hospital revoking or otherwise affecting adversely the staff appointment or clinical privileges of a medical staff member will be sustained when, as an element of fair hearing procedures, there is substantial evidence supporting that decision.

Some of the more egregious incidents supporting the hospital's decision in this case include the following.

Dr. Mahmoodian interfered with a lymph node biopsy being performed by his archrival, another obstetrician/gynecologist, Dr. Rahimian. When Dr. Mahmoodian thought he had discovered evidence that Dr. Rahimian was performing a surgical procedure for which he was not privileged, he (Dr. Mahmoodian) strode into the operating room suite and demanded that a nurse, who was the operating room coordinator, stop Dr. Rahimian's surgery. Dr. Mahmoodian did not follow the appropriate procedure of complaining before the surgery to the chief of surgery or to the chief of the medical staff. Dr. Mahmoodian waited until the case was in progress before demanding of the nurse that the procedure be stopped. The danger to patient care is obvious.

In the case of a patient named Virginia Edgell, one of the hospital's family practice residents called Dr. Mahmoodian at 1:30 a.m. and requested a caesarean section evaluation on this patient, who had been in labor for fifteen to sixteen hours and had had no progress for about eight hours. Dr. Mahmoodian did not come to the hospital to see the patient but advised that the patient could wait until morning. The physician supervising the family practice residents suggested that it was reasonable to obtain a second opinion. Dr. Rahimian was consulted, came to the hospital, evaluated the patient and performed a caesarean section. The next morning, when Dr. Mahmoodian learned that Dr. Rahimian had done a caesarean section on the patient, he (Dr. Mahmoodian) wrote a consultation note in the chart, the accuracy of which the family practice resident disputed. In the note Dr. Mahmoodian stated that he had told the resident he would come to the hospital in the morning and do a section, or, if the resident wanted him before then, he could call and Dr. Mahmoodian would come in. The resident testified that Dr. Mahmoodian had told him not to call back unless a prob-

lem developed with the fetal heart monitor and that the patient could wait until morning. Dr. Mahmoodian's actions in this case prompted the chief of the medical staff to warn Dr. Mahmoodian in writing to come to the hospital to evaluate patients when called by a resident. Again, the threat to patient care is obvious.

The obstetrical department nurse manager testified that Dr. Mahmoodian refused to give verbal orders to the registered nurses with whom he was feuding. Instead, he would give such orders to licensed practical nurses only, who, as he knew, were not authorized under hospital policy to accept verbal orders from a physician. That practice made it necessary for a registered nurse to whom he would speak to call back to Dr. Mahmoodian to receive formally the order. The impact of this circuity was that orders were delayed and quality patient care was implicated.

The record also documents the loss of at least one obstetrician/gynecologist candidate recruited by the hospital, due to Dr. Mahmoodian's behavior and remarks. This fact evinces the threat Dr. Mahmoodian represents to the continued viability of this critical health service at UHC.

The record is replete with other evidence supporting the hospital's decision to revoke Dr. Mahmoodian's staff appointment privileges. In short, there was substantial evidence supporting that decision. Such decision was reached reluctantly by the hospital, but the record establishes that this drastic action was based upon the informed recommendation of the medical peers after fair hearing procedures and was within the sound discretion of the hospital.

Accordingly, this Court reverses the final order of the Circuit Court of Harrison County granting Dr. Mahmoodian's request for a permanent injunction against the hospital's revocation of his medical staff appointment privileges.

Reversed.

Discussion Questions

1. The court states that the hospital's decision "is subject to limited judicial review." Is this statement consistent with the *Leach* court's view of its role?

2. Do you understand the "basic, common-law procedural protections" that a medical staff member should be accorded? What are they?

3. Do you agree that the incidents outlined in the opinion constituted unprofessional conduct?

4. After reading *Patrick v. Burget* in Chapter 15, compare the peer review processes used in the two cases. Can you explain the differences in the two outcomes?

15

Peer Review and Professional Ethics

Formalized peer review had its beginnings in the early parts of the twentieth century, but not until the malpractice crisis of the 1970s did it begin to assume the importance that it now exhibits. Further, as Southwick points out, peer review is only one aspect of the larger concept of quality assurance (also referred to with terms such as *total quality management*, or *continuous quality improvement*, or some similar rubric), which has come into vogue in recent years.

Programs of quality assurance are now the standard of care, being dictated by the Joint Commission for Accreditation of Healthcare Organizations, various state and federal laws, and judicial precedent. A focus on quality is valuable for its own sake, of course, but it is also driven by concerns for limiting hospital liability and for containing the cost of health care, the hope being that such programs can improve the standard of practice rendered within the facility and identify costly providers and practices.

Three major areas of legal concern have arisen as a result of peer review activities: (1) the confidentiality of peer review records, (2) the liability of persons participating in peer review functions, and (3) antitrust. The following cases demonstrate some of the issues that have surfaced in the litigation surrounding peer review.

Medical professionals exercise significant influence on their patients. Due to educational qualifications, training, licensing, and practice, physicians are in a position of dominance and superior knowledge when dealing with most patients and their families. This creates an environment of potential patient vulnerability and requires that physicians and related health professionals recognize their position of trust. This imposes a fiduciary duty on the part of the physician in the physician-patient relationship. The Oath of Hippocrates states that a physician will "do no harm." The

Nurembourg Code and the Declaration of Helsinki recognized in formal documentation the ethical obligations of the physicians in positions of trust where clinical research is involved. Additionally, physicians must be aware of the civil, criminal, and professional sanctions that might result from improper sexual activities and advances with patients and their families. The emerging legal doctrines focusing on the new rules and regulations involving sexual harassment are future areas for which the medical professional must be alert. Again, the Oath of Hippocrates notes that physicians will "remain free . . . of sexual relations . . . " with their patients.

The Health Care Quality Improvement Act (Title IV of Pub. L. No. 99-660, as amended) was passed in 1986 to encourage the identification and disciplining of unprofessional, substandard physicians, dentists, and others. The act provides a limited immunity for persons acting in good faith to conduct peer reviews. It also created a "National Practitioner Data Bank," the purpose of which is to collect and disseminate information concerning adverse actions affecting health care practitioners' hospital privileges, credentials, licenses, medical malpractice histories, etc. Thus, the data bank is to be a clearinghouse for activities relating to peer review and medical staff privileges.

Because of the act, hospitals are required to query the data bank when a provider initially applies for privileges and every two years after that to determine whether any adverse information regarding the individual's professional performance has been reported. In addition, hospitals must report to the data bank such matters as malpractice judgments and settlements, licensure actions, the restriction or termination of medical staff privileges and credentials, and other matters relating to professional competence or conduct that may adversely affect the welfare of future patients.

The act has obvious implications for hospital liability. Failure to comply with the act's requirements will undoubtedly be cited by plaintiff-patients as evidence of a breach of the standard of care in future medical malpractice cases. At the time this book went to press, however, litigation had not yet reached the appellate courts to clarify the uncertainties surrounding details of the act's requirements. Students will wish to follow developments in this area closely in the next few years.

DiMiceli v. Klieger
58 Wis. 2d 359, 206 N.W.2d 184 (1973)

Hansen, J.

FACTS.

On January 18, 1971, the plaintiff, Ettore DiMiceli, M.D., commenced this action for libel against defendant, Jack A. Klieger, M.D. Both are staff members of St. Joseph's Hospital in Milwaukee, the plaintiff a specialist in anesthesiology, the defendant a specialist in obstetrics.

The plaintiff's complaint alleges that, on or about June 24, 1970, the defendant wrote a letter to the president of the medical staff of the hospital, reading:

"On Saturday morning June 12th Dr. E. DiMiceli called the labor room and arbitrarily indicated to the nurse that although he was responsible for obstetrical anesthesia on that day he would not be available for the patients of Doctors Klieger or Massart. Should their patients require anesthesia they could 'just call Dr. Schoeneman.' Dr. DiMiceli did not inform Dr. Klieger of this fact, nor did he call Dr. Massart, nor did he call Dr. Schoeneman or even insure the fact that Dr. Schoeneman would be available. This placed in jeopardy a group of obstetrical patients completely unprotected from the standpoint of anesthesia, and without their doctors knowledge. This hostile act, according to Dr. DiMiceli's own admission, was a 'reprisal' for having called Dr. Schoeneman to assist us with some surgical procedures during the past several weeks. The record will indicate that since Dr. Schoeneman's appointment to the Staff our office has performed 90 surgical procedures. Dr. Schoeneman was invited to participate in only 12 instances; the remainder was shared by the other members of the Department of Anesthesiology including Dr. DiMiceli.

"It was our opinion, and I believe this is factual, that Dr. Schoeneman was approved by the Credentials Committee and that his application was supported by a letter of recommendation from Dr. Robert Schuyler. The Executive Committee recommended him for Staff appointment and the Board of Governors agreed. Dr. Schoeneman was not placed on rotation in the Department [of Anesthesiology] and hence his only opportunity for work was of necessity by personal invitation. Normal, kindly, human and professional interrelationships made it mandatory that he be given a case occasionally and this is precisely what we did in good faith. It appears to me that this kind of conduct hardly warrants reprisals of any kind.

"The Department of Obstetrics is covered by nurse anesthetists almost completely. On rare occasions it becomes necessary to enlist the help of the Department of Anesthesiology. This occasional coverage, in the absence of a nurse anesthetist, is not merely a courtesy on the part of the anesthesiologist, but an obligation that grows out of the luxury of being permitted to practice medicine at St. Joseph's Hospital.

"Conduct which would permit a doctor to place his own personal prejudices ahead of the safety of patients and the security and reputation of a hospital must be labeled as reprehensible. Such behavior is diametrically opposed to the high moral and ethical standards and traditions which are synonymous with the name of St. Joseph's Hospital. Dr. DiMiceli has violated his own Hippocratic Oath, and since he has indicated that he intends to continue in this fashion I have no alternative but to ask that the Executive Committee send him a severe letter of censure. I ask too that the Executive Committee undertake to resolve the problem immediately and with the same forthrightness that has been typical of the Committee's activities during stressful times in the past. This I ask in the name of good patient care and hospital unity."

The plaintiff's complaint alleges the letter to be false, libelous and maliciously written. The plaintiff further alleges that, as a result of such letter, the executive committee of the hospital, on October 26, 1970, issued an order reading in part:

"That Dr. Di Miceli be reprimanded by letter for conduct that does not fit in with the modern concept of team effort in the practice of medicine in a modern hospital today."

Alleging damage in his professional capacity and humiliation, the plaintiff seeks damages in the amount of $10,000 compensatory damages and $50,000 punitive damages.

The defendant answered, denying that the letter was false, libelous or actuated by malice. Defendant further alleges that the order or letter of the hospital executive committee was issued after and as a result of hearings and investigation. Defendant contends that the letter was a good faith effort to protect the interests of his patients and of the hospital. Defendant's answer further contends that the letter, written to the executive committee of the hospital, was a privileged communication involving patient care and staff conduct.

On June 21, 1971, the defendant filed a motion for summary judgment. On October 4, 1971, the court issued an order denying the motion for summary judgment. On January 5, 1972, the defendant filed notice of appeal to this court from such order.

. . . .

This is an appeal from an order denying defendant's motion for summary judgment in a libel action. Two issues are raised. Three will be discussed.

THE TEST. Not raised, at least at the summary judgment stage, is the question of whether the letter sent was or could be considered defamatory. In this state and elsewhere, a communication is defamatory " * * * if it tends so to harm the reputation of another as to lower him in the estimation of the community or to deter third persons from associating or dealing with him." The test is whether the communication is capable of such meaning. If reasonable men might differ as to whether a communication is defamatory, the question is for the jury. To save a return trip on this issue, we join the trial court in seeing the question here as one for a jury to determine.

THE TRUTH. Defendant contends that his motion for summary judgment should have been granted because the statements contained in his letter are true. Truth of a statement is a defense in an action for libel. In fact, it is enough if the statement is "substantially true." Since this case is at the summary judgment stage, a definite procedure is to be followed in determining whether there are issues of fact presented which require trial. Steps in that procedure are:

1. Pleadings are to be examined to determine whether a cause of action has been stated, and, if so, whether material issues of fact are presented. If so,—

2. Affidavits and proof of the moving party are to be examined to determine if a prima facie defense has been established. If so,—

3. Affidavits and proof of the party opposing the motion for summary judgment are to be examined to determine if there are disputed material facts (or undisputed material facts from which reasonable alternative inferences may be drawn) sufficient to entitle the opposing party to go to trial.

In the case before us, we find, exactly as did the trial court, disputes as to material facts sufficient to entitle the plaintiff to go to trial. For example, there is a basic disagreement as to whether or not the plaintiff stated that he would not be available for the patients of the defendant doctor. The statement of a nurse at the hospital is that: " * * * Dr. DiMiceli told me that Dr. Schoeneman should be called, but that he would not come." As to the conversation with the nurse, plaintiff submits an affidavit by a doctor, including the statement that: "* * * at no time, in the presence of affiant, did the plaintiff state that he would not administer anesthetics for the defendant, Dr. Klieger." On the defense of truth, this dispute as to what actually occurred is not peripheral. Since the summary judgment procedure is "not to be a trial on affidavits," such dispute makes entirely proper the trial court's denial of the motion for summary judgment on this point.

A PRIVILEGE? Additionally, defendant contends that his motion for summary judgment should have been granted because the hospital executive committee was, to quote his brief, "a quasi-judicial body," and the letter sent is therefore "absolutely privileged."

As to judicial proceedings, it is true that defamatory words published or spoken by parties, witnesses and counsel in judicial proceedings are thus privileged when the statements bear a proper relationship to the issues. And such absolute privilege has been extended to quasi-judicial proceedings, including petition to a governor for removal of a sheriff, town board proceedings concerning a tavern license, a complaint to the state real estate brokers' board. Also, it is true that there seems to be "no clear definition" of what constitutes a quasi-judicial proceeding before a quasi-judicial body.

However, we find nowhere cases cited which extend or define a "quasi-judicial body" to come close to including the meeting of the executive committee of the medical staff of a private hospital. The case before us concerns a letter of complaint related to the internal affairs and operation of a private medical facility. It is true that the hospital here was required to have an organized medical staff, and such staff was given jurisdiction in matters of disciplinary procedures for infraction of hospital and medical policies. In terms of the possible impact upon the right to practice medicine or use the facilities of a certain hospital, a public interest is involved. But this falls short of transforming an executive committee of staff members of a private hospital into a quasi-judicial body.

As to the claim of absolute privilege, this court has held that even school board members " * * * do not fall within the category of high ranking executive officials of government whose defamatory acts should be accorded absolute privilege. * * *" In that case its court discussed the "competing values" that exist as to " * * * determining the scope of the privilege to be accorded public officials while acting in an executive or administrative capacity. * * *" Here we do not reach, much less cross, the threshold of finding the committee, which here received the defendant's letter, to be a "quasi-judicial body." It is not such, and the letter sent to it by a staff member can not [sic] be accorded "absolute privilege" as is here sought.

On this record and on the issues raised, the trial court properly denied defendant's motion for summary judgment.

Order affirmed.

Discussion Questions

1. In the absence of a statutory provision of immunity for peer review (and there was none in *DiMiceli*), how would you feel about participating in peer review activities?

2. In its discussion of privilege, the court places considerable weight on the concept of *quasi-judicial body*. What exactly does that expression mean? Would a board of trustees functioning in its capacity of approving medical staff privileges be a quasi-judicial body?

3. The law draws a distinction between absolute privilege and a "qualified privilege" for peer review conducted in good faith. What does this case say about how a qualified defense shall be determined?

4. What do you think was really going on between doctors DiMiceli and Klieger? Why did the matter get to court, and why should not the hospital administration be required to deal with it before it goes to litigation? How

would you have dealt with this situation had you been the hospital CEO?

State ex rel. Grandview Hosp. and Medical Center v. Gorman
51 Ohio St. 3d 94, 554 N.E.2d 1297 (1990)

Per curiam.

The record indicates that Anthony Melling ("Melling") and his wife, Marilyn, brought a malpractice action against relator-appellant, Grandview Hospital and Medical Center ("Grandview"), in February 1989. Melling alleged that surgeons Laszlo Posevitz, D.O., and Bruce Rank, D.O., negligently removed Melling's chest tumor, releasing excessive blood and eventually causing Melling to go blind. Melling claims Grandview negligently approved the credentials of Posevitz. In the course of discovery, Melling sought to obtain various Grandview records. Grandview resisted, asserting the medical review committee privilege under R.C. 2305.25 and 2305.251. Eventually respondent, Barbara P. Gorman, trial judge, ordered Grandview to produce "all documents concerning the credentialing and recredentialing of Dr. Po[s]evitz" for an *in camera* inspection to ascertain the applicability of the claims of privilege.

On July 31, 1989, Grandview sought a writ of prohibition in the court of appeals to restrain Judge Gorman from enforcing the orders to produce the documents. Grandview contends Judge Gorman lacked judicial authority to order an *in camera* inspection. The court of appeals dismissed Grandview's complaint. Grandview appeals.

. . . .

The court of appeals determined that Grandview's complaint failed to state a claim in prohibition upon which relief could be granted. Grandview did not set forth facts showing that the common pleas court lacked jurisdiction in this situation. We agree and hold that a trial court, in the course of regulating discovery, has authority to direct an *in camera* inspection of hospital records despite claims of the medical review committee privilege under [a certain Ohio statute].

"For a writ of prohibition to issue, a relator must ordinarily establish: (1) that the court against whom it is sought is about to exercise judicial power, (2) that the exercise of such power is unauthorized by law, and (3) that, if the writ is denied, he will suffer injury for which no other adequate remedy exists."

Grandview can not [*sic*] meet the second element of this test. Judge Gorman has complete inherent authority to direct an *in camera* inspection of the disputed hospital records. Trial courts have extensive jurisdiction and power over discovery. . . .

The scope of pretrial discovery is broad. "Parties may obtain discovery regarding any matter, not privileged, which

is relevant to the subject matter * * * ." Privilege must rest upon some specific constitutional or statutory provision.

Ohio law does provide a comprehensive privilege for hospital committee proceedings and records. R.C. 2305.251 reads in part:

"Proceedings and records of all review committees described in [R.C. 2305.25] * * * shall be held in confidence and shall not be subject to discovery or introduction in evidence in any civil action against a health care professional or institution arising out of matters which are the subject of evaluation and review by such committee. * * * Information, documents, or records otherwise available from original sources are not to be construed as being unavailable for discovery or for use in any civil action merely because they were presented during proceedings of such committee * * * ."

This statutory privilege does not extend to "[i]nformation, documents, or records otherwise available from original sources * * * ." Ohio courts have recognized this exclusion as a major exception.

Here, Melling sought records essential to his claim that Grandview negligently approved the credentials of Posevitz. Grandview responded with claims of the medical review committee privilege under R.C. 2305.251. Yet the statute itself contains a major exclusion. Faced with this claim of privilege, and its exception, Judge Gorman clearly had authority to inspect the documents, *in camera*, to determine if and how the privilege applied and to separate out nonprivileged portions. Applying this . . . privilege to actual documents is not necessarily easy. An *in camera* inspection is only a minimal first step.

In various contexts, Ohio courts have explicitly recognized the inherent authority of trial courts to order *in camera* inspections and the usefulness of doing so. In *Peyko v. Frederick* (1986), the defendant asserted an attorney-client privilege over an insurance claims file. In that case, we directed the trial court to determine "by *in camera* inspection which portions of the file, if any, are so privileged. * * * "

In *Henneman v. Toledo* (1988), we reaffirmed that trial courts could use *in camera* inspections to weigh claims of privilege. There, Justice Douglas said:

"In camera inspection of the documents by the trial judge is the most appropriate method of dealing with claims of executive privilege. By conducting such an inspection in chambers away from the jury and without the presence or participation of counsel for either party, the trial judge may make the necessary determination without compromising the confidentiality of any information he finds to be privileged. * * *"

. . . .

Thus, Grandview has failed to establish any illegality whatever in Judge Gorman's order. Its underlying claim of unreasonable intrusion into the hospital record also lacks merit. Judge Gorman's review of the record causes no conceivable injury, let alone irreparable injury. Grandview's claims of injury are thus premature.

For the foregoing reasons, the judgment of the court of appeals is affirmed.

Discussion Questions

1. Who is the defendant in this case? Why?

2. What is an *in camera* inspection?

3. The immunity of peer review records is a major worry of hospital counsel. Do you believe the balance the court struck in this case is a reasonable one?

4. Why do hospitals worry about keeping peer review records immune? Is this not akin to covering up vital information that would be useful to ascertain the truth at trial?

5. What are the public policy arguments favoring immunity? What are the differences in those arguments as they relate to pretrial discovery versus the trial phase of a case?

Patrick v. Burget
486 U.S. 94 (1988)

Marshall, J.

The question presented in this case is whether the state-action doctrine of *Parker v. Brown* protects physicians in the State of Oregon from federal antitrust liability for their activities on hospital peer-review committees.

I

Astoria, Oregon, where the events giving rise to this lawsuit took place, is a city of approximately 10,000 people located in the northwest corner of the State. The only hospital in Astoria is the Columbia Memorial Hospital (CMH). Astoria also is the home of a private group-medical practice called the Astoria Clinic. At all times relevant to this case, a majority of the staff members at the CMH were employees or partners of the Astoria Clinic.

Petitioner Timothy Patrick is a general and vascular surgeon. He became an employee of the Astoria Clinic and a member of the CMH's medical staff in 1972. One year later, the partners of the Clinic, who are the respondents in this case, invited petitioner to become a partner of the Clinic. Petitioner declined this offer and instead began an independent practice in competition with the surgical practice of the Clinic. Petitioner continued to serve on the medical staff of the CMH.

After petitioner established his independent practice, the physicians associated with the Astoria Clinic consistently refused to have professional dealings with him. Petitioner re-

ceived virtually no referrals from physicians at the Clinic, even though the Clinic at times did not have a general surgeon on its staff. Rather than refer surgery patients to petitioner, Clinic doctors referred them to surgeons located as far as 50 miles from Astoria. In addition, Clinic physicians showed reluctance to assist petitioner with his own patients. Clinic doctors often declined to give consultations, and Clinic surgeons refused to provide backup coverage for patients under petitioner's care. At the same time, Clinic physicians repeatedly criticized petitioner for failing to obtain outside consultations and adequate backup coverage.

In 1979, respondent Gary Boelling, a partner at the Clinic, complained to the executive committee of the CMH's medical staff about an incident in which petitioner had left a patient in the care of a recently hired associate, who then left the patient unattended. The executive committee decided to refer this complaint, along with information about other cases handled by petitioner, to the State Board of Medical Examiners (BOME). Respondent Franklin Russell, another partner at the Clinic, chaired the committee of the BOME that investigated these matters. The members of the BOME committee criticized petitioner's medical practices to the full BOME, which then issued a letter of reprimand that had been drafted by Russell. The BOME retracted this letter in its entirety after petitioner sought judicial review of the BOME proceedings.

Two years later, at the request of respondent Richard Harris, a Clinic surgeon, the executive committee of the CMH's medical staff initiated a review of petitioner's hospital privileges. The committee voted to recommend the termination of petitioner's privileges on the ground that petitioner's care of his patients was below the standards of the hospital. Petitioner demanded a hearing, as provided by hospital bylaws, and a five-member ad hoc committee, chaired by respondent Boelling, heard the charges and defense. Petitioner requested that the members of the committee testify as to their personal bias against him, but they refused to accommodate this request. Before the committee rendered its decision, petitioner resigned from the hospital staff rather than risk termination.

During the course of the hospital peer-review proceedings, petitioner filed this lawsuit in the United States District Court for the District of Oregon. Petitioner alleged that the partners of the Astoria Clinic had violated §§ 1 and 2 of the Sherman Act. Specifically, petitioner contended that the Clinic partners had initiated and participated in the hospital peer-review proceedings to reduce competition from petitioner rather than to improve patient care. Respondents denied this assertion, and the District Court submitted the dispute to the jury with instructions that it could rule in favor of petitioner only if it found that respondents' conduct was the result of a specific intent to injure or destroy competition.

The jury returned a verdict against respondents Russell, Boelling, and Harris on the § 1 claim and against all of the respondents on the § 2 claim. It awarded damages of

$650,000 on the two antitrust claims taken together. The District Court, as required by law, trebled the antitrust damages.

The Court of Appeals for the Ninth Circuit reversed. It found that there was substantial evidence that respondents had acted in bad faith in the peer-review process. The court held, however, that even if respondents had used the peer-review process to disadvantage a competitor rather than to improve patient care, their conduct in the peer-review proceedings was immune from antitrust scrutiny. The court reasoned that the peer-review activities of physicians in Oregon fall within the state-action exemption from antitrust liability because Oregon has articulated a policy in favor of peer review and actively supervises the peer-review process. The court therefore reversed the judgment of the District Court as to petitioner's antitrust claims.

We granted certiorari to decide whether the state-action doctrine protects respondents' hospital peer-review activities from antitrust challenge. We now reverse.

II

In *Parker v. Brown* this Court considered whether the Sherman Act prohibits anticompetitive actions of a State. Petitioner in that case was a raisin producer who brought suit against the California Director of Agriculture to enjoin the enforcement of a marketing plan adopted under the State's Agricultural Prorate Act. That statute restricted competition among food producers in the State in order to stabilize prices and prevent economic waste. Relying on principles of federalism and state sovereignty, this Court refused to find in the Sherman Act "an unexpressed purpose to nullify a state's control over its officers and agents." The Sherman Act, the Court held, was not intended "to restrain state action or official action directed by a state."

Although *Parker* involved a suit against a state official, the Court subsequently recognized that *Parker*'s federalism rationale demanded that the state-action exemption also apply in certain suits against private parties. If the Federal Government or a private litigant always could enforce the Sherman Act against private parties, then a State could not effectively implement a program restraining competition among them. The Court, however, also sought to ensure that private parties could claim state-action immunity from Sherman Act liability only when their anticompetitive acts were truly the product of state regulation. We accordingly established a rigorous two-pronged test to determine whether anticompetitive conduct engaged in by private parties should be deemed state action and thus shielded from the antitrust laws. First, "the challenged restraint must be 'one clearly articulated and affirmatively expressed as state policy.' " Second, the anticompetitive conduct "must be 'actively supervised' by the State itself." Only if an anticompetitive act of a private party meets both of these requirements is it fairly attributable to the State.

In this case, we need not consider the "clear articulation" prong of the Midcal test, because the "active supervision" requirement is not satisfied. The active supervision requirement stems from the recognition that "[w]here a private party is engaging in the anticompetitive activity, there is a real danger that he is acting to further his own interests, rather than the governmental interests of the State." The requirement is designed to ensure that the state-action doctrine will shelter only the particular anticompetitive acts of private parties that, in the judgment of the State, actually further state regulatory policies. To accomplish this purpose, the active supervision requirement mandates that the State exercise ultimate control over the challenged anticompetitive conduct. The mere presence of some state involvement or monitoring does not suffice. The active supervision . . . test requires that state officials have and exercise power to review particular anticompetitive acts of private parties and disapprove those that fail to accord with state policy. Absent such a program of supervision, there is no realistic assurance that a private party's anticompetitive conduct promotes state policy, rather than merely the party's individual interests.

Respondents in this case contend that the State of Oregon actively supervises the peer-review process through the State Health Division, the BOME, and the state judicial system. The Court of Appeals, in finding the active supervision requirement satisfied, also relied primarily on the powers and responsibilities of these state actors. Neither the Court of Appeals nor respondents, however, have succeeded in showing that any of these actors reviews—or even could review—private decisions regarding hospital privileges to determine whether such decisions comport with state regulatory policy and to correct abuses.

Oregon's Health Division has general supervisory powers over "matters relating to the preservation of life and health," including the licensing of hospitals, and the enforcement of health laws. Hospitals in Oregon are under a statutory obligation to establish peer-review procedures and to review those procedures on a regular basis. The State Health Division, exercising its enforcement powers, may initiate judicial proceedings against any hospital violating this law. In addition, the Health Division may deny, suspend, or revoke a hospital's license for failure to comply with the statutory requirement. Oregon law specifies no other ways in which the Health Division may supervise the peer-review process.

This statutory scheme does not establish a state program of active supervision over peer-review decisions. The Health Division's statutory authority over peer review relates only to a hospital's procedures; that authority does not encompass the actual decisions made by hospital peer-review committees. The restraint challenged in this case (and in most cases of its kind) consists not in the procedures used to terminate hospital privileges, but in the termination of privileges itself. The State does not actively supervise this restraint unless a state official has and exercises ultimate authority over private privilege determinations. Oregon law does not give the

Health Division this authority: under the statutory scheme, the Health Division has no power to review private peer-review decisions and overturn a decision that fails to accord with state policy. Thus, the activities of the Health Division under Oregon law cannot satisfy the active supervision requirement of the state-action doctrine.

Similarly, the BOME does not engage in active supervision over private peer-review decisions. The principal function of the BOME is to regulate the licensing of physicians in the State. As respondents note, Oregon hospitals are required by statute to notify the BOME promptly of a decision to terminate or restrict privileges. Neither this statutory provision nor any other, however, indicates that the BOME has the power to disapprove private privilege decisions. The apparent purpose of the reporting requirement is to give the BOME an opportunity to determine whether additional action on its part, such as revocation of a physician's license, is warranted. Certainly, respondents have not shown that the BOME in practice reviews privilege decisions or that it ever has asserted the authority to reverse them.

The only remaining alleged supervisory authority in this case is the state judiciary. Respondents claim, and the Court of Appeals agreed, that Oregon's courts directly review privilege-termination decisions and that this judicial review constitutes active state supervision. This Court has not previously considered whether state courts, acting in their judicial capacity, can adequately supervise private conduct for purposes of the state-action doctrine. All of our prior cases concerning state supervision over private parties have involved administrative agencies or State Supreme Courts with agency-like responsibilities over the organized bar. This case, however, does not require us to decide the broad question whether judicial review of private conduct ever can constitute active supervision, because judicial review of privilege-termination decisions in Oregon, if such review exists at all, falls far short of satisfying the active supervision requirement.

As an initial matter, it is not clear that Oregon law affords any direct judicial review of private peer-review decisions. Oregon has no statute expressly providing for judicial review of privilege terminations. Moreover, we are aware of no case in which an Oregon court has held that judicial review of peer-review decisions is available. The two cases that respondents have cited certainly do not hold that a physician whose privileges have been terminated by a private hospital is entitled to judicial review. In each of these cases, the Oregon Supreme Court assumed, but expressly did not decide, that a complaining physician was entitled to the kind of review he requested.

Moreover, the Oregon courts have indicated that even if they were to provide judicial review of hospital peer-review proceedings, the review would be of a very limited nature. The Oregon Supreme Court, in its most recent decision addressing this matter, stated that a court "should [not] decide the merits of plaintiff's dismissal" and that "[i]t would be unwise for a court to do more than to make sure that some sort of reasonable procedure was afforded and that there was evidence from which it could be found that plaintiff's conduct posed a threat to patient care." This kind of review would fail to satisfy the state-action doctrine's requirement of active supervision. Under the standard suggested by the Oregon Supreme Court, a state court would not review the merits of a privilege termination decision to determine whether it accorded with state regulatory policy. Such constricted review does not convert the action of a private party in terminating a physician's privileges into the action of the State for purposes of the state-action doctrine.

Because we conclude that no state actor in Oregon actively supervises hospital peer-review decisions, we hold that the state-action doctrine does not protect the peer-review activities challenged in this case from application of the federal antitrust laws. In so holding, we are not unmindful of the policy argument that respondents and their amici have advanced for reaching the opposite conclusion. They contend that effective peer review is essential to the provision of quality medical care and that any threat of antitrust liability will prevent physicians from participating openly and actively in peer-review proceedings. This argument, however, essentially challenges the wisdom of applying the antitrust laws to the sphere of medical care, and as such is properly directed to the legislative branch. To the extent that Congress has declined to exempt medical peer review from the reach of the antitrust laws, peer review is immune from antitrust scrutiny only if the State effectively has made this conduct its own. The State of Oregon has not done so. Accordingly, we reverse the judgment of the Court of Appeals.

Discussion Questions

1. Do you think Dr. Patrick was the victim of anticompetitive activity? On what facts do you base your conclusion?

2. What are the implications of this case for quality assurance in health care?

3. Do you suppose this decision has had a chilling effect on the peer review function?

4. What effect did this litigation have on Astoria Clinic and its physicians?

5. How should physicians and others involved in peer review protect themselves from antitrust (and other) liability for making peer review decisions?

6. Compare *Patrick* to *Mahmoodian v. United Hospital Center* in the previous chapter. Can you reconcile the outcomes?

Moore v. Regents of the Univ. of Calif.

51 Cal. 3d 120, 793 P.2d 479, 271 Cal. Rptr. 146 (1990)

Panelli, J.

I. INTRODUCTION

We granted review in this case to determine whether plaintiff has stated a cause of action against his physician and other defendants for using his cells in potentially lucrative medical research without his permission. Plaintiff alleges that his physician failed to disclose preexisting research and economic interests in the cells before obtaining consent to the medical procedures by which they were extracted. The superior court sustained all defendants' demurrers to the third amended complaint, and the Court of Appeal reversed. We hold that the complaint states a cause of action for breach of the physician's disclosure obligations, but not for conversion.

II. FACTS

. . . .

The plaintiff is John Moore (Moore), who underwent treatment for hairy-cell leukemia at the Medical Center of the University of California at Los Angeles (UCLA Medical Center). The five defendants are: (1) Dr. David W. Golde (Golde), a physician who attended Moore at UCLA Medical Center; (2) the Regents of the University of California (Regents), who own and operate the university; (3) Shirley G. Quan, a researcher employed by the Regents; (4) Genetics Institute, Inc. (Genetics Institute); and (5) Sandoz Pharmaceuticals Corporation and related entities (collectively Sandoz).

Moore first visited UCLA Medical Center on October 5, 1976, shortly after he learned that he had hairy-cell leukemia. After hospitalizing Moore and "withdr[awing] extensive amounts of blood, bone marrow aspirate, and other bodily substances," Golde confirmed that diagnosis. At this time all defendants, including Golde, were aware that "certain blood products and blood components were of great value in a number of commercial and scientific efforts" and that access to a patient whose blood contained these substances would provide "competitive, commercial, and scientific advantages."

On October 8, 1976, Golde recommended that Moore's spleen be removed. Golde informed Moore "that he had reason to fear for his life, and that the proposed splenectomy operation * * * was necessary to slow down the progress of his disease." Based upon Golde's representations, Moore signed a written consent form authorizing the splenectomy.

Before the operation, Golde and Quan "formed the intent and made arrangements to obtain portions of [Moore's] spleen following its removal" and to take them to a separate research unit. Golde gave written instructions to this effect

on October 18 and 19, 1976. These research activities "were not intended to have * * * any relation to [Moore's] medical * * * care." However, neither Golde nor Quan informed Moore of their plans to conduct this research or requested his permission. Surgeons at UCLA Medical Center, whom the complaint does not name as defendants, removed Moore's spleen on October 20, 1976.

Moore returned to the UCLA Medical Center several times between November 1976 and September 1983. He did so at Golde's direction and based upon representations "that such visits were necessary and required for his health and well-being, and based upon the trust inherent in and by virtue of the physician-patient relationship * * *." On each of these visits Golde withdrew additional samples of "blood, blood serum, skin, bone marrow aspirate, and sperm." On each occasion Moore travelled to the UCLA Medical Center from his home in Seattle because he had been told that the procedures were to be performed only there and only under Golde's direction.

"In fact, [however,] throughout the period of time that [Moore] was under [Golde's] care and treatment, * * * the defendants were actively involved in a number of activities which they concealed from [Moore]. * * *" Specifically, defendants were conducting research on Moore's cells and planned to "benefit financially and competitively * * * [by exploiting the cells] and [their] exclusive access to [the cells] by virtue of [Golde's] ongoing physician-patient relationship * * *."

Sometime before August 1979, Golde established a cell line from Moore's T-lymphocytes. On January 30, 1981, the Regents applied for a patent on the cell line, listing Golde and Quan as inventors. "[B]y virtue of an established policy * * *, [the] Regents, Golde, and Quan would share in any royalties or profits * * * arising out of [the] patent." The patent issued on March 20, 1984, naming Golde and Quan as the inventors of the cell line and the Regents as the assignee of the patent. (U.S. Patent No. 4,438,032 (Mar. 20, 1984).)

The Regent's patent also covers various methods for using the cell line to produce lymphokines. Moore admits in his complaint that "the true clinical potential of each of the lymphokines * * * [is] difficult to predict, [but] * * * competing commercial firms in these relevant fields have published reports in biotechnology industry periodicals predicting a potential market of approximately $3.01 Billion Dollars by the year 1990 for a whole range of [such lymphokines] * * *."

With the Regents' assistance, Golde negotiated agreements for commercial development of the cell line and products to be derived from it. Under an agreement with Genetics Institute, Golde "became a paid consultant" and "acquired the rights to 75,000 shares of common stock." Genetics Institute also agreed to pay Golde and the Regents "at least $330,000 over three years, including a pro-rata share of [Golde's] salary and fringe benefits, in exchange for * * * exclusive access to the materials and research performed" on the cell line and products derived from it. On June 4, 1982,

Sandoz "was added to the agreement," and compensation payable to Golde and the Regents was increased by $110,000. "[T]hroughout this period, * * * Quan spent as much as 70 [percent] of her time working for [the] Regents on research" related to the cell line.

III. DISCUSSION

A. *Breach of Fiduciary Duty and Lack of Informed Consent*

Moore repeatedly alleges that Golde failed to disclose the extent of his research and economic interests in Moore's cells before obtaining consent to the medical procedures by which the cells were extracted. These allegations, in our view, state a cause of action against Golde for invading a legally protected interest of his patient. This cause of action can properly be characterized either as the breach of a fiduciary duty to disclose facts material to the patient's consent or, alternatively, as the performance of medical procedures without first having obtained the patient's informed consent.

Our analysis begins with three well-established principles. First, "a person of adult years and in sound mind has the right, in the exercise of control over his own body, to determine whether or not to submit to lawful medical treatment." Second, "the patient's consent to treatment, to be effective, must be an informed consent." Third, in soliciting the patient's consent, a physician has a fiduciary duty to disclose all information material to the patient's decision.

These principles lead to the following conclusions: (1) a physician must disclose personal interests unrelated to the patient's health, whether research or economic, that may affect the physician's professional judgment; and (2) a physician's failure to disclose such interests may give rise to a cause of action for performing medical procedures without informed consent or breach of fiduciary duty.

To be sure, questions about the validity of a patient's consent to a procedure typically arise when the patient alleges that the physician failed to disclose medical risks, as in malpractice cases, and not when the patient alleges that the physician had a personal interest, as in this case. The concept of informed consent, however, is broad enough to encompass the latter. "The scope of the physician's communication to the patient * * * must be measured by the patient's need, and that need is whatever information is material to the decision."

Indeed, the law already recognizes that a reasonable patient would want to know whether a physician has an economic interest that might affect the physician's professional judgment. As the Court of Appeal has said, "[c]ertainly a sick patient deserves to be free of any reasonable suspicion that his doctor's judgment is influenced by a profit motive." The desire to protect patients from possible conflicts of interest has also motivated legislative enactments. Among these is Business and Professions Code section 654.2. Under that section, a physician may not charge a patient on behalf of, or

refer a patient to, any organization in which the physician has a "significant beneficial interest, unless [the physician] first discloses in writing to the patient, that there is such an interest and advises the patient that the patient may choose any organization for the purposes of obtaining the services ordered or requested by [the physician]." Similarly, under Health and Safety Code section 24173, a physician who plans to conduct a medical experiment on a patient must, among other things, inform the patient of "[t]he name of the sponsor or funding source, if any, * * * and the organization, if any, under whose general aegis the experiment is being conducted."

It is important to note that no law prohibits a physician from conducting research in the same area in which he practices. Progress in medicine often depends upon physicians, such as those practicing at the university hospital where Moore received treatment, who conduct research while caring for their patients.

Yet a physician who treats a patient in whom he also has a research interest has potentially conflicting loyalties. This is because medical treatment decisions are made on the basis of proportionality—weighing the benefits to the patient against the risks to the patient. As another court has said, "the determination as to whether the burdens of treatment are worth enduring for any individual patient depends upon the facts unique in each case," and "the patient's interests and desires are the key ingredients of the decision-making process." A physician who adds his own research interests to this balance may be tempted to order a scientifically useful procedure or test that offers marginal, or no, benefits to the patient. The possibility that an interest extraneous to the patient's health has affected the physician's judgment is something that a reasonable patient would want to know in deciding whether to consent to a proposed course of treatment. It is material to the patient's decision and, thus, a prerequisite to informed consent.

Golde argues that the scientific use of cells that have already been removed cannot possibly affect the patient's medical interests. The argument is correct in one instance but not in another. If a physician has no plans to conduct research on a patient's cells at the time he recommends the medical procedure by which they are taken, then the patient's medical interests have not been impaired. In that instance the argument is correct. On the other hand, a physician who does have a preexisting research interest might, consciously or unconsciously, take that into consideration in recommending the procedure. In that instance the argument is incorrect: the physician's extraneous motivation may affect his judgment and is, thus, material to the patient's consent.

We acknowledge that there is a competing consideration. To require disclosure of research and economic interests may corrupt the patient's own judgment by distracting him from the requirements of his health. But California law does not grant physicians unlimited discretion to decide what to disclose. Instead, "it is the prerogative of the patient, not the physician, to determine for himself the direction in which he believes his interests lie." "Unlimited discretion in the physician is irreconcilable with the basic right of the patient to make the ultimate informed decision * * * ."

Accordingly, we hold that a physician who is seeking a patient's consent for a medical procedure must, in order to satisfy his fiduciary duty and to obtain the patient's informed consent, disclose personal interests unrelated to the patient's health, whether research or economic, that may affect his medical judgment.

1. Dr. Golde

We turn now to the allegations of Moore's third amended complaint to determine whether he has stated such a cause of action. We first discuss the adequacy of Moore's allegations against Golde, based upon the physician's disclosures prior to the splenectomy.

Moore alleges that, prior to the surgical removal of his spleen, Golde "formed the intent and made arrangements to obtain portions of his spleen following its removal from [Moore] in connection with [his] desire to have regular and continuous access to, and possession of, [Moore's] unique and rare Blood and Bodily Substances." Moore was never informed prior to the splenectomy of Golde's "prior formed intent" to obtain a portion of his spleen. In our view, these allegations adequately show that Golde had an undisclosed research interest in Moore's cells at the time he sought Moore's consent to the splenectomy. Accordingly, Moore has stated a cause of action for breach of fiduciary duty, or lack of informed consent, based upon the disclosures accompanying that medical procedure.

We next discuss the adequacy of Golde's alleged disclosures regarding the postoperative takings of blood and other samples. In this context, Moore alleges that Golde "expressly, affirmatively and impliedly represented * * * that these withdrawals of his Blood and Bodily Substances were necessary and required for his health and well-being." However, Moore also alleges that Golde actively concealed his economic interest in Moore's cells during this time period. "[D]uring each of these visits * * * , and even when [Moore] inquired as to whether there was any possible or potential commercial or financial value or significance of his Blood and Bodily Substances, or whether the defendants had discovered anything * * * which was or might be * * * related to any scientific activity resulting in commercial or financial benefits * * * , the defendants repeatedly and affirmatively represented to [Moore] that there was no commercial or financial value to his Blood and Bodily Substances * * * and in fact actively discouraged such inquiries."

Moore admits in his complaint that defendants disclosed they "were engaged in strictly academic and purely scientific medical research * * * ." However, Golde's representation that he had no financial interest in this research became false,

based upon the allegations, at least by May 1979, when he "began to investigate and initiate the procedures * * * for [obtaining] a patent" on the cell line developed from Moore's cells.

In these allegations, Moore plainly asserts that Golde concealed an economic interest in the postoperative procedures. Therefore, applying the principles already discussed, the allegations state a cause of action for breach of fiduciary duty or lack of informed consent.

We thus disagree with the superior court's ruling that Moore had not stated a cause of action because essential allegations were lacking. We discuss each such allegation. First, in the superior court's view, Moore needed but failed to allege that defendants knew his cells had potential commercial value on October 5, 1976 (the time blood tests were first performed at UCLA Medical Center) and had at that time already formed the intent to exploit the cells. We agree with the superior court that the absence of such allegations precludes Moore from stating a cause of action based upon the procedures undertaken on October 5, 1976. But, as already discussed, Moore clearly alleges that Golde had developed a research interest in his cells by October 20, 1976, when the splenectomy was performed. Thus, Moore can state a cause of action based upon Golde's alleged failure to disclose that interest before the splenectomy.

The superior court also held that the lack of essential allegations prevented Moore from stating a cause of action based on the splenectomy. According to the superior court, Moore failed to allege that the operation lacked a therapeutic purpose or that the procedure was totally unrelated to therapeutic purposes. In our view, however, neither allegation is essential. Even if the splenectomy had a therapeutic purpose, it does not follow that Golde had no duty to disclose his additional research and economic interests. As we have already discussed, the existence of a motivation for a medical procedure unrelated to the patient's health is a potential conflict of interest and a fact material to the patient's decision.

. . . .

. . . [W]e hold that the allegations of Moore's third amended complaint state a cause of action for breach of fiduciary duty or lack of informed consent . . . .

. . . .

Discussion Questions

1. The court in *Moore* looks to the fiduciary duty of the physician to the patient and to the informed consent doctrine to impose an obligation to fully disclose research and economic interests. What does the court say about potential impairment of the patient's medical treatment by the physician's financial interests in the research project?

2. What professional and legal standards might be applied today to Dr. Golde?

Mazza v. Huffaker
61 N.C. App. 170, 300 S.E.2d 833 (1983)

Hedrick, J.

In the present case, plaintiff presented evidence tending to show the following:

Plaintiff suffers from manic depressive psychosis. Since 1975, he had received ongoing treatment of his illness from defendant Huffaker, a psychiatrist. As part of his treatment, plaintiff was prescribed medication by defendant Huffaker and participated in frequent and regular sessions at Huffaker's office, during which plaintiff was encouraged to have very intimate, self-revelatory, and uninhibited discussions with Huffaker. The treatment was described as "insight therapy" and "psychoanalysis." Plaintiff, in many of his sessions, for example, one on 4 May 1979, expressed to Huffaker serious concern about maintaining a healthy marital relationship with his wife, Jacqueline Mazza. Plaintiff had come to think of defendant Huffaker as his best friend. In May 1979, Jacqueline requested that she and plaintiff separate, and on 28 May 1979, plaintiff moved out of the Woodhaven Road house, in Chapel Hill, in which he, his wife, and family had lived. On 6 July 1979, plaintiff was entertaining one of his and Jacqueline's sons, with her prior agreement. Upon calling his wife at the Woodhaven Road home, at 10:40 p.m., to check with her as to whether he could bring the son back to her the next morning, plaintiff became concerned about his wife's welfare after noticing her conduct over the telephone. Plaintiff thereupon drove over to the Woodhaven Road house "to make sure everything was okay." Plaintiff observed his psychiatrist's automobile parked near the Woodhaven Road house and saw some of his psychiatrist's clothing strewn about the family room. Upon approaching and entering the locked master bedroom, plaintiff discovered his psychiatrist, Robert Huffaker, and his wife, Jacqueline Mazza, together in bed. Huffaker was naked and putting on his undershorts, and Jacqueline was naked and putting on a light housecoat.

Plaintiff also presented expert testimony tending to show the following:

Psychiatrists are physicians. The first duty of a physician to a patient is to do no harm; the second is to maintain the patient's trust and confidence in the physician. These basic duties apply and are even more stringent with psychiatrists, since a psychiatrist's patient reveals his innermost thoughts, feelings, worries, and concerns. Psychiatrists, therefore, have a strict duty not to breach the trusting relationship and must be very careful about what they say and how they influence patients. Psychiatrists have to take great care in the termination of a relationship with a patient so that the psychiatric patient, who is very sensitive, does not feel that he is abandoned or rejected. Especially in light of the intimate relationship between psychiatrist and patient, the psychiatrist's duty

once the psychiatrist-patient relationship has been established extends beyond the hospital or consulting room and includes social situations. The psychiatrist must endeavor to assure that the patient does not forget that the doctor is a doctor. A patient can be seriously harmed if the relationship changes from a therapeutic one to a social one. Special duties exist in the practice of medicine not to ruin a doctor and patient relationship, and those duties are more critical in psychiatry than in other areas of medicine. If the relationships are not terminated properly, but too abruptly, great harm can result to a patient. The psychiatrist's duty to advance his patient's interests is violated if the psychiatrist has sex with the patient's spouse; such sexual relations are not therapeutic. Sexual relations between a psychiatrist and his patient's wife would destroy the patient's trust in the psychiatrist and would destroy the doctor-patient relationship. Covert sexual relations between a psychiatrist and a patient's wife, if discovered by the patient, would make it extremely difficult for the patient to establish ever again a necessary trusting relationship with any psychiatrist, would render previous treatment useless, and would do harm to the mental well-being of the patient. A psychiatrist who becomes sexually involved with a relative of a patient is not exercising the requisite amount of skill, learning, and ability that a psychiatrist in any community in the United States ought to exercise. All the aforementioned standards and duties of physicians and psychiatrists are applicable in Chapel Hill.

There is ample evidence in the present case that the relevant standard of care applicable to Chapel Hill psychiatrists included the negative imperative that they not have sexual relations with their patients' spouses. The expert testimony tended to establish an obligation on the part of psychiatrists, as a part of their duties within the patient-psychiatrist relationship, to conduct themselves in a certain way and this obligation applies even beyond the office, clinic, hospital, or laboratory.

There was abundant evidence that defendant Huffaker did not refrain from having sexual relations with the plaintiff's wife. Hence, there was expert evidence defining the applicable standard of care and evidence that defendant Huffaker violated such standard. Contrary to defendants' assertions, plaintiff thus presented sufficient evidence of the professional malpractice element of his claim.

. . . .

The evidence and instructions in the present case placed central focus on the sexual relations between defendant Huffaker and the plaintiff's wife during the term of Huffaker's and plaintiff's psychiatrist-patient relationship. In light of that central focus, the instruction challenged here must also be deemed to pertain to the sexual relations between defendant Huffaker and the plaintiff's wife, with the added issues of transference and counter-transference. Hence, if the jury based its finding of malpractice on the instruction that it find malpractice if it determined defendant

Huffaker reacted improperly to transference or counter-transference, then the jury necessarily found that defendant Huffaker had sexual relations with plaintiff's wife during the course of the psychiatrist-patient relationship, since such sexual relations are of what the improper reaction to transference or counter-transference consisted. This assignment of error is meritless.

In their final assignment of error directed to the court's charge to the jury on liability, defendants challenge the court's instructions that the jury must find malpractice if it found defendant Huffaker abandoned plaintiff as a patient or if it found defendant Huffaker continued to treat plaintiff after becoming emotionally and sexually involved with plaintiff's wife. Defendants contend this charge "was tantamount to a virtual peremptory instruction on the malpractice issue" in that it compelled the jury to find malpractice by requiring it to do so whether it found one set of facts as true or whether it found the opposite set of facts as true. The court's instructions on abandonment and continued treatment do not pose a situation in which the jury must find malpractice if it finds that either of two mutually exclusive events occurred. The two prongs of the challenged instruction do not call for opposite determinations by the jury; rather, each may be answered in the affirmative since each deals with defendant Huffaker's having sexual relations with plaintiff's wife prior to an appropriate, gradual, and careful cessation of the psychiatrist-patient relationship between defendant Huffaker and plaintiff. The jury would have to find that the same essential set of facts occurred to answer either prong in the affirmative, and that set of facts, i.e. Huffaker's sexual relations with plaintiff's wife on 6 July 1979, sufficed as a predicate for malpractice liability. This assignment of error is without merit.

Defendants next assign error to the court's failure to submit an issue of plaintiff's contributory negligence with respect to the malpractice claim. Defendants first contend there was sufficient evidence to warrant the submission of such issue because of evidence that (1) prior to discovering his wife and defendant in bed together on 6 July 1979, plaintiff suspected the two were having an affair, (2) prior to his breaking down the door of the bedroom occupied by the two on 6 July 1979, plaintiff was aware of the possibility defendant Huffaker was in the house with plaintiff's wife, since plaintiff had seen Huffaker's clothing in the family room and his automobile parked nearby, and (3) plaintiff was sufficiently informed about his psychological vulnerabilities to have reason to know he would be very distressed if he were to see his wife and his psychiatrist in bed together. Defendants contend this evidence shows that plaintiff, in entering the bedroom, did not exercise ordinary care for his own safety in light of a foreseeable danger and unreasonable risk and that his conduct contributed to his injury. Defendants also contend the issue of contributory negligence should have been submitted on the basis of evidence tending to show that plaintiff had led

defendant Huffaker to believe their psychiatrist-patient relationship was terminated.

We have carefully perused the record in light of defendants' imaginative contentions with respect to an issue of contributory negligence and conclude the trial court did not err in failing to submit such an issue. We can hardly perceive of a situation where an issue of contributory negligence would be less appropriate.

. . . .

In their next assignment of error, defendants argue, "[t]he Court erred in permitting the [expert] witnesses * * * to express their opinions as to professional ethics for reason that breaches of professional ethics are not civilly actionable as malpractice, and this error * * * permitted * * * [the jury] to impose liability upon defendants for a breach of professional ethics."

As previously discussed, the professional malpractice element of an actionable malpractice claim is satisfied if it is shown that the health care provider violated the relevant standard of practice for his profession, and such standard of practice may be supplied by expert testimony. In the present case, expert testimony supplied such standard of practice and equated it with the standards of professional ethics. According to such expert testimony, the accepted standards of care are coterminous with the relevant standards of professional ethics. Hence, it was not improper for the expert witnesses to give content to the accepted standards of care by referring to the ethical standards of the profession, since expert testimony asserted that both standards are the same. Although defendants may be correct in arguing that breaches of professional ethics are not actionable in a malpractice suit when such standards differ from the reasonable standard of care imposed by tort law, their argument is unavailing in the present case, where expert testimony equated the two sets of standards. This assignment of error is overruled.

. . . .

The evidence in the present case, taken in the light most favorable to plaintiff, tends to show that on 6 July 1979 defendant Huffaker proceeded to have sexual relations with his patient's wife despite an awareness of the special vulnerabilities of his patient if the patient were to discover such a rendezvous. Evidence of such conduct by a psychiatrist towards his patient, in the face of the trusting relationship which develops between psychiatrist and patient, is evidence of more than mere inadvertence on the part of the psychiatrist. The evidence tends to show a wilful act by defendant Huffaker of having sex with his patient's wife, and an awareness, although disregarded, of the risks such an act posed towards his patient, Dr. Mazza. This evidence was sufficient to support an inference by the jury that defendant Huffaker acted with conscious disregard of the mental well-being of Dr. Mazza, the very mental well-being with which defendant Huffaker had been entrusted. Hence, the evidence was sufficient to support submission of a punitive damage issue in the medical malpractice case.

    . . . .

    . . . [T]he judgment will be affirmed in all respects.
No error.

Discussion Question

1. The physician's duty to a patient is spelled out in *Mazza* as, first, to do no harm. Secondly, the physician is to maintain the patient's trust and confidence. Increasingly, medical malpractice cases have arisen when physicians engage in sexual relations with patients or members of the patient's family. *See generally* Annotation, *Civil Liability of Doctor or Psychologist for Having Sexual Relationship with Patient*, 33 A.L.R.3d 1393 (1970). Discuss the ethical and moral issues that arise in *Mazza* in light of existing common-law and professional standards. Under what various legal theories might the patient seek redress?

Table of Cases

About the Editors

J. Stuart Showalter, J.D., is vice president of the Catholic Health Association in St. Louis, Missouri. He is a member of the Missouri and District of Columbia bars and teaches in the Washington University Medical School, Department of Health Administration in St. Louis, Missouri.

Bernard D. Reams, Jr., J.D., Ph.D., is a professor of law, a professor of technology management, and the director of the law library at Washington University School of Law in St. Louis, Missouri, where he teaches health law and policy. Dr. Reams is a member of the Kansas, Missouri, and federal bars. He is the author of numerous books, including *Human Experimentation, Industry-University Research Partnerships,* and *The Health Care Quality Improvement Act of 1986: A Legislative History of Pub. L. No. 99-660.*